VIDEOTAPE TECHNIQUES IN PSYCHIATRIC
TRAINING AND TREATMENT

Videotape Techniques

in

Psychiatric Training and Treatment

REVISED EDITION

Edited by MILTON M. BERGER, M.D.

"O wad some Power the giftie gie us
To see oursels as ithers see us!"

ROBERT BURNS

BRUNNER/MAZEL *Publishers* • New York

Library of Congress Cataloging in Publication Data

Berger, Milton Miles.
   Videotape techniques in psychiatric training and treatment.
   Bibliography: p. 373
   Includes index.
   1. Video tapes in psychotherapy.   2. Psychiatry—Study and teaching—Audio-
visual aids.   I. Title.   [DNLM: 1. Television. 2. Psychotherapy. 3. Psycho-
therapy, Group. 4. Cognition. 5. Self concept. 6. Audio-visual aids—Utilization.
WM18 V652] RC455.2.T45B47 1978   616.8'9'0028   78-1782
ISBN 0-87630-163-4

Copyright © 1978 by Milton M. Berger

Published by
BRUNNER/MAZEL, INC.
19 Union Square, New York, N.Y. 10003

MANUFACTURED IN THE UNITED STATES OF AMERICA

*This book is dedicated
to my wife and cotherapist*

LYNNE FLEXNER BERGER, A.T.R.

PREFACE TO THE REVISED EDITION

Reading this book gives one the feeling of watching the opening up of a new frontier. In a smaller compass, it arouses sentiments similar to the start of the space age explorations. The frequently remodelled but still familiar psychiatric landscape is being drastically enlarged to include the videoscape, with its freeze-frames, instant replays, split images, voice overlays, multi-angles, and other cyclopean-eye views of human encounters. Yet another technological revolution may change, and in a startling fashion, the way we practice our profession.

The fact that a revised edition of this book is being published only seven years after its first appearance indicates that the advocates of the new technology—the innovators—have just about passed through their pioneer stage. The period of covered wagons and isolated settlements is ending. For this is a "how to" book, written by the growing number of technologically sophisticated therapists, trainers and researchers for those who are incipiently curious, definitely interested, or wishing to be instructed.

Although still colored by the ambiguous appeal of novelty, the field of videotape techniques in psychiatric treatment and training is about ready to take stock of what has been accomplished and of what the future holds in store. While such a goal is not emphasized by the editor, nor by his contributors, it emerges from between the this-is-what-we-are-doing lines of the text.

First and foremost is the contribution of videotaping to the openness of psychiatric procedures. What was formerly transacted behind closed doors is now made available for scrutiny. Communications between therapists and patients, in private practice or in public facilities, in individual, group, or family therapy, in supervision or in other training contexts, is *there*, preserved for cognitive processing and learning through repeated viewing. The patient can learn how he presents himself to others; the

vii

therapist can learn how he presents himself to the patient. Likewise for supervisor and supervisee. The event is retrievable, sealed on tape, unless it is erased because of someone's objections.

Related to seeing and hearing what actually transpires is the opportunity for confrontation with the unexpected—the existential surprise. If to some extent all of us know not what we do or how we do it, what we communicate or conceal, what games we play, what roles we take outside of awareness, the videotape is *there* to show us, with fantastic clarity. Self-confrontation is an emergent and inescapable property of videotaping and viewing. Thus the "Rashomon" aspect of interpersonal events is transformed into something under personal rather than theatrical control. "Know thyself" becomes less an abstract principle, more a demand property of "See thyself"—in action, through one's own eyes rather than through the interpretations or responses of others.

Finally, what emerges from this preliminary stock-taking is an unexpected version of the "repetition compulsion." If neurotic behavior is (partly) the result of unconsciously repeating an event for the sake of mastery, but without new learning, the videotape offers the opportunity to repeat, by oneself or with others, what one actually did, with improvements. It is everyone's, or anyone's, ideal "staircase" reaction. The multilevel and mixed messages inherent in any event involving conflict or contradiction of motives can be reviewed over and over again so that the various aspects can be sorted out, placed in perspective, and gradually put at an emotional distance. We know that the learning of tasks and facts requires repetition; we know that emotional learning requires repeated "working through" to modify unconscious factors—but we have not previously realized how much repeated audiovisual viewing of one's self in action speeds up this process by aborting selective inattention and defense by denial.

These potentially enduring contributions of videotaping are interlaced in the text with a series of "what-it-is-not" comments—constraints against the unrealistic expectations and instant myth-making apt to accompany new technologies. Videotaping is *not* a form of therapy, in and of itself. Rather, it is conceived as a supplement to the standard approaches. Videotaping is *not* the child of any one theoretical approach or treatment modality but is adaptable to any type of uncovering therapy. Videotaping technique is *not* picked up by reading a paper or scanning a brochure. A fairly complex technique, it requires the kind of training and practice for which this book is an introduction.

If one is ready to incorporate the videoscape into one's professional experience for a generation of consumers and trainees reared on television viewing, the chapters that follow will make the journey easier. Even if one is not prepared to go to the time, trouble and expense of acquiring a new technique, the insights here provided into the therapeutic learning experience are well worth a perusal of this book.

JOHN P. SPIEGEL, M.D.
Florence Heller School
Brandeis University

March 16, 1978

PREFACE TO THE FIRST EDITION

Today, technological advance is recognized as a major contributor to the development of science, the control of the human environment and the material well being of men. New knowledge, made possible through the power of new technological advances, has brought to light data that have required the abandonment of long-held theories. Their abandonment often has necessitated the construction of more pertinent hypotheses. But, to bring about its effects, the discovery of a new technology requires its ready availability, its acceptance by the culture into which it is introduced and the presence of men and facilities capable of its operation and maintenance. The spread of a new technology demands that its acquisition and operation fall within the fiscal means of those who may desire its functions.

Beyond all other sciences and professions, those concerned with behavior have been handicapped by the lack of a readily available, easily operative and relatively inexpensive instrumentation to allow quick recording of the totality of organismal response. This instrumental deficiency has been most conspicuous where psychiatrists and psychologists have wished to study man—and that complex totality of his behavior designated "personality," best revealed in his ongoing transactions with others—that is, in a social matrix.

To be sure, the cinema has been available for decades. But its cumbersome operation, its operative intrusion into natural settings and its high cost have defeated its use as the technology which might provide the instrumentation needed to push forward investigation and teaching in the sciences.

The enormous potential contained in the evolution of high quality, portable and relatively inexpensive television cameras, closed circuit reproduction and, later, tape recording devices which have allowed both permanent recording and immediate playback was recognized a decade ago—particularly by various psychiatric educators—as the major technological advance that might bring to the study of personality the solid basis for its future evolution. In the easily and inexpensively developed audio television tape recording, behavior scientists for the first time

perceived means of gaining a permanent record of spontaneously interacting men, women and children for later studied review and scientific
analysis. So too, the new television technology was foreseen as the opportunity of recording for educational purposes all the experiences to which
students in psychiatry were exposed in their teaching sessions in class-
rooms or clinics. The educators foresaw, as of particular importance, the
use of the technique in the teaching of psychotherapy which, up till
then, had been largely dependent upon the seminar or individual supervisory technique. In such teaching sessions the students reported their
recollections of transactions with their patients; the supervisor interpreted, commented upon, and attempted to bring out the hidden communication he presumed to perceive in the verbal abstraction of the
patient encounter, variously recollected and distorted by the student
therapist.

I find myself enthusiastically surprised and delighted with the contents
of this book, arranged and edited by Dr. Milton M. Berger. As one of
those immediately fascinated by the potential perceived for psychiatrists
and the behavioral sciences in the new television technology, as one who
threw himself into the development of a behavioral laboratory specifically
constructed around the acquisition and use of the improved instruments,
as one who personally participated in some of the early educational experiments in psychiatry using both closed circuit and taped television
recording, Dr. Berger, in his editorial selections, reveals the enormous
development and creative application of the technology that have come
about within a few years time.

One will find here, well brought together, the summary of a decade of
application and innovation of the new television technology in the field
of psychiatric education and treatment. In addition, the editor wisely has
seen to it that the reader will consider the emerging legal, moral and
ethical issues consequent to the increasing exposure of patients and their
families to wider audiences than that of their treating physicians. Also,
in the final section on "Technical and Artistic Considerations" there is
much of value for those who propose now to apply the technique to
their areas of interest. The selected bibliography and the glossaries also
give the interested reader the means to comprehend and further explore
the field.

I commend to the reader Dr. Berger's chapter on "The Use of Videotape in the Integrated Treatment of Individuals, Couples, Families and
Groups in Private Practice." He, particularly, has been responsible for the
application and trial of television recording in the private practice of
psychiatry. Nowhere else will one discover today a record of the many

novel ways in which one may use the instrumentation to foster patient participation, self-awareness and deepening insight. Dr. Berger interprets the television exposure of an individual's behavior to that individual, if a patient, as one means of application of the confrontation technique in psychotherapy. So, too, he conceives of the confrontation as revealing to the individual consciousness denial of hidden aspects of his image of his body.

Within the next decade, we may expect an even more widespread use of videotape recording as educational and therapeutic aids. One may foresee a progressive evaluation and eventual definition of its most powerful and effective application. As the educational and therapeutic applications of videotape expand and grow, we shall also expect its wider use in research concerned with human behavior.

The editor and the contributors are to be congratulated in making available this important and timely volume.

LAWRENCE C. KOLB, M.D.

CONTRIBUTORS

IAN ALGER, M.D. is Training Analyst and Supervisory Psychoanalyist, New York Medical College; Visiting Associate Professor of Psychiatry, Einstein College of Medicine, Bronx, New York.

MILTON M. BERGER, M.D. is Clinical Associate Professor of Psychiatry, Downstate Medical Center, Brooklyn, New York; Director of Education and Training, South Beach Psychiatric Center, Staten Island, New York; Chairman of the Video Subcommittee of the American Psychiatric Association Program Committee since 1970.

EUGENE CHERNELL, M.D. is in private practice in Anchorage, Alaska.

PATRICK M. CORBITT is Media Director, Department of Education and Training, South Beach Psychiatric Center, Staten Island, New York.

DAVID N. FIELDS, LL.B. is a former legal staff member of the New York State Department of Mental Hygiene; Special Counsel to the Commissioner of Mental Health, Commonwealth of Pennsylvania; and has lectured on Law and Psychiatry under the auspices of New York University Law School and New York State University Medical School at Stony Brook, New York.

HERBERT FREED, M.D. was Clinical Professor of Psychiatry, Temple University School of Medicine, Philadelphia. (Now deceased.)

ROBERT E. FROELICH, M.D. is Professor and Chairman of Psychiatry, University of Alabama School of Primary Medical Care, Huntsville, Alabama.

HARRY H. GARNER, M.D. was Professor and Chairman, Department of Psychiatry and Neurology, The Chicago Medical School. (Now deceased.)

MARCIA KRAFT GOIN, M.D. is Associate Clinical Professor at the University of Southern California School of Medicine.

PETER GRUENBERG, M.D. is Assistant Professor of Psychiatry, U.C.L.A. School of Medicine, Los Angeles; Member of Faculty, Los Angeles Psychoanalytic Society/Institute, California.

HERMAN HIRSH, M.D. is Associate Clinical Professor of Psychiatry and Community Medicine, Temple University School of Medicine, Philadelphia, Penn.

NORMAN KAGAN, Ph.D. is Professor of Education, College of Education, and Professor of Medical Education, College of Human Medicine, Michigan State University, Lansing, Michigan.

FRANK KLEIN, M.D. is Professor of Psychiatry, University of California at Irvine; Chief of Psychiatry, Long Beach, Veterans Administration Hospital; Vice Chairman and Director, Veterans Administration Affairs, University of California at Irvine.

LAWRENCE C. KOLB, M.D. is former Commissioner of New York State Department of Mental Hygiene; former Director, New York State Psychiatry Institute; Past-President American Psychiatric Association.

EDWARD H. LISTON, JR., M.D. is Associate Professor, Department of Psychiatry, U.C.L.A. School of Medicine; Chief, Adult Inpatient Services, The UC.L.A. Neuropsychiatric Institute, Los Angeles, California.

HUGH JAMES LURIE, M.D. is Clinical Associate Professor, Department of Psychiatry and Behavioral Sciences, University of Washington, School of Medicine, Seattle, Washington.

EDWARD MESSNER, M.D. is Assistant Clinical Professor, Harvard Medical School, Boston, Mass.

RICHARD J. METZNER, M.D. is Chief, Audiovisual Education System, Brentwood Veterans Administration Hospital; Assistant Professor of Psychiatry, U.C.L.A.

PHILIP C. MORSE, Ph.D. is Adjunct Professor in Clinical Psychology, Long Island University, New York; Director of South Richmond Partial Hospitalization Program, South Beach Psychiatric Center, Staten Island, New York.

FLOY JACK MOORE, M.D. is Founding Editor: *TV In Psychiatry Newsletter;* Medical Consultant, Douglas County Vocational Rehabilitation Division, Roseberg; Vice-Chairman of Board of Directors, Douglas County Council on Alcoholism; Member, Mental Health Committee, Oregon.

CONSTANCE B. NELSON, Ph.D. is Clinical Psychologist, M.H.C. of the Veterans Administration Hospital, Denver, Colorado.

NAZNEEN SADA MAYADAS, D.S.W., is Professor of Social Work, the University of Texas at Arlington.

DONALD E. O'BRIEN, A.C.S.W. is Chief Social Worker, Consultation Service, Mental Hygiene, U.S. Army Hospital, Tehran, Iran.

NANCY A. ROESKE, M.D. is Professor and Director, Undergraduate Curriculum; Coordinator of Medical Education, Department of Psychiatry, Indiana University School of Medicine, Indianapolis, Indiana.

MAX ROSENBAUM, Ph.D. is Editor, *Journal of Group Psychoanalysis and Process*; Clinical Professor, Department of Psychiatry, New York University; Clinical Professor, Adelphi University.

DAVID D. SCHMIDT, M.D. is Associate Professor, Department of Family Medicine, School of Medicine, Case Western Reserve University, Cleveland, Ohio.

FREDERICK H. STOLLER, Ph.D. was Co-Director, Group Studies Center, University of Southern California, Los Angeles; Associate Editor of Comparative Group Studies. (Now deceased.)

JOHN WALDRON, M.D. is Professor and Head, Department of Psychiatry, Queens University Medical Center, Kingston, Ontario, Canada.

GEORGE J. WAYNE, M.D. is Clinical Professor of Psychiatry, University of California School of Medicine, U.C.L.A. Center for Health Sciences, Los Angeles, California.

W. DOUGLAS WEIR, M.D. is Associate Professor of Psychiatry and Associate Professor of Family Medicine, Institute of Psychiatry and Human Behavior, Department of Psychiatry, University of Maryland, School of Medicine.

MAXWELL J. WEST, M.B., B.S., D.T.M. & H., M.A.N.Z.C.P., M.R.C. Psych. is Visiting Psychiatrist at the Royal Newcastle Hospital and the Mater Misericordiae Hospital, New South Wales, Australia.

CARL A. WHITAKER, M.D., is Professor of Psychiatry and Family Therapy, University of Wisconsin School of Medicine, Center for Health Sciences, Madison, Wisconsin.

HARRY A. WILMER, M.D., Ph.D. is Professor of Psychiatry, The University of Texas Medical School, Health Science Center at San Antonio, Texas.

CONTENTS

SECTION III

TREATMENT

Section IV

LEGAL, MORAL AND ETHICAL CONSIDERATIONS

Section V

TECHNICAL AND ARTISTIC CONSIDERATIONS

SECTION VI

BIBLIOGRAPHIES AND GLOSSARIES

INTRODUCTION

The use of videotape in psychiatry is no longer new and it is used in every medical school and psychiatric training setting in this country. We find installations in public and private facilities which range in scope from single camera, videorecorder, monitor and microphone units costing $2,000 to media departments costing $250,000 staffed with five or more personnel manning multiple cameras, videorecorders, microphones, microphone mixers and special effects generators to create, record and compose elaborate sophisticated video productions comparable to what the commercial and public educational television broadcast stations bring to us daily in our television-centered society. The use of videotape for learning and for treatment has increased as the cost of simple equipment has gone down and the availability of mobile equipment has expanded. At the same time, as the present generation, which has often been called the "television generation," has come of age, the people involved in the mental health field as helpers have been increasingly exposed to the values of television as an adjunct to psychiatry through exposure to video special sessions at annual meetings of the American Psychiatric Association, the American Group Psychotherapy Association,* the American Orthopsychiatric Association and other national, regional or local groups.

It has at long last been well documented and acknowledged that the absence of early clinical experience is a source of disappointment and disillusionment to the student whose first "patient" is a cadaver. As patients and doctors are experienced through television more as persons and less as objects to and for each other, the relationship between patient and doctor is coming into the foreground of training and treatment. It is hoped that sensitive, gifted, bright, humanitarian and idealistic

---

* For over a decade the Annual Training Institute conducted by the American Group Psychotherapy Association just prior to its Annual Convention has held two-day group process videotape groups in which the focus on equipment and techniques useful in group approaches for training, therapy and growth has been equally as important as the focus on group process.

medical students who formerly had to become hardened, detached and alienated in order to avoid becoming overly emotional or identified with their patients will no longer have to repress or deny their reactions as troubling emotions come into awareness and are made available for clarification, discussion and resolution. (See chapters 5-13.)

The historic report in 1947 regarding the innovative use of closed circuit television in medicine described the transmission of five surgical operations from the operating rooms of Johns Hopkins to a group of physicians at a nearby medical meeting. In the following years a few articles were published reporting on intramural and extramural closed circuit television in surgery and as an aid in teaching physiology, anatomy and the basic sciences.

In what is perhaps the earliest report on closed circuit television as a new tool in psychiatric education,* Wittson and Dutton in 1956 reviewed their experiences with small and large groups of medical students, psychiatric residents and nurses. In 1957, Tucker and his colleagues** reported on closed circuit television as an effective medium in the treatment of the mentally ill. Further impetus to interest in television in the teaching of psychiatry came from the 1960 report of Ruhe, Gundel and their colleagues† at the University of Kansas School of Medicine on their four years of integrating television into the regular curriculum.

In 1961, Moore, Hanes and Harrison‡ reported in the *Journal of Medical Education* on "Improved television, stereo and the two-person interview." By 1964 Kornfeld and Kolb§ were reporting on the use of closed circuit television facilities for teaching purposes at the New York State Psychiatric Institute since 1960. They commented on the superiority of closed circuit television over the one-way screen, use of the sound tape recorder, and the encouraging promises of television as an aid in teaching interviewing techniques, psychotherapy and group therapy.

---

* Wittson, C., and Dutton, R.: A New Tool in Psychiatric Education. *Ment. Hosp.,* 7:11-14, 1956.

** Tucker, H., Lewis, R. B., Martin, G. L., and Over, C. H.: Television Therapy: Effectiveness of Closed Circuit TV for Therapy and Treatment of the Mentally Ill. *Archives of Neurology and Psychiatry,* 77:57-69, Jan., 1957.

† Ruhe, D. S., Gundel, S., Laybourne, P. D., Forman, L. D., Jacobs, M., and Eaton, M. T.: Television in Teaching Psychiatry. *J. Med. Educ.,* 35:916-927, 1960.

‡ Moore, F. J., Hanes, L. C., and Harrison, C. A.: Improved Television, Stereo and the Two-Person Interview. *J. Med. Educ.,* 36:162-166, 1961.

§ Kornfeld, D. S. and Kolb, L. C.: The Use of Closed Circuit TV in the Teaching of Psychiatry. *J. Nerv. Ment. Dis.,* 138:452-459, 1964.

A year later Ryan,* writing in *Mental Hospitals* on teaching by video-tape, gave outlines of courses in psychotherapy, psychopathology, psychogenics, neuroanatomy, hypnosis and psychology at the New York State Psychiatric Institute, and presented the reactions of patients as well as viewers to this new instructional modality. Meanwhile, in another direction, Cornelison and Arsenian,** in their trend-setting approach to views and confrontation, reported in 1960 on a study of the response of psychotic inpatients to a photographic self-image experience at the Boston State Hospital.

My interest in the communicational problems of patients developed during my post World War II years as clinical director of Stony Lodge when Glueck and I wrote an article on the use of the telephone as a psychiatric treatment adjunct.† Patients improved considerably when again trusted with what perhaps they should never have been deprived of in the first place—a direct, albeit supervised, communication line with family members and friends via the telephone. It decreased their distrust of the hospital staff when this evidence of respect for them, as individuals possessed with health, not only sickness residing in them, was manifested. In the following years the nonverbalized behaviors of patients in groups and families interested me and the recent development and availability of video has continued to stimulate my interest in understanding and improving communication. The numerous exciting potential uses for videotape as I have personally experienced them led me to develop the theme of this book—a book which represents the varied contributions of many workers in different settings to the growing field of video.

The first edition of this book created international ripples immediately when it was delivered "hot off the press" in Vancouver, British Columbia, the second week in May 1970 at the First Television in Psychiatry Conference hosted by Drs. John and Libba Tyhurst at the Health Sciences Centre of the University of British Columbia. The occasion of the Conference and the arrival of the published book signaled to all that television in psychiatry had truly come of age.

In 1970, John Ewing, who was then Chairman of the Program Committee of the American Psychiatric Association, invited me to develop and serve as Chairman of a Video Task Force for the Program Com-

---

*Ryan, J.: Teaching and Consultation by Television: II. Teaching by Videotape. *Ment. Hosp.*, 16:101-104, 1965.

** Cornelison, F. S. and Arsenian, J.: A Study of the Response of Psychotic Patients to Photographing Self-Image Experience. *Psychiat. Quart.*, 34:1-8, 1960.

† Berger, M. M. and Glueck, B. C., Jr.: The Telephone—Its Use as a Psychiatric Treatment Adjunct. *Psychiat. Quart.*, 23:522-529 (July) 1949.

mittee to screen, create, solicit and present quality video programs at the annual meetings of the Association. At the same time, the APA asked Ed Mason to review films. We have both been at the task for APA since then and some of our experiences may be instructive to others planning video presentations.

In the first years of APA Continuing Education Video Special Sessions we allowed individual presenters a full three hours to cover a theme and we projected our pre-taped and live closed circuit programs onto a 15' × 20' screen while producing live programs and discussions from the brightly-lit curtained stage area with three commercial quality color cameras and an experienced video producer in charge. All the live closed-circuit pictures and sound projected beautifully to audiences ranging from 1000 to 2000 but some of the pre-taped material which had looked good to us in previewing sessions on standard-size monitors tended to fall apart when projected with such magnification. We met our "Waterloo" in Anaheim, California at the 1975 Annual APA Meeting in the Disneyland Arena. The room was *vast* with 9000 seats of which we planned to use up to 3000, the screen was *vast*—20' × 30'—and the huge sound speakers were located on the ceiling two hundred feet overhead. When we projected tapes that had looked good on 19" monitors but had been made on one-half inch reel to reel recorders, the pictures broke up and the sound broke up, too, causing such an exodus of viewers from the arena that I was on the edge of requiring "crisis therapy." Tapes that had been technically made with meticulous attention to sound and lighting on one inch or two inch recording equipment came through okay when magnified in the arena. However, the following year, 1976, we turned to a smaller room seating 300 people in Miami's Convention Center and broadcast to five 21" color monitors, did no live production with color cameras and no large screen projection. We encouraged presenters and producers to state their objectives succinctly on the tape, and to edit tightly in fulfilling those objectives. As a result we had a very successful week of programming, with overflow audiences. At the 1977 Annual Meeting in Toronto, the carefully edited and selected continuing education programs were received with great satisfaction and acceptance by APA registrants. We had learned and demonstrated that we had reached the stage where "home-movie" type productions were passé and we could insist on accepting only programs that could meet more stringent criteria in terms of content, production, light, sound and video quality (see Chapter 29, this book).

An important development was the fact that for a few years, from 1973-75, only the video special sessions portion of the entire annual APA program was acceptable as meeting the criteria for Category I Continuing Education Credit of the AMA for the Physicians Recognition Award. In the past seven years, the video special sessions have drawn about 75,000 viewers and have served to introduce the value of video as a self-learning, teaching and treatment auxiliary to many who now have video installations for their own use.

The APA Video Subcommittee has assiduously struggled to educate video producers who apply for participation in video special sessions with regard to what is required in the way of clearly stated learning objectives, content that fulfills those objectives, and summary. Wrap-up statements, graphics or messages presented for viewers to grasp and incorporate as newly learned material significant for treatment, training or expansion of knowledge must be given serious attention to be effective. Accompanying written materials or guides containing self-assessment questions and references must be succinct.

The *Television in Psychiatry Newsletter* originally created by Floy Moore for those involved in using video in psychiatric settings has been carried on despite many logistic and financial difficulties by Libba Tyhurst who has served as editor since the first conference in 1970. The *Newsletter* serves as the main source for: sharing news of meetings; new work and papers; reprints of significant articles; requests for information and help. The editor has also been the main force in continuing to organize international conferences on television in psychiatry.*

In 1974 the officers of the American Board of Psychiatry and Neurology accepted the idea that the development of a library of carefully created videotaped interviews for showing to board candidates seeking certification as specialists in psychiatry was a necessity because the thousands of live patients required for examinations were becoming increasingly difficult to obtain. The October 1976 policy of the board was to have each candidate examine one patient in a live interview and see one videotaped patient interview before being examined orally by a board examiner to assess his knowledge and practice of clinical psychiatry.** The use of videotaped interviews allows for a more standardized, less expensive, less cumbersome and more controlled examination procedure.

---

* *Ed. Note*: Anyone interested in this publication devoted to the use of video in psychiatry should send a $10 check to Dr. Libba Tyhurst, Editor, *TV in Psychiatry Newsletter*, Department of Psychiatry, University of British Columbia, Vancouver, B.C., Canada V6T 1W5.

** See the two films produced by M. M. Berger in 1975 for Merrell-National Laboratories on "Insight into the Examination of the American Board of Psychiatry and Neurology, Inc." These are available for showing at psychiatric facilities through local Merrell representatives without charge.

The initial videotapes accepted for use by the board were produced by Richard Metzner* and were presented over color monitors in a room in which about 20 candidates and examiners sat together prior to pairing off for private oral examinations in adjacent rooms. According to Metzner a survey given to the one thousand candidates in psychiatry and neurology and the several hundred examiners who participated in the first audiovisual board examination showed that candidates gave high rating to the technical quality of the videotapes and the interview itself. They showed a high preference for the videotape over the live patient examination. This fact doesn't make this way of examining better but may simply indicate that this method decreases anxiety in the board candidates who are experiencing peak-anxiety at this crucial moment of their professional lives when they symbolically are moving from "student-child" to "certified psychiatrist-adult." There was a high correlation between the scores achieved by individual candidates with their live and videotaped patient interviews.** The ABPN is planning to expand its use of audiovisual examinations to include an audiovisual written examination in neurology for psychiatrists to replace the live patient examination in neurology previously required. It is also working on plans to standardize written examinations in psychiatry.

At the 20th winter meeting of the American Academy of Psychoanalysis in 1976 the two-day workshop of family interviews showed videotapes of the work of Ian Alger, Virginia Satir, Salvador Minuchin and Carl Whitaker. The room was packed with psychoanalysts eager to see and discuss the working styles and approaches of these well-known colleagues through pre-taped consultations.

A developing trend which deserves attention is the collaboration of two or more medical facilities in the production of highest quality videotapes. A project currently in process was initiated by Loren Mosher and Walter Clark of the National Institute for Mental Health when they requested me as producer of the "Beyond the Double Bind" Conference†

---

* Richard J. Metzner, M.D. is Chief of the AVES Learning Resources Laboratory at the Brentwood Veterans Administration Hospital in Los Angeles, Calif.

**The average length of pretaped interviews was 20 minutes and the standard format was a single medium close-up shot of the patient as seen by the interviewer. A zoom lens was used sparingly to provide opening and closing wide shots of patients and interviewer and occasional close-ups of the patient during the interview.

† *Ed. Note*: The "Beyond the Double Bind" Conference was held March 3, 4, 1977 at the Barbizon-Plaza Hotel in New York City. This Conference brought together on one podium the three living authors of the original double-bind presentation "Towards a Theory of Schizophrenia," Gregory Bateson, Jay Haley and John Weakland with such other pioneering figures in family systems theory, therapy and communications theory as Murray Bowen, Albert Scheflen, Carl Whitaker and Lyman Wynne.

tapes to improve their continuing education teaching value, having in mind broadcasting them via satellite to 22 cities in Alaska and the United States. They suggested we add voice-over narrations and freeze-frame special effects, as well as introductory and summary statements to clarify the intent and meaning of the interventions made by Murray Bowen, Carl Whitaker and Lyman Wynne as they conducted consultations with families in order to highlight their individual clinical approaches and theories. This was done with the cooperation of the crew of the excellent video studio at Walter Reed Hospital in Washington, D.C. in allowing us to use their two-inch quad hardware for taping additional segments with Murray Bowen. This example of collaboration allows for a better usage of talent and equipment in video production units supported by public funds.

At the time of this writing, October 1977, the Video Subcommittee of the Scientific Program Committee of the American Psychiatric Association is reviewing 38 videotapes submitted by members and nonmembers for presentation at the 1978 APA Annual Meeting in Atlanta. The tapes submitted for our consideration cover most major concerns of psychiatry:

> Normal development in infancy through three years of age; development of self-image in the first two years; psychiatric evaluation of a child and family; anorexia nervosa; family theory and therapy of psychotic families to resolve multigenerational transmission of emotional problems; the relationship between family functioning and individual psychopathology; community and family therapy with drug users; sexuality and intimacy in early marriage; the marriage contract; transexualism and gender identity; multiple personalities; a cognitive theory and therapy of depressed patients; timelessness and forgetting in frontal lobe defect; diagnosis and management of tardive dyskinesia; the interrelationship between high hypnotizability states and certain kinds of psychotic or otherwise seriously disturbed behavior; hypnosis in psychotherapy; the marathon session as a part of long-term dynamic psychotherapy; the psychotherapy of patients with frozen affect; art videotherapy treatment of psychotic patients; the use of videotape techniques in individual psychotherapy; assessing suicidal risk in depression; the psychiatric evaluation of criminal responsibility and the preparation of the psychiatrist to testify as an expert witness; use and misuse of various interviewing techniques; testing the psychiatric skills of medical residents; continuing medical education video review groups in a psychiatric hos-

Videotapes of papers, family interviews and workshops were made on 2″ quad recorders, with three color cameras and other "hardware" supplied by the Rimith Corp. of New York City at a cost of $20,000 which was paid for by conference registration fees.

pital; the psychology of aging; attitudes toward and differentiation of acute and chronic organic brain syndromes; various forms of depression in the aging; late-onset paranoid states; behavioral problems and issues in management and care of the elderly; issues in death and dying.

Kubie stated in 1952, "The effects of facing an auditory and visual image of one's own psychological activities have never been examined systematically. We do not know if it would be therapeutic or noxious, and whether it would bypass the resistances to insight or increase them. Many considerations suggest that it would put certain psychoanalytic assumptions to searching tests. Here again the intial focus of the inquiry would be on the influence of these technical maneuvers on the patient's spontaneous and free production of material from conscious, preconscious and unconscious levels of his personality."*

In 1969, Kubie, after some experience with a psychoanalytical patient who had been involved with videotape self-confrontation, made the point that the self-image which each person carries around has many layers. Kubie states, "Among these, which rise to the surface depend upon many transplanted residual relationships which are modified by disturbing identifications, guilt feelings and buried conflicts which have been carried over from the past to add their own complexities to the current image."**

Kubie is in the avant-garde of our psychoanalytic colleagues when he notes, "It is impossible for anyone to process so many layers of identifications in a single moment of exposure. This is the simple psychophysiological reason why the exposure to one's own TV-image must be provided in a form which can be repeated for study. If psychiatrists are going to explore the effects of confronting human beings with their own images as a method for communicating to them about themselves and for enabling them to study themselves, then psychiatry must make it possible to reexpose the subject repeatedly in different moods and states of mind, in different periods of stress or peace. As is true of a single exposure to anything, a single transitory exposure to the self-image on TV cannot be more than a weighted, unrepresentative and statistically inadequate sample of what a total experience can be."

---

* Kubie, L. S.: Problems and Techniques of Psychoanalytic Validation and Progress. In Pampian-Mindlen, E. (Ed.), *Psychoanalysis as Science. Second ed.* New York: Basic Books, 1956, p. 175.

** Kubie, L. S.: Some Aspects of the Significance to Psychoanalysis of the Exposure of a Patient to the Televised Audiovisual Reproduction of His Activities. *J. Nerv. Ment. Dis.,* 148:301-309, 1969.

In this volume the reader will find the beginnings of answers to many of the questions posed by Kubie and others.

In conclusion, it is obvious that since the first edition of this book was published in 1970, the use of video in psychiatry as well as the implications of television for psychiatric health and illness of our species has grown to substantial if not immense proportions. In the individual introductions to the sections of this volume, as well as in the contents of each section, a comprehensive overview of the use of videotape techniques in psychiatric training and treatment is presented. A large majority of the chapters in this revision are new although a few of the original chapters and historical articles have been kept. The panoramic psychiatric domain which video has touched from teaching medical students and other students in the social and human sciences to video playbacks with sexually dysfunctional and terminal persons has been covered or touched upon and so the book should be of interest to all in the helping profession. Its contents can be a springboard for additional creative uses of video in treating patients of all kinds and ages and training mental health workers in all settings at various stages of their professional growth.

ACKNOWLEDGMENTS

To all those colleagues and people called patients who have explored the use of television to expand our awareness and understanding of just what in human interpersonal relationships fuels the pump for the multilevel interactions and systems operating in and between people. To Floy J. Moore and to L. Tyhurst for creating and continuing the dialogue of the *TV in Psychiatry Newsletter*.

Specific appreciation is acknowledged and given to Donald Cisky and Millie Montagna of our South Beach library staff, to Patrick Corbitt for his loyal friendship and creative contributions to the technical know-how in this book, and to his steadfast crew at the South Beach media department; to Debbie Rozanski and Henrietta Wise for their help with manuscript preparation; to Susan Barrows of Brunner-Mazel, Inc. for her editorial guidance and help.

SECTION I

Confrontation: History, Theory and Techniques

EDITOR'S INTRODUCTION

Confrontation has become perhaps the most significant concept of this decade as anxiety and alienation were the most common in the preceding one. The confrontational aspects of videotape techniques became a necessity when it was realized that methods used in psychiatric training and treatment previously were not adequate enough in view of the pressing socio-psychological needs of our times. But in addition to the desire to reduce human suffering by shortening the duration of psychotherapeutic treatment there have been economic pressures to find ways to reduce the time and dollars spent for psychiatric treatment. Such issues as third-party payments, with pressure for greater accountability, and the need to find more rapid ways to help patients gain understanding and insight leading to change have also increased interest in confrontational approaches and accordingly in the use of video playback.

Undoubtedly the rapid growth of family therapy approaches in the 60s and 70s has also been fostered by the use of video in almost all family training and treatment centers. Of course we must also keep in mind that the most outstanding family therapists have not only been innovators but also have personalities which lend themselves to the more active confrontational approaches which video provides opportunities for. I refer here to family therapists such as Nathan Ackerman, Carl Whitaker, Virginia Satir, Norman Paul, Salvador Minuchin, Donald Bloch, Ian Alger, and Peter Hogan.

The increasing experience and body of knowledge developed in the 50s and 60s showed that patients were not as fragile as some therapists and trainees believed. The age-old concept that "the truth will set you free" was seen by more and more therapists as being true even in the domain of psychotherapy which had prided itself on being the torch-bearer for truth. Now, video playback and other more direct confrontational approaches were seen less as "gimmicks" and were accepted more as ancillary tools to aid in the difficult process of "working-through."

1

Garner spent many years reviewing historical approaches to confrontation as they have been tried and altered by pioneers in our field and his chapter in this section includes a distillate of his findings as well as providing his version of a successful problem-solving technique through confrontation. His assessment of confrontation goes up to the era of videotape.

In the following chapter confrontation via videotape has been presented with detailed findings from some of the most creative research workers in this fast-evolving field—Carrere, Cornelison, Arsenian, Paredes, Geertsma, Reivich—as well as my own clinical data from work with patients in private practice and institutions. And then a brief review chapter on video feedback confrontation methodology is included. This shows how data for confrontation can be presented for feedback confrontations and what video feedback offers to patient (s) who have an opportunity to experience it.

Individual, couple, family and group confrontations via videotape lead to the challenge of assumptions and of double-binding, confused, ambiguous, contradictory, perplexing communications. They thus allow for the development of more open and truthful communications with greater clarity, directness, adequacy, and mutuality, as well as for negotiation, compromise and, it is hoped, changed and improved relationships.

1

A REVIEW OF CONFRONTATION IN PSYCHOTHERAPY FROM HYPNOSIS TO THE PROBLEM-SOLVING TECHNIQUE

Harry H. Garner, M.D.

Modifications of orthodox psychoanalysis, and of psychoanalytically oriented psychotherapy, were directed at reducing the shortcomings of a technique which restricts therapy to a group of patients with certain limiting specifications. These in fact constitute a very small segment of the total number of patients needing and wanting care. It is true that the number and types of patients considered capable of benefiting from psychotherapy have gradually increased as basic psychoanalytic and other psychotherapeutic methods have been modified and developed. However, one should demonstrate that the therapeutic course and effects of such usage can be understood in terms of an internally consistent theoretical system. Therapeutic results, in order to be scientifically acceptable as a method of treatment, must be understandable on more than trial and error, or empirical grounds.

For example, the range of possible systematic procedures in the treatment of a neurosis conceived theoretically as a reaction to unsuccessful repression would be: 1) strengthening of the defenses, 2) increasing repression, 3) supporting the ego, and 4) increasing problem solving effectiveness and capacity. The strengthening of defenses which may impoverish the individual's adaptive capacity and decrease the possibility of controlling drives by diminishing biologic intensity for expression has a limited potential and would probably not be too rewarding for the individual. The treatment of choice by the psychoanalytically oriented therapist is to produce a permanent readjustment in the total personality. These readjustments should be such that the individual is enabled to integrate within himself and to direct into more acceptable channels drives which

3

had previously required unsuccessful defensive measures, as well as developing an increased capacity to solve stressful environmental problems.

Management of patients by means consistent with psychoanalytic technique and theory has been modified from time to time as certain operational concepts and practices were developed, first by Freud (1, 2, 3), and then by Jung (4), Adler (5), Rank (6), Reich (7), Alexander (8), Horney (9), Fromm (10), and Sullivan (11). Certainly, major modifications in therapeutic technique have resulted from the theories of these therapist-theoreticians as to the nature of the neuroses and the methods best designed for their "cure."

Freud himself suggested activity in therapy as a change from standard analytic technique to be especially suitable for overcoming the protection and adaptive service which a phobia affords patients with hysteria. He believed that only when the therapy had induced phobic patients to relinquish such protective measures did the anxiety-producing material become accessible for achieving dissolution of the hysteria and the phobia. Freud, however, warned against an indiscreet use of such activity. By inducing the patient to accept the thought, or consummate the act which is irrationally feared, the analyst was expected to actively bring about an increased awareness of the conflict, greater insight, a weakening of repressive forces and a strengthening of the patient's adaptive capacity. The patient sees in such activity of the therapist the fulfillment of his wish to be cared for actively, loved and protected by mother or father. Thus, activity may have an important influence in shortening treatment by deepening the transference relationship early in therapy. This will be particularly true in patients possessing strong dependent needs which are being mobilized at the time they are seeking help.

More than any other, Ferenczi's (12) name is associated with the concept of "activity therapy" because of his energetic efforts toward modification of what were considered to be the non-variables in standard psychoanalytic technique. Later Ferenczi repudiated his efforts. He believed that he had been mistaken about the usefulness of active techniques. His thinking was dominated by a concept of "energy flow." As an example of his use of "activity therapy" Ferenczi mentions the command to a patient to abstain from masturbation because he felt treatment was being delayed by the discharge of his psychic energies in the onanistic act. He regarded any sudden change in the patient as an expression of the flow of energy into new channels. Ferenczi also actively intervened by interjecting prohibitions against free associations offered by the patient in the form of a defensive logorrhea. He also suggested that the patient produce phantasy material when resistance was encountered to spontaneous productions. In Discontinuous Analyses, he indicated that the interruption of treatment, as yet another type of activity, was disadvantageous. It is my judgment that Ferenczi was originally correct in principle, but that he failed to carry activity far enough to effect any real change in the patient. His writing about activity did not express much about how significant this activity can become in terms of transference phenomena. A form of activity less significant historically was suggested by Bjerre (13), who recommended ethical education of the patient during psychoanalysis.

Alexander and French (8) have recommended the deliberate use of a variety of active techniques, handled in a flexible manner, with the analyst shifting tactics as the particular needs of the moment arise. They have divided such therapeutic activity into (a) environmental manipulation, and (b) attempts to modify the personality.

General modifications of standard techniques in the direction of more active role for the therapist are suggested as necessary in the increased acceptance of "brief psychotherapy." Such modifications include face to face interviews with content of a more directive nature, manipulating the frequency of interviews, giving advice, employing long- and short-duration interruptions and regulating the intensity of transference feelings to meet the specific needs of the case. Alexander and French emphasize the imperative need for a highly flexible use of known principles of psychodynamics. Neither the use of "empirical" psychotherapy, nor prolonged orthodox psychoanalytic procedures fulfills this need. They stress as the paramount therapeutic process in therapy the importance of a "corrective emotional experience" with the therapist as against a genetic reconstruction of the past. In this, they follow the attempts of Ferenczi and others to add activity to the basic technique.

It has been suggested that a revolution is taking place in efforts at conceptualizing psychotherapy. Social reinforcement and behavior control have been described as key concepts in this new approach. Investigations into influences on attitudes, placebo effects, hypnosis, psychotherapy, sensory deprivation, "brain washing," role-taking and operant conditioning are characteristic areas of study. The effects of reward and manipulation of environmental stimuli are emphasized.

Beginning with Mesmer, the hypnotist psychotherapist took a role in which there was an implied confrontation (14). The patient is threatened with danger of losing the help of an omnipotent and omniscient helper if improper behavior follows upon the failure to fulfill the therapist's expectation. The patient improves, loses symptoms, changes behavior, controls thoughts in keeping with the predictions of the therapist. Hypnosis usually represents a confrontation approach which is at one end of a continuum. The continuum involves confrontation approaches in which problem solving is not expected and may in fact be discouraged at one end of the continuum. The middle section includes therapies in which there is implied problem solving interest on the part of the therapist and includes many of the visual and auditory playback confrontations. At the opposite end of the continuum is the confrontation problem-solving technique which will be described in detail.

That a confrontation approach to the patient has been characteristic of almost every type of psychotherapy endeavor is sometimes overlooked. Certainly, suggestion, persuasion, questioning, advice, reassurance, clarification and actions taken in a two-party system of healer and to-be-healed are seen by the patient as confrontations. There is an implied—"look here, there is something wrong with how you perceive, think or act and I will show you what's wrong and how to correct it." The confrontation aspects of interpretations made in psychoanalytic therapy are evident in that the patient responds as if there were some element of criticism in every interpretation offered. John Rosen's use of a psychoanalytically-oriented approach to the treatment of schizophrenia certainly was associated with rather direct confrontations of a sort (15). A specific role related to a significant figure in the past life of the patient was important for the technique.

The existential therapists in their emphasis on "being" and "becoming" are certainly involved in a confrontation dealing with the values, ethics and morality of the patient. Viktor Frankl, Medard Boss, and Ludwig Binswanger are described as the best known in Harper's book (16). The paradoxical intention intervention used by Frankl represents an overt intervention of a confrontation type.

Suggestion, persuasion, commanding and forbidding, clarification, selective attention and inattention, manipulation, and control are all terms used to describe actions by a therapist intended to influence the behavior of a patient. Learning theory, social theory or conditioning theory refer to the broader hypotheses covering such organized programs of therapy.

TECHNIQUES DIRECTED TOWARD CREATING AN INFLUENCING PROCESS DURING PSYCHOTHERAPY

Experimental methods for verbal and other methods of control of human behavior have been important areas of research by the Russian psychologists for some time. The work of Luria (17) was particularly noted by American psychologists interested in conditioning techniques. Lesse

(18), in describing Russian psychiatry in June of 1956, was impressed by the work on "the second signal system." Experiments in conditioning and deconditioning in which words and language were significant were being carried out by Bykov at the Pavlov Institute of Physiology. He describes Bykov as asserting that cortical control of visceral functions is possible on the basis of laboratory work in animals and man. There is considerable information substantiating this reciprocal relationship in medical literature. Salter's conditioned reflex therapy approach (19) was published sometime before the more familiar publications of Wolpe (20). Instructing, provoking, and instigating confrontations were evident in the techniques described for reconditioning the patient.

Thorne's directive psychotherapy (21) seemed to represent an attempt at an alternative to the emphasis on the so-called "client-centered psychotherapy" of Rogers (22). In offering directions suggesting constructive alternatives to the sick role, Thorne proceeded along the lines of many directive psychotherapists and learning theory psychologists such as Dollard and Miller (23). Basically, the interventions represent confrontations in which the therapist is saying: Your previous experiences have taught you to face situations which cause you so much distress and to experience them with lesser and lesser distress until you have learned that they can be gratifying rather than distressing.

Assuming the role of an important parental figure was also used with the assumption that specific effects would be produced. Rintz and I. M. Rosen (24) worked with manic-depressive psychoses. I. M. Rosen (25) in group therapy found a non-directive approach unrewarding and changed to provocative and more directive interventions, stopping short of anything offensive to society. He worked primarily with chronic schizophrenics and found that certain attempts to contact a patient tended to be somewhat specific in that the repetition of the attitude or action could re-elicit the previous response. As an example, Rosen describes telling a patient, "You are crazy," and continuing to repetitively assert the statement and found that improvement occurred. Some specificity can be determined for the individual patient based on other than intuitive or empirical methods of treatment and determined by peculiar attitudinal needs from other persons.

Wolpe (20) has applied techniques of desensitization, reciprocal inhibition or basically what is described by him as equivalent to unlearning something previously learned. The neurotic anxiety and symptoms having been learned through conditioning but being unadaptive are inhibited by a deconditioning psychotherapy. The psychotherapy has the elements of a method in which behavior is controlled through use of techniques which the therapist suggests, urges or persuades the patient to adopt. He lists several forms of anxiety and suggested responses, or lines of action calculated to decrease anxiety:

1. Assertive responses where the patient who feels anxiety because of an inhibited desire to express resentment is encouraged to such expression.

2. Sexual responses where the patient with a partial sexual inhibition is advised to refrain from sexual activity until he has developed a powerful need to do so.

3. Utilizing the progressive relaxation concepts of Jacobsen, he believes that persistent relaxation implies some measure of reciprocal inhibition of the effects of such anxiety-producing stimuli as may appear.

4. Conditioned avoidance responses where a patient imagines a fall and is simultaneously shocked with a mild faradic current, thereby deconditioning a fear of falling.

5. Feeding responses may be used by having the anxiety-provoking food given under so intense a state of hunger that in the act of eating there will be an inhibition of the anxiety. Possibilities similar to those for feeding responses may be developed for other psychophysiological anxiety reactions in order to stimulate the psychological response and similarly induce an inhibition of the anxiety.

6. If the emotional response evoked by the interviewer is antagonistic to anxiety and of sufficient strength, it may be supposed that it will reciprocally inhibit anxiety responses evoked by the subject matter of the interviews. In abreaction, improvement is produced by the reciprocal inhibition of the anxiety evoked by the emotional reaction to the material brought up in the interview. Emotional responses produced by the sympathetic attitude of the therapist create the reciprocal inhibition.

Ewen Cameron (26) introduced an interesting psychotherapeutic procedure which he referred to as "psychic driving." The procedure essentially consists of repeating to the patient 1) his own verbal cues, "autopsychic driving"; and 2) cues verbalized by others but based on known psychodynamics, "hetero-psychic driving." The repetition is accomplished through playbacks of recorded material. An example is given of a patient who felt intensely rejected by her husband and had experienced a childhood situation in which she felt threatened with abandonment by her mother. As the recording was repeated in subsequent visits, the patient seemed to develop progressive insight and a significant abreaction to the "autopsychic" driving. One must identify a major problem in selecting the key statement for driving. It should not be a long statement and should not contain a multiplicity of topics. This technique is directed at 1) penetration and exploration of the defenses; 2) a continuous activation and expansion of a given area of the patient's experience, that is, making accessible previously unaccessible material; and 3) the setting up of a dynamic implant. Other examples of confrontations of patients by their verbal productions or combinations of hearing or seeing a sample production of their own behavior have been described. Cornelison and Arsenian (27) use a photographic self-image. Moore et al. (28) consider a television taped interview as having therapeutic value when shown to the patient. These aspects of confrontation will be elaborated in more detail by others. (See Chapters 2, 9, 11, 12, 13)

In attempting to influence the withdrawn psychotic patient to establish communication, studies have been made of the use of objects supposedly having symbolic significance for the patient. Azima and Wittkower (29) used such symbols as finger paints, bean bags, balls and baby bottles.

Stevenson (30) investigates chiefly three kinds of new behavioral responses called communicative, assertive, and affiliative responses and attempts to instigate in the patient new behavioral responses to current stressful persons and situations. The patient is encouraged to substitute immediate, direct, and verbal communications with other people for delayed, indirect, and nonverbal communications. He is encouraged to assert his legitimate needs and express, at the moment of arising, his important emotions. When his social contacts were insufficient he was encouraged to increase them, partly for the greater gratification he could obtain and partly to increase his interaction with other people. In general, he uses indirect techniques to stimulate new behavior. Since patients try to change to please the therapist in every psychotherapy, it is better from the beginning to assist the patient to change for his sake, rather than to please the therapist. In any case, direct instructions are not often needed. Stevenson raises questions with the patient about his failure to make different responses. Such a question as, "Why didn't you discuss this matter with your wife when she came home?" arouses in the mind of the patient the possibility that he ought to have done this. When the patient seemed to have denied emotions which could be inferred or which reached expression later or indirectly, he attempts to evoke the original emotions more strongly and to help the patient discover that he had inhibited more appropriate behavior. "Well, I think nearly everyone in your place would have felt angry." "What thoughts did you have when your father said you were lazy?" Stevenson indicates that once inhibited behavior occurs, it tends to be reinforced by misperceptions the patient acquires about himself. False generalizations about himself, e.g., "I am a failure, a coward, or an alcoholic," tend to inhibit further constructive action. Finally, he helps the patient correct his misperceptions of other people. Stevenson spends considerable time working with ideas the patient has of himself. Behavior toward the therapist is discussed under two circumstances only: when such behavior glaringly demonstrated some important trait which the patient practiced to his own detriment with other people, and whenever the patient's attitude interfered with his progress in the interviews. This most commonly happened when the patient relaxed to await discovery of "what the cause was."

E. Lakin Philips' (31) confrontations are in the nature of assaults on the patient's assertions about himself which put him in the position of fulfilling an expectation of himself as a loser. Teaching substitute patterns that hold greater probability of being confirmed by experiences in living represents the confrontation intervention.

Ellis (32), in describing a "rational therapy," expressed his therapeutic endeavors as making a concerted attack on the irrational positions of the patient. The therapist was seen as a frank counter-protagonist who directly contradicts and denies the self-defeating propaganda originally learned and perpetuated through repetition. The therapist encourages, cajoles, and at times commands the patient to engage in activity which will act as a forceful counter-propagandistic agent. The patient in effect is the object of confrontations directing attention to self-defeating perceptions, thoughts and behavior, and is obliged to respond positively to confrontations which suggest a new orientation and behavior.

The terms complementary or symmetrical are descriptive for the relationship of two people in communication with each other. It is assumed that the individuals are constantly trying to define and influence the nature of their relationship. Jackson et al. (33) and Haley (34, 35), state in essence, that a person may be in a complementary relationship if he does what he is told or if he tells others what to do. A symmetrical relationship is one in which two people exchange the same sort of behavior: one asks for something and the other asks for something, one gives and the other gives. The problem of psychotherapy and patient or therapist control is expressed by Haley as follows: Although psychotherapy involves many factors such as support, encouragement of self-expression, and so on, it is crucial that the therapist determine whether he or the patient is to control what is to happen in their relationship. No form of therapy can avoid this problem because if the patient gains control, he will perpetuate his difficulty, particularly if he gains it by his usual symptomatic means. If one describes psychotherapy as a process whereby the therapist maintains control of the relationship he will have with a patient, then it becomes necessary for one person to gain control of another person's behavior and, therefore, his emotions. The approach offered by him has emphasized how the hypnotic relationship is a useful model for the exploration of such tactics.

Erikson's technique mentioned by Haley includes encouraging the subject to resist him after having asked him to cooperate. The patient is now in a peculiar position, and cannot easily gain control of what is going to happen. "If the subject resists, he is doing what the hypnotist asks, and if he cooperates he is doing what the hypnotist asks." In the control interview he is encouraged to talk and also to withhold material. During treatment, instructions typically involve doing something he is doing anyway, but under direction. For instance, a patient seeking to lose weight, although a compulsive eater, is encouraged to gain weight in keeping with her personality needs. Erikson finally compromises with the patient after she has gained weight against her protest and then permits her to stop gaining weight. In essence, the basic rule of brief psychotherapy described by Haley is to encourage the symptom in such a way that the patient cannot continue to utilize it.

Mowrer (36) sees the prime action of the therapist as self-disclosure of unresolved personal guilt. He starts with the premise that deviant behavior has been concealed by the patient. It is the possibility of being found out, being called to account by his reference group, or the disapproval of an active, well-developed conscience which he sees as the essence of what has been called a neurosis. He swings from a center of emphasis on abnormal emotions to abnormal or deviant behavior. The individual's sense of identity and his social integration will be restored. Behavior therapies are divided by him into three classes. Type I is that exemplified by the desensitization techniques of Wolpe (20), Type II by the operant conditioning methods of Skinner (37) and Type III by the social integration therapy of Mowrer (36). In Type III therapy, the therapist models the behavior he expects the patient to learn. The behavior modification is expected to come from the patient as he learns that his duplicitous behavior is where his real problem lies.

OPERANT CONDITIONING CONCEPTS ARE APPLICABLE TO CONFRONTATION TECHNIQUES

In operant conditioning the therapist is seen as being in a position to manipulate the patient's behavior. The presence of the therapist is in itself a factor in controlling the nature of the verbal productions. Sex, prestige, socio-economic factors, role expectancies transmitted to the patient, the role the patient feels he is to assume, and the conditioning situation when structured in a positive way are all determinants of the significance of the therapist as a "social reinforcement machine" (38). Karno (39) questions psychotherapeutic effect as being the result of a patient's acceptance of a model of more mature or healthy behavior following upon logical and verbal rationale or insight. "The large part of such persuasion is the person of the therapist, whose skillful communications form an elaborate system of operant conditioning."

Operant conditioning methods as a basis for treatment have been used in a variety of psychiatric problems and settings. Operant conditioning as a concept was used by Skinner (37) to explain the whole range of the child's learned behavior. He has referred to the parental responses which indicate attention, affection, and approval as general reinforcers. It is this earlier behavior which determines that relationship of the patient to the therapist and makes the operant conditioning of psychotherapy possible. The extensive experimental work with animals needs no elaboration here. The use of operant conditioning techniques in treatment was recently reviewed by Krasner (40). Krasner cites the work of Ayllon in using nurses as "behavioral engineers," of Thomas and Goldiamond to reinstate verbal behavior in psychotics, and Saslow and Matarazzo to enhance generalization of newly learned behavior, Slack to reinforce desirable behavior in delinquents and Richard Dignam and Horner in rewarding non-delusional thinking.

In operant conditioning, the concepts of general and specific reinforcers in learning theory have a built-in acceptance of the implied compliant attitude of the patient. Behavioral change can be recognized by its compliant, non-compliant and problem-solving significance, whether the therapist is seen as a "social reinforcement machine," a teacher, or a parent whose influencing action is directed at increasing the maturational needs for being a problem-solver. The author (41-45) has indicated that operant conditioning experimenters seem to influence toward compliance; teachers may waiver between seeking compliance or problem-solving. The intent in confrontation problem-solving is to recognize and utilize problem-solving potential whenever the situation permits. Confirmatory evidence of the significance of compliance is found in abundance in the literature. The following evidence mentioned demonstrates this point but is far from an inclusive report of the literature. Dreams have been described frequently as showing the influence of compliant tendency and in helping to establish the evidence for compliance and the operant conditioning concepts to psychoanalysis. "Confirmatory dreams" come about according to Freud during analytic sessions by the analyst suggesting repressed material to the patient based on symptoms, associations and other signs and, shortly thereafter, the patient reports a dream which contains the repressed material. The analyst interprets, constructs and propounds, and the patient confirms the validity of the suggestion by the subsequent dream material. The analyst's suggestions are seen as successful because an unconscious force in the patient derived from a positive transference yields a "compliance toward the analyst" which, in turn, aids the treatment process. It follows that "if anyone wishes to maintain that most of the dreams that can be made use of in analysis are compliant dreams and owe their origin to suggestion, nothing can be said against the opinion from the point of view of analytic theory." Certainly, the approval sensed by the patient for producing dream material may be a general reinforcer. More specific reinforcement resulting from "successful" dream interpretation is obvious evidence of the operant conditioning elements in psychoanalysis on dream interpretation. Ritter (46), using a form of indirect suggestion patterned after verbal conditioning, was able to influence the ratio of male and female figures in dream material and, Zubin (47), in referring to the possible implication of verbal conditioning for psychotherapy, wrote, "reinforcement may be the reason why Freudians get freudian dreams, Jungians get jungian dreams, Rogerians get no dreams at all!" Fisher's experimental work with dreams on patients in analysis is likewise confirmatory.

The experiments of Sloane et al. (48) confirm the desirability of the use of a technique which would tend to act as a process for deconditioning. Their results indicate that psychoneurotic patients are more easily conditioned than normal subjects. Their results are also in keeping with what has been termed the greater responsiveness to suggestion of the psychoneurotic or the individual in a situation in which he seeks help. The importance of compliance as a basis for bringing about social improvement in chronically ill schizophrenic patients is verified by studies such as the following. Cohen (49) treated 28 chronically regressed schizophrenics by focusing on specific behavioral patterns, demanded improved behavior, exerted group pressure on recalcitrants and rewarded improvement publicly. Of the 28 patients whose average length of current hospitalization had been 12 years, only five failed to show some improvement. It seems self-evident in this study that behavioral change is brought about as a result of compliant attitudes out of fear of loss of love or punishment. The compliant attitude of the patient was recognized as important by Freud and is expressed in the following quote: "If the patient does not show compliance enough to respect the necessary conditions of the analysis, we can not regularly succeed in giving all the symptoms of the neurosis a new transference-coloring and in replacing his whole ordinary neurosis by a transference neurosis of which he can be cured by therapeutic work."

The author described the successful utilization of the confrontation problem-solving technique in psychiatric treatment for the first time at a meeting of the Illinois Psychiatric Society in 1954. This technique has a problem-solving rather than a permissive or coercive approach. It has been used on hundreds of patients with diverse psychiatric, medical, and surgical problems. The application of the confrontation technique as a tool to be used extensively and intensively throughout the therapeutic process is based on the difficulty with which old learned patterns, which once had adaptive value, are unlearned. In the learning process, motivational pressures and the subjective needs of the individual have created goal-seeking directed at satisfying the needs of hunger, love, and urge toward mastery. The responses that brought satisfaction were repetitively carried out until they become automatic responses no longer requiring problem-solving. The person accepts his adaptations, when effectively repeated over a significant period, as unalterable. Indeed, he reacts with resistance to alteration even when the pattern of behavior becomes obviously maladaptive.

The techniques of therapy applied in confrontation problem-solving psychotherapy include the presentation of a statement and a question. A problem which is crucial but only vaguely recognized or not recognized may be used as a therapeutic focus. It is then clearly stated: "Stop believing that you have nothing to look forward to. What do you think or feel about what I told you?" The frequent reiteration of the statement is intended to create the atmosphere or feeling that the status quo is unacceptable, and a solution is found by continuous searching. It is as if the therapist's repetitious question acts as a continuous pressure to force the acceptance of a need to explore and solve a problem.

The confrontation technique has developed within the framework of uncovering psychotherapy in which interpretations and questions are intended to overcome resistances and bring about varying degrees of reconstruction of the past. An understanding of the nature of the pathological defenses and an awareness of the personality structure in concepts expressed by terms such as drives, needs, desires, anxiety, controls, social conformity, superego, conscience, adaptive functions and reality-testing are necessary. An awareness of the influence of past on present interpersonal relations and their importance for transference phenomena is essential. The basic psychotherapeutic framework in which the technique has evolved might, therefore, be described as psychodynamically oriented psychotherapy. When insight is not involved because of the technique used or because the goals for the treatment of the patient are limited, transference interpretations, or dealing with the relationship of past and present, may be totally avoided. The goal is then to bring about a change in symptoms or to improve social functioning rather than focusing on alteration of personality structure.

Authoritarian directives intensify transference phenomena and the tendency to repeat a behavior pattern previously executed without questions as to its significance. However, the patient is invited to work out a mutually satisfactory solution to conflicts, rather than being simply instructed or left to wander on alone by the question, "What do you think or feel about what I told you?" The question creates a desire in the patient to test the significance of the controls and to evaluate these further on a realistic basis. In other words, it fosters reality-testing instead of fostering transference neurosis.

Choosing the statement with which the patient is confronted will vary in light of the clinical picture of the patient and the nature of the relationship at the initial use of the confrontation. The area of conflict selected will vary from case to case. It is a question of the therapist's acuity in ascertaining the area of core conflict or immediate struggle, whether it is sexual, sibling rivalry, or some other disequilibrium. The patient may be confronted with a prohibitive statement: "You must never, under any circumstances, masturbate!" or an expressive or permissive statement: "It would be better if your husband dies," or an adaptive statement involving a mature value orientation: "I want you to continue to work at your job." By and large, all of the confrontation statements may be classified in one of these three categories. The confrontation, once stated, is used continuously. The process of developing self-assurance through mastery and achievement is not inhibited by fear of punishment, shame, failure, or fear of loss of love because of the noncondemning nature of the relationship and the encouragement to seek a solution suggested by the repetitive question.

In the natural sciences, predictive hypotheses are made with the assurance that the matter being studied will not be influenced to change by the prediction of the investigator. In interpersonal relations, one cannot be certain that the authority of the therapist will not overwhelm the patient. Patients will often do that which was predicted for them. The boundary line between prediction and suggestion, which is of no consequence in the natural sciences, is difficult to maintain in any of the social sciences. A psychotherapy which can enable the therapist to predict the outcome of an intervention and then check on the prediction would be one which might offer possibilities for creating a science of psychotherapy. The confrontation statements as used in the psychotherapy and followed by the question, "What do you think or feel about what I told you?" are repeated frequently. The patient's responses offer an opportunity of studying the degree to which suggestion or problem-solving dominates the patient's attempt to understand the significance of the statement. By constant observation of the patient's verbal responses, behavior and propensity for exploring alternatives, one can reach some conclusions with reasonable certainty. For example, one may conclude that the patient is being compliant (showing the responses expected to a suggestion); critically compliant (his behavior suggests that compliance was recognized as being in his best interest); non-compliant (his behavior, affect, thoughts are appropriate for rejecting a suggestion); or problem-solving in his behavior (attitudes, thoughts and affect are appropriate for decision-making).

REFERENCES

1. Freud, S.: The Future of Psychoanalytic Therapy. *Coll. Papers,* 2:285-296. London: Hogarth Press, 1946.
2. Freud, S.: Remarks Upon the Theory and Practice of Dream Interpretation. *Coll. Papers* 5:136-149. London: Hogarth Press, 1950.
3. Freud, S.: Further Recommendations in the Technique of Psychoanalysis: Recollection, Repetition and Working Through. *Coll. Papers* 2:366-376. London: Hogarth Press, 1946.
4. Jung, C. G.: *Contributions to Analytical Psychology.* New York: Harcourt Brace & Co., 1928.
5. Adler, A.: A Study of Organ Inferiority and Its Psychical Compensation. (Trans. by E. J. Smith) *Nerv. & Ment. Dis. Mono. Series* #24, 1917.
6. Rank, O.: *The Trauma of Birth.* New York: Harcourt Brace & Co., 1929.
7. Reich, W.: *Character-Analysis: Principles and Technique for Psychoanalysts in Practice and Training.* (Trans. by P. Wolpe). New York: Orgonne Inst. Press, 1949.
8. Alexander, F. and French, T. M.: *Psychoanalytic Therapy: Principles and Application.* New York: Ronald Press, 1946.
9. Horney, K.: *The Neurotic Personality of Our Time.* New York: W. W. Norton and Co., 1937.
10. Fromm, E.: *Escape from Freedom.* New York: Farrar and Rinehart, 1941.
11. Sullivan, H. S.: *Conceptions of Modern Psychiatry.* Washington, D. C.: William Alanson White Psychiatric Foundation, 1947.
12. Ferenczi, S.: *Further Contributions to the Theory and Technique of Psychoanalysis.* London: Hogarth Press, 1952.
13. Bjerre, P.: *The History and Practice of Psychoanalysis.* (Trans. by E. Barrow). London: Gorham Press, 1920.
14. Sweig, S.: *Mental Healers.* London: Cassel, 1933.
15. Rosen, J. N.: *Direct Analysis: Selected Papers.* New York: Grune & Stratton, 1953.
16. Harper, R. A.: *Psychoanalysis and Psychotherapy: 36 Systems.* New York: Prentice Hall, 1960.

17. Luria, A. R.: *The Nature of Human Conflict: An Objective Study of Disorganization and Control of Human Behavior.* (Trans. & Ed. by W. Horsly Gantt). New York: Liveright, 1932.
18. Lesse, S.: Current Clinical and Research Trends in Soviet Psychiatry. *Amer. J. Psychiat.* 114:1018-1022, 1958.
19. Salter, A.: *Conditioned Reflex Therapy.* New York: Creative Age Press, 1949.
20. Wolpe, J.: Reciprocal Inhibition as the Main Basis of Psychotherapeutic Effect. *Arch. Neur. Psychiat.* 72:205-226, 1954.
21. Thorne, F.: *Principles of Psychotherapy Counseling.* Brandon, V. J.: J. Clin. Psychol., 1950.
22. Roger, C.: *Client-Centered Therapy.* Boston: Houghton, 1951.
23. Dollard, J. and Miller, N.: *Personality and Psychotherapy.* New York: McGraw-Hill Book Co., 1950.
24. Rintz, N. D. and Rosen, I. M. Psychotherapy of Manic-Depressive Patients in the Manic Phase. *Psychiat. Quart.*, 26:462-471, 1952.
25. Rosen, I. M.: Specificity in the Psychotherapeutic Approach to the Psychotic Person. *Arch. Gen. Psychiat.*, 2:350-355, 1960.
26. Cameron, D. E.: Psychic Driving. *Amer. J. Psychiat.*, 112:502-509, 1956.
27. Cornelison, F. S., Jr., and Arsenian, J.: A Study of the Responses of Psychotic Patients to Photographic Self-Image Experience. *Psychiat. Quart.*, 34:1-8, 1960.
28. Moore, F. J., Chernell, E., and West, M. J.: Television as a Therapeutic Tool. *Arch. Gen. Psychiat.*, 12:217-220, 1965.
29. Azima, H. and Wittkower, E. D.: Gratification of Basic Needs in Treatment of Schizophrenics. *Psychiatry*, 19:121-129, 1956.
30. Stevenson, I.: Direct Instigation of Behavioral Change in Psychotherapy. *Arch. Gen. Psychiat.*, 1:99-107, 1959.
31. Philips, E. L.: *Psychotherapy: A Modern Theory and Practice.* Englewood Cliff., N. J.: Prentice Hall, 1956.
32. Ellis, A.: *How to Live with a Neurotic.* New York: Crown, 1957.
33. Jackson, D. D., Riskin, J., and Satir, V.: A Method of Analysis of a Family Interview. *Arch. Gen. Psychiat.*, 5:321-339, 1961.
34. Haley, J.: Control in Brief Psychotherapy. *Arch. Gen. Psychiat.*, 4:139-153, 1961.
35. Haley, J.: Control in Psychotherapy with Schizophrenics. *Arch. Gen. Psychiat.*, 5:340-353, 1961.
36. Mowrer, O. H.: The Behavior Therapies with Special Reference to Modeling and Imitation. Presented at the Guthiel Memorial Lectures, New York, October, 1965.
37. Skinner, B. F.: *Science and Human Behavior.* New York: MacMillan Press, 1953.
38. Ekman, P., Krasner, L., and Ullman, K. P.: The Interaction of Set and Awareness as Determinants of Response to Verbal Conditioning. *J. Abnorm. Soc. Psychol.*, 66:387-489, 1963.
39. Karno, M.: Communication, Reinforcement and "Insight"—the Problem of Psychotherapeutic Effect. *Amer. J. Psychother.*, 19:467-479, 1965.
40. Krasner, L.: The Therapist as a Social Reinforcement Machine. In H. H. Strupp and L. Luborsky (Eds.): *Research in Psychotherapy*, Amer. Psychol. Assoc., 2:61-64, 1962.
41. Garner, H. H.: A Confrontation Technique Used in Psychotherapy. *Amer. J. Psychother.*, 13:18-34, 1959.
42. Garner, H. H.: A Nascent Somatic Delusion Treated Psychotherapeutically by Confrontation Technique. *J. Clin. & Exper. Psychopath.*, 20:135-143, 1959.
43. Garner, H. H.: A Confrontation Technique Used in Psychotherapy. *Progr. in Psychother.*, 5:94-98, 1960.
44. Garner, H. H.: A Confrontation Technique Used in Psychotherapy. *Compr. Psychiat.*, 1:201-211, 1960.

45. Garner, H. H.: Interventions in Psychotherapy and the Confrontation Interview. *Amer. J. Psychoanal.*, 22:47-58, 1962.
46. Ritter, W.: The Susceptibility of Dream Recall to Indirect Suggestion Patterned After Verbal Conditioning. *Amer. J. Psychother.*, 19:87-98, 1965.
47. Zubin, J.: Criteria for Evaluation of Results in Psychotherapy. *Amer. J. Psychother.*, 18 (Suppl. 1): 138-144, 1964.
48. Sloane, R. B., Davidson, P. O. and Payne, R. W.: Anxiety and Arousal in Psychoneurotic Patients. *Arch. Gen. Psychiat.*, 13:19-23, 1965.
49. Cohen, L.: How to Reverse Chronic Behavior. *Ment. Hosp.*, 15:39-41, 1964.
50. Fisher, C.: Studies on the Nature of Suggestion, Part I. *J. Amer. Psychoanalyt. Assoc.*, 1:222-255, 1953.
51. Gordon, R. E.: Sociodynamics and Psychotherapy. *Arch. Neur. Psychiat.*, 81:486-503, 1959.
52. Greenson, R.: The Working Alliance and the Transference Neuroses. *Psychoanalyt. Quart.*, 34:155-181, 1965.
53. Loewald, H.: On the Therapeutic Action of Psycho-analysis. *Int. J. Psychoanal.*, 41:16-33, 1960.

2

CONFRONTATION THROUGH VIDEOTAPE

Milton M. Berger, M.D.

As Garner in the preceding chapter has so well pointed out in his historical review of confrontation in the pre-television period, techniques evolved ranging from psychotherapeutic approaches like those of Mesner which demanded change without insight to those methods replete with opportunities for insight and/or directed or non-directed corrective emotional experiences which might lead to change.

However it was not until the recent development of video facilities for immediate and later replay confrontations with one's own self-image, alone or in interaction with others, that the depth of exploration, understanding and self-knowledge possible to achieve now marked another milestone in psychotherapeutic approaches. The margins of our knowledge of self-image(s) and self-concept(s) have been expanding profoundly by videotape confrontations.

The understanding and undermining of measures used by therapists as well as patients which have served to protect and maintain crippling maladaptive neurotic and psychotic systems of functioning have been profoundly enhanced by the development of various confrontational methods including videotape playback. My advocacy of the flexibly integrated use of psychodynamic theory and the multiple confrontational methods we now have available is in the service of offering patients the corrective emotional experience necessary to bring about real change and not just intellectual insight into the genesis and perpetuation of their neurotic patterns.

Confrontation in treatment is a form of psychotherapeutic intervention. However, whether it serves as more of an interference or intrusion than a constructive intervention will depend upon the scientific and artistic skill of the therapist, his intuitive sense of timing, and the goals for confrontation envisioned by the therapist.

Rogers used photographs with phonograph recordings to improve psychotherapy in 1942.* Self-image or self-confrontation techniques in American psychiatry have been used by Cornelison, one of our major pioneers, since 1954. Carrère in 1954 published a report in a French journal on the principles and techniques of applying cinematography to the treatment of patients with delirium tremens (1, 2). The report by Cornelison and Arsenian in 1960 (3) has become an historical breakthrough and stimulus to other workers to use photographs, motion pictures or videotape for self-image confrontation with patients. They reported on a self-confrontation study using polaroid pictures of themselves shown to patients one minute after being taken, and sound motion pictures shown to patients in intermittent sessions. They studied the use of this self-confrontation technique for investigative research and therapy. Their basic procedure consisted of the following steps: 1) A photograph was taken of the subject; 2) the photograph was shown to the subject; 3) the experience was discussed with the subject; 4) the subject's response to seeing the photographic self-image was observed.

They focused on the patient's self-perception by asking the following questions: 1) Who is the person in the picture? 2) What do you like about the picture? 3) What do you dislike about the picture? 4) What would you like to change? 5) Do you think that future pictures will show any change? 6) Does the picture remind you of anyone else?

All patients in their study were acutely ill psychotics selected from the reception service at Boston State Hospital in 1958 and were without gross organic involvement or recent electric shock treatment or drug therapy. They ranged from 19 to 50 years of age and were mostly diagnosed as schizophrenic. One was in a manic state and another in an involutional psychotic depression.

Cornelison and Arsenian concluded that there were certain noticeable sex differences in patient responses. 1) Women expressed interest in cosmetic aspects of appearance, especially that of face and hair. If men showed an interest in the face, it was to note the presence or absence of a smile. 2) Male patients were more concerned with qualities of strength or weakness, for example, fatigue, inactivity or laziness. 3) Greater intensity as well as quality of feeling was expressed by women than men. Women complained more vigorously than men about pictures they did not like. Two women tore up pictures of themselves. Men did not. Women also expressed positive feelings for their pictures more readily than the men.

---

* Rogers, C. R., The Use of Electrically-Recorded Interviews in Improving Psychotherapeutic Techniques. *Amer. J. of Orthopsychiatry*, 12:429-434, 1942.

They also found that self-image confrontations were influential in bringing about rapid changes in psychotic states. In my private practice I find the same acceleration in the process of change (see Chapter 16). They conjectured that self-confrontation may bring a psychotic individual into better contact with the realistic self. They quote Freud that psychosis is a withdrawal of libido from the world of external objects. The photograph of self may be a means of redirecting libido outward as the image does present a familiar object.

They also state that individual differences in the degree and kind of narcissism may affect a psychotic person's response to photographic self-images. "The early existence of primary self-love and the gradual acquisition of secondary narcissism are steps in normal ego development" (4).

Geertsma and Reivich in their first report on repetitive self-observation by videotape playback in 1965 (5) indicated that repeated playbacks "occasioned changes in self-concept and induced intense affective reactions." In an article in 1968 (6) the same authors report that they applied a systematic feedback technique to 64 hospitalized psychiatric inpatients at the University of Kansas Medical Center and elicited a wide variety of responses. Prior to a structured videotaped interview each patient was instructed to describe himself as he generally felt himself to be (his Self-As-Is description) and as he would ideally like to be (his Ideal-Self description). Following the structured interview he was instructed to rate himself according to how he remembered himself in the interview (his Remembered-Self description). A videotape playback of the interview then followed immediately and the patient was instructed to rate himself in terms of what he had just observed of himself on the television monitor (his TV-Self description). The next phase of their carefully worked out experimental project was to have each patient fill out a completion-type questionnaire designed to elicit a subjective account of his self-viewing experience. This questionnaire consisted of six completion items preceded by the instruction: "Try to fill in the following phrases as accurately as possible." The six items were: 1) "While watching the videotape playback, I felt. . . ." 2) "My appearance. . . ." 3) "I was surprised by. . . ." 4) "I was reminded of. . . ." 5) "The experience of watching myself was. . . ." 6) "Further comments: . . ."

The entire protocol, from initial self-rating to completion of the questionnaire, required from 45 to 90 minutes depending largely on how fast the patient could work. Of the original 64 patients in this research study, 26 (41%) randomly selected patients were re-exposed to another standardized interview and videotape self-observation experience, along with the identical testing regimen, two to three weeks after the initial experimental session and just prior to the patients' dismissal from the hospital.

Reivich and Geertsma found that the initial videotape self-observation experience evoked anxiety in 77% of their patients and caused temporary disorganization in a few. Subsequent exposure induced less anxiety. Sixty-eight percent of the patients responded favorably to the questionnaire item, "The experience of watching myself was" with comments such as, "eye-opening," "interesting," "enlightening," "reassuring," "enjoyable," "rewarding," "exciting," "profitable," "helpful," "informative," "relaxing," "educational," "thrilling," and "fun." Twenty-three percent expressed mixed or guarded attitudes such as, "suprising" and "different," while 17% were openly negative about the experience, considering it "disgusting," "not very encouraging," "sickening," "heartbreaking," "depressing," "dumb," and "awful." Of the 26 patients who repeated the experience twice only six reported unfavorable responses on either occasion. In general those patients who were more upset by the experience tended to dislike it but there was in no patient evidence of sustained negative effect.

In regard to identifications, it was found in their study that most patients recognized and identified with their self-image, although there were a few notable exceptions such as one patient who had burst into tears twice during the structured interview but watched the playback without apparent affect. She commented, "It doesn't seem real. It doesn't seem like me. It seems as if I've been watching somebody else. I didn't experience any of the emotions while watching that I experienced in the tape. It made me feel it wasn't true." She described the experience as a "weird unreality." Five other patients expressed similar feelings stating, "It was like watching a stranger"; "It was not really me and yet it was"; "It was not me at all but a stranger"; "It was like watching . . . someone else who was rather withdrawn and casual or indifferent." Reivich and Geertsma reflect that these statements probably represent effects of disturbed ego functioning such as the utilization of extreme denial or some other defense mechanisms. To me the reactions of these hospitalized, acutely disturbed patients are a reflection of their profound alienation-from-self as described by Horney (7).

It is only in a passing observation that they mention in their 1968 paper the reaction in some patients to recognition of an unconscious identification with a significant relative, such as a woman who suddenly recognized her similarity to her despised and hated grandmother whom she had discussed with great feeling in several previous interviews. In my experience with videotape in private practice, I have seen such a recognition trigger startling shock reactions which were important milestones for therapeutic insight and progress. For example, Clara, an overweight, quiet, passive-aggressive, 35-year-old married mother of two school children was taken aback by experiencing a selected videotape playback of herself in interaction during a group session. She had been reared in an unloving home with a double-binding, inconsistent mother and a cruel, intermittently absent ne'er-do-well alcoholic father. She said: "I looked at myself and saw my mother, I nearly dropped dead! It's like a look of distaste or suspicion and as if she smelled something bad. God, I never realized that I had this look—that I looked like this in repose and when I was just looking at somebody. And I also noticed this real ploppy-blobby expression—and with a real double chin. I never knew that. And I realized that I looked a lot like Mary—like organic—like a sleepwalker—like one-half asleep and dopey. (Mary is a former alcoholic group member who dropped out of the group and was in a sanitarium at this time). My husband has been telling me that for years. I look sleepy and all doped up and I thought of my father, too—ugh! It was quite a surprise—I never knew I looked that way! And oh! my voice (pause) it's this high little girl voice with a definite pattern of rrr-rrr-rrr-rrr—an up and down singsongy effect."

Though the video playback brought forth many painful expressions of her self-hate and awareness of ways she had unconsciously incorporated her mother and father into her character structure, she definitely became more clearly motivated following this disturbing confrontation to work more actively toward giving up her alienation, her resignation and her passivity in her group and in her home life.

Selections used for focused confrontational feedback may range from a few moments of audiovisual playback to the playback of a single visual behavior without sound in order to trigger insight, awareness or free associations in a patient or family or group. It is often necessary to play back segments of the preceding complex social interaction taking place over a period of minutes in order to confront and then review with people the arrangements they unconsciously make with others through their nonverbalized communications. There is no longer a necessary reliance upon the patient's or therapist's ability to recall as we now have a system of recall much more reliable and better than his memory or the therapist's memory or notes or even audiotapes, because it provides para and meta communications as well as context.

The study made by Reivich and Geertsma also revealed that 44% of their patients openly disparaged some aspect of their appearance, there being no striking difference between men and women in this regard. A larger proportion of their patients, 50%, were favorably inclined toward the way they looked on the monitor although half of these made critical comments about specific points such as weight, facial features or baldness. They found that a person's reaction to his appearance is significantly related to his total affective response to the self-viewing experience.

In reporting my experience with the use of videotape playbacks with psychotherapy groups in a community mental health service program* in 1968, it was noted that videotape playback confrontations can serve as a crucial part of the therapeutic process with inpatients (8). Remarkable self-image reactions occur which circumvent some of the overprotective experiences encountered in psychotherapy or on the ward. Seeing oneself and reflectively reexperiencing meaningful interactions frequently allows a person to acknowledge something about himself which he has not previously been ready to accept from either therapist or other patients who have themselves been more or less ambivalent about making the necessary but perhaps painful confrontation. Once this self-perception has taken place the patient is much more open to validation by his group, which can become more caring, meaningful and constructive and is less likely to be experienced as criticizing or attacking.

For example, Lydia, who had been repeatedly told of her sullenness and anger, was able to share her shocked reaction with her group after confronting her self-image during a playback session. She acknowledged that she was now aware that she had indeed been displaying exactly those behaviors group members had been trying to point out to her and which she had previously been denying. It is as if a group member is now able to see himself almost as if he were another member of the group whom he can view more objectively. This kind of experience is important for growth and maturing through the expanding of one's observing ego.

The first playback session of a group is extremely important, primarily as a self-image confrontational experience. It is almost as if other members are not noticed during this session as each individual fixes on his own ongoing image. Some of the self-confrontations occurring during the first playback sessions had profound and long-lasting effects on subsequent behavior. Here are some examples of patients' reactions immediately during and following this experience:

Ron, an extremely childish 29-year-old chronic schizophrenic, reacted with more spontaneity and appropriate affect than ever before. In a subdued and choked voice he said, "I haven't changed since I was six years

* This work was done on the Washington Heights Community Mental Health Service at the New York State Psychiatric Institute.

old. I thought I was growing up, but I am acting there as if I were a six-year-old boy. I haven't grown up at all."

Mary, a withdrawn, 19-year-old, unmarried high school dropout who had been hospitalized for more than a year, said, "I always thought I was involved in the group and a part of things. I'm not involved. I'm not here! I'm never involved with anyone in any group!" Following exposure of this blind spot to Mary, she was motivated to make strenuous and successful efforts to actively involve herself differently with various people and to give up her detachment. The changes in her interpersonal relationships were marked and have been maintained. She has intermittently referred to the impact of her first playback experience, almost as if to remind herself to continue to move her growing edge forward.

George, a 31-year-old, single, compulsive, intellectual, obsessional schizophrenic, who functioned as an emotional illiterate, said, "When I told Lydia she was blocking her emotions, I was projecting. That's me —I block my emotions—I don't know what they are."

May, a 26-year-old mother of twin boys, with a disposition to feeling abused and collecting rejections, commented: "First of all, Susan, Tom and I dominated the group. Then I was amazed how sad I looked. Either I was looking sad or I was being a know-it-all. We all talked on a high plane, but we really didn't talk about anything."

It has been my experience that in group psychotherapy with predominantly character-neurotic patients in private practice the initial videotape playback reactions are more often positive than with psychotic inpatients; there are reactions such as, "I look prettier than I thought I did," or "Gee, I didn't know I had such a sexy voice and nice smile." Others are primarily self-critical such as, "God, I come through with such a sickening smile," or "I didn't realize I look like such a mouse. I hardly ever moved my body or changed my tone." In general, the majority of initial playback reactions with both neurotic and psychotic patients includes remarks indicating preoccupation with appearance and sex appeal in women and masculinity or its absence in men.

The continued effects of videotape confrontation in groups are somewhat different from the primarily self-image preoccupation which occurs initially. Subsequent playbacks lead to a more profound awareness of pathological interaction and characteristic styles of being and relating. Repeated confrontations enable patients to identify their own self-defeating patterns and to become more quickly identified with and to join the therapist in a protherapeutic position as they see and hear their overreactions and underreactions and inappropriate ways of reacting. It is as if the process of awareness through the playback itself tends to demand the giving up of denial systems. Further, where change is achieved, patients are often best able to see it in the playback session, when they can be more objective and less interactionally or defensively involved than in the ongoing experience of a regular group session.

Playback sessions are also valuable in either precipitating therapeutic crises or effectively confronting patients in crises. For example, Selena, an extremely disorganized manic-depressive, unmarried, artistic woman of 38, with a history of many prior hospitalizations, was shocked during one of her relatively quiescent periods to confront herself during the playback of the previous week's tape of her group meeting during which she had been explosively manic. At first she sat silently, in stunned disbelief, then she asked the therapist to turn off the tape. The therapist and other group members urged her to continue watching. Selena began to weep and scream, insisting that she could not bear the ugliness of herself. Another group member took her hand and together the group helped Selena confront and accept the irrational, disproportionate and inappropriate way she had been driven to function. She wanted to know more of what was behind all this. Although the playback session was extremely charged, painful and difficult, Selena said at the end, "Thank you. Now I know what it means when people say I'm high. I never understood. I always felt the same. I never could have gone through this if all of you weren't here, and I never realized before that you must really care about me to put up with all of this." Having visually perceived herself go through a "high" she could now be helped by the therapist to understand and acknowledge that her "high" behavior was the way she dealt with emotionally-charged thoughts and feelings she did not yet know how to live with or respond to. This helped her to accept that getting "high" was something she would continue to be driven to unless she learned to own what went on in her and to develop more appropriate ways of responding to or living with it.

Some patients, during very upset periods, refused to attend playback sessions despite urging by therapists, nurses or their peer group members. It was as if they were saying they were too raw and vulnerable inside to risk further confrontation at that moment. Such self-encapsulating actions need to be responded to individually with empathy and deep understanding of the dynamics in operation at such a moment in order to work through such blockages.*

* Permission to include the above material which was originally contained in "The Use of Videotape with Psychotherapy Groups in a Community Mental Health Service Program," published in *Int. J. of Group Psychotherapy* (Vol. XVIII, No. 4, October 1968, pp. 504-15), has been given by Harris B. Peck, M.D., Editor.

CLARIFICATION OF MULTI-LEVEL MESSAGES

A very attractive, 24-year-old, intelligent, single, college graduate, whom I have treated in my private practice, was plagued by her inability to establish a significant relationship with a moderately mature male, although she was able to meet such men quite often in her business and social network. Her first self-confrontation experience helped her to become aware of how she sent a series of messages whose essential theme was, "Don't take me seriously; I'm just a silly kid." Her mother was an infantile, "cute," narcissistic woman who drowned her self-hate in an intermittent alcoholic state and who used her flip sense of humor to appeal to others for recognition and acknowledgment.

During videotape playback the daughter, Karen, experienced herself as coming through like a 16-year-old teenager who repeatedly laughed and giggled in the middle of what she was saying and thus wiped out with these meta-communications the possibility of really being taken seriously. She could see the basis for her date's not believing it when she said, "No. Stop. I don't want to go any further." She commented on the self-effacing impact of her voice, smile, facial, shoulder and hand mannerisms and said, "I come through as if I'm not really sure that I know what I mean or what I want."

She was helped to understand the confusing and negating effect her statements have when she shakes her head in a "no" fashion while talking. After first making typically self-critical remarks she was able to smile softly after a few minutes of the playback experience and say in a pleased fashion, "You know, I look good. I'm pretty."

Winn has emphasized that "One concomitant of confrontation is interpersonal competence" (9). Confrontation in psychotherapy groups alters the expectations one has of himself and others about what is legitimate behavior with other people.

Paredes, Cornelison and their associates at Eastern Pennsylvania Psychiatric Institute have focused in recent years on the value of audiovisual self-image confrontation in the study and treatment of alcoholics (10). They have added clarity to the definitions of roles and attitudes. "Implicit in social interchanges is the portrayal of roles. . . . Roles are portrayed through acts such as verbal communication, accent, intonation, facial expressions, posture, movements, gait, dress, adornments, grooming and visible emblems such as tattoos, uniforms or silver badges. These behaviors may be perceived and organized by observers into role concepts" (11). "Enactment of roles may be used to indicate what is to be expected of an individual, his position in a hierarchy and to affect others in a particular way. It is also a way to conceal or deny feelings to oneself or to others. The degree of awareness and intensity of the role played varies widely from one person to another and in differing social contexts." (Chapter 16, p. 193, re roles.)

Unlike the shock effect which was to be the basis of the curative goal of Carrière in France (1, 2), who first used playbacks of alcoholics' self-images filmed during episodes of delirium tremens, Paredes and Cornelison aimed to bring into awareness for the alcoholic the nature and context of his role conflicts. Their playback of sound motion pictures served to confront the alcoholic with certain aspects of his behavior in order to help him examine the characteristic roles he enacts as he talks about his life problems and hopefully to understand the self-destructive devices he has used to escape from uncomfortable conflictual personal issues.

Spelling out the anatomy of an attitude which serves not only as a response to social expectations but also to affect others in particular ways, they state, "Attitudes are composed of a variety of individual actions including facial expressions, posture, gestures, mannerisms, etc. They possess qualities such as mood, fluidity (ease of flow of the sequence of movements or actions) and social appeal. They indicate ascendancy and gender and have functions such as: affective (indicating of feeling); attributive (e.g., pointing with a finger); mimicking (imitation of a person, animal, or mechanism); preening (smoothing the hair with one's hand); courting (e.g., rubbing the sides of the thighs, hips, and waist with the palm of both hands); autistic (seemingly idiosyncratic movements, probably unconsciously determined); coping or instrumental (such as grabbing a glass) and postural" (10).

In their confrontation study of alcoholics who were filmed while being interviewed after the experimental administration of alcohol, they found that this alcohol intake did not act as a triggering mechanism for alcoholic craving, leading to the inference that greater importance has to be attributed to the role of the social setting in bringing out craving. The social setting may also be critical in determining or triggering disruptive behavior patterns in alcoholics. In their study of 66 patients they also found that alcohol did not favorably affect their mood. They infer, therefore, that the alcoholic does not drink to ease anxiety or depression but rather to express feelings which are unacceptable during sobriety. Patients who adopted a consultative-receptive attitude more easily disclosed significant personal data, invited empathy from the interviewer and gained more from confrontation with their problems while making possible exploration of new solutions. Many patients became more receptive to the interviewer and to the prospect of collaboration with psycho-therapy and rehabilitation after being confronted with their evasive, casual-impersonal, reluctant and hostile attitudes. This recognition plus the recognition of the low degree of self-esteem revealed in the playback contributed to heightened motivation for many as well as assisting in the development of a better relationship with the therapist who was working with them so they could now accept help.

Paredes and Cornelison emphasize that it is not audiovisual self-confrontation itself which is claimed to be of specific curative value for alcoholism. It is, however, emphasized that what is protherapeutic is that such *self-confrontation in the presence of and with the assistance of a trained therapist may help patients to better understand the self-deceiving and self-defeating mechanisms they have been using to deny or conceal their conflicts and low self-esteem. Following such understanding they may be motivated to work toward finding ways of handling or solving their conflicts other than through drinking.*

TELEVISION MAGNIFIES

Television magnifies. There is an immediacy, intimacy and powerful confrontational impact from seeing the closeup of a portion of a face, or of hands anxiously twisting a kleenex or matches, or of a woman unconsciously taking off and putting on alternatingly her wedding band while talking about the difficulties in her marriage. The impact of magnification is equally at home in treatment as it is in training.

Ann, a 40-year-old married woman I saw in my private practice, repeatedly fiddled with her marriage ring, taking it off and putting it on, during one session from which the following dialogue was taken. It had been a frustrating experience working with her over a period of time because she so often reacted as if she were a brick wall. In this session Ann discussed her reactions to a videotape playback. (Let's talk about your reaction to you, what you really picked up about you during this playback.) "I react so poorly emotionally, so poorly. I don't react emotionally at all. (What stands out for you?) My voice; I feel it is a sort of studied calmness, my hands and my emotions are sort of studied. There's a sort of restraint. I don't show anger. In my opinion when I react my voice is held back, everything is held down. Voice, emotions, everything. I know my husband is very explosive. But I always feel so flat . . . especially when I am with him. (Does anything come to you about the fact that this is how you are?) I used to feel like dead, incapable of feelings. I sort of feel like I died inside. There is no life anymore, there is no enthusiasm. No great sadness, no great happiness. (Do you really see it? Do you finally feel it?) I do. (Do you have some reactions about that, how you are, do you feel anything about that?) I was familiar with it. I remember once talking about it to a friend. She said she was the same way. I'm not capable of feeling great happiness, great enthusiasm, great sadness, I have just lost feeling. It is just like being a thing—you are existing. (Who is existing?) I am existing. (She laughs) (Yes, but Ann, you have found some moments of joy in your life?) Yes. (a minute of silence) (So it is possible.) But that does not solve this problem. (But it shows you are capable of feeling.) I'd like no strains, obligations or responsibilities, just to be carefree and happy is the way I guess I want to feel. This is something I could not talk about with my husband. (Is it possible that the fact that this is how you are really, that is, that you don't come through with strong feelings is also the way you are in bed with your husband?) It could be. (Therefore, the lack of this masculine output which you complain of in him may be a response which is in relationship to your lack of response. Maybe you both feed each other a similar message.) H'm. I was not unaware of this. When we were first married I didn't have those kinds of feelings. I was just terribly modest and very uncomfortable and then when I started to respond, Jack started having a problem with impotency when we were married for a few years and that was on our minds for a long time. There was always a reticence on both of our parts. I'm very conscious of the way he looks. He looks like a big fat Buddha. I guess I don't love his soul enough. I am sure what you say is true. How do you discuss this with somebody? I am not free to tell Jack even certain things that I wanted him to do when we were making love. It was not possible to tell him. I have always been very reticent. (How come? Maybe if you felt you had the right to feel, you could look for more. You have the right to ask him to help you really feel—to give you what you want, the opportunity to feel.) I have always put on such an act that I could not let him think that I was not feeling. The way he came through I thought I was a pretty good actress. (You have been practicing disguising your real feelings and you really are a great actress. La Rochefoucauld said that one who spends his life disguising himself to others winds up having disguised himself to himself.) That is true. (You've been putting on an act sexually.) For so many years I never was able to have any kind of real orgasm and I didn't want him to know so I pretended that I did to show how good I was. Later I couldn't say perhaps if he would try this or that I might. When he lost a lot of weight some years back I remember I would look at him and find him attractive. I would look at the side of his head, the way his hair fell, and I would feel very affectionate. I haven't this feeling now. I don't find him attractive. Of course, it has to be deeper than this. Maybe I'm very immature. It has to be something. I really feel I don't want him to make love to me and when I do I suppose it has to show. So many times he too comes to me without really feeling like it, like he feels it is something he should do rather than something he wants to do. (He gives you what you give him.) I always have to — well, he is lying in bed and is waiting for me and I have to touch and start caressing him. Because when he is waiting for me he's not really aroused, maybe he has the thought in his mind that he wants to — but I can't start him when I am not aroused. I can't tell him 'I do not want to come to you and find you soft and waiting.' This is the way I feel. I want to be soft and waiting. Every time I come to him I sort of hope maybe I'll feel he is hard and wants me but he's not. He used to get hard. And after I caress him I can make him aroused but it is just not the same thing. And it annoys me. When I come to him and I feel that it is soft I feel annoyance and my frame of mind is not affectionate really. I put on an act again. (So, hopefully, somewhere, there's going to be some truth emerging?) What am I going to say to him? (I'm not going to tell you exactly what to say to him.) I didn't mean for you to tell me what to say to him, it was just an expression. (Really? Maybe someday you can say to him, 'you know, if you aren't really aroused you don't have to make the effort. Wait until you're aroused and really want me.') He says, 'well, I want you.' He said this on our anniversary. As soon as I start to kiss or caress him he puts my hand down to touch him and he becomes aroused. He feels this is perfectly normal. I cannot make him have an erection by wishing it or telling him. I want it to happen. (The problem seems to be in that, whatever your feelings are, you right away deny them because you feel maybe you have no right to say them to him. Do you know what I am saying?) It's true. The feelings that I have when I come to him I don't say. I'd like to say, 'put your arms around me and hold me tight, let me feel the pressure, let me feel the strength of your arms.' (What blocks you from that?) The feeling that he would take it that I feel that he is not loving. (But you're editing, you are writing the whole script. I would say you spend your life with scripts instead of being natural. For you it's, 'I will say this and I will think that and he will have to say this because I will think that and he knows what.' You are so on guard you have to push your feelings down . . . like you said ten minutes ago, 'I've been pushing my feelings down like I'm dead.') I'm really not living, I am really not hot, I'm really not anything. (Because you're so busy writing the script.) I feel I know him so well. (Can't you see how important it then becomes for you to look or fantasy elsewhere than your marriage for excitement and aliveness and spontaneity and creativity? You yourself contribute a major share of the deadness to this relationship and then you have to look outside.) Yes, I do. (Don't you see then your role in creating a situation which requires that which has new problems associated with it? The place to begin is at home. I guess that's what they mean by 'charity begins at home.' That remark must have meaning.)

PROCESSES INVOLVED IN CONFRONTATION

Processes involved in confrontation are those of encountering or meeting and bringing face to face: people with themselves, people with people, and people with issues or situations. In psychotherapy the nuances and subtleties of bringing patients face to face with themselves require the combined resources of many approaches of people to people. A list of overlapping, interdigitating processes involved in confrontational approaches used by therapists hopefully to bring about change has to include:

Communicating	Deconditioning	Role-playing
Interpreting	Desensitizing	Instigating
Questioning	Advising	Directing
Exploring	Anticipating	Looking without
Analyzing	Predicting	answering
Clarifying	Implanting	Frustrating
Activating	Nonconventionalism	Challenging
Suggesting	Repeating	Altering
Urging	Demonstrating or	Permitting
Persuading	modeling	Helping
Encouraging	Mimicking	Assuring
Commanding	Reinforcing	Reassuring
Cajoling	Depriving	Acting
Forbidding	Inhibiting	Symbolizing
Silencing	Silence	Expressing
Limit-setting	Explaining	Touching
Catalyzing	Teaching or instructing	Pressuring
Reminding	Offering examples,	Coercing
Insisting	analogies, metaphors,	Restricting
Controlling	images, similes, and	Giving
Opposing	fantasies.	Praising
Manipulating	Being authentic	Rewarding
Minimizing	Evaluating	Stimulating
Influencing	Criticizing	Exhorting
Discounting	Emphasizing	Prodding
Contradicting	Intervening	Demanding
Repeating	Provoking	Reality-testing
Conditioning		

The use of operant learning principles and behavioral feedback via television has been reported of value by Bernal in training mothers in child management (13). Several intervention or instruction sessions were held during which the mothers' management behaviors were gradually shaped. Direct instruction on what operants to emit contingent on the boys' behaviors, teaching of reinforcement principles, social reinforcement of the mothers' successful management behavior and playback of videotaped mother-son interaction sessions were used in the shaping. When necessary, the mothers were trained in management of the problem child in the presence of another child such as a playmate or sibling. Both children involved in this project, male "brats" aged five and eight years, improved markedly within a period of 25 weeks from the point of first contact with the parents.

Wilmer has stated that video is "a new electronic communicational environment in which the patient is provided with a metaphorical experience" (14). As accurately as video can reflect a person like he is, there is no modality to reproduce a person exactly as he is.

When, during videotape playback, a patient experiences himself in interaction with his therapist he has an opportunity to more comprehensively become aware of the degree to which he functions in a compliant fashion. More of what is subliminally in operation can be brought into the open and examined to assess whether its basis is in positive transference towards the therapist or based on other values.

Clarence, aged 34, is the self-effacing, compliant son of a shrewd, dominating, overprotective, smothering, infantilizing mother and an absentee father. Unable to be angry with his mother, he gets drunk and turns to sexual deviations instead. Following self-image confrontation during his first videotape playback, he excitedly said: "Watching myself as I said the words is like an actor reading words—it's like I'm casual— it's just chitchat—I smooth it all out, the level I show has nothing to do with my real feeling inside, like moments when I talked of getting her pregnant, or going to Boston to see her, which I'm very nervous about. I saw how I wiped my brow with my hand, but I did'nt really say how I feel scared and tense inside about going with her—because if she likes it or not, it could change my life.

"I'm kind of awed by the application of this machinery. I realize when I flip with anger in my office, I make it into a long script and dramatize it comedy fashion and summarize it and make it more acceptable—like ripping a telephone out of a wall in a humorous fashion." Finally, he laughingly says: "You know, I like the picture of myself—I look likable."

AUDIO CONFRONTATION

Prior to the use of television in psychotherapy, there was a keen interest by many serious workers in using audio playbacks for treatment.* There is no need to discard audio usage in therapy simply because video is now available. The new inexpensive, lightweight, portable, cassette recorders are ideally suited for taping sessions by patient as well as therapist. For those patients whose recall of what goes on during a psychotherapy session is practically nil, I have found it of marked value not only to analyze this amnesia in the usual manner but also to suggest they purchase a tape recorder and tape some or all of their individual sessions. This technique, like all others espoused in this volume, requires that the therapist not apply it automatically with all patients, but use it according to skilled judgment concerning appropriateness and timing for each individual patient-person.

A 30-year-old single, female, office administrator who had already experienced herself on a few occasions with video self-image confrontation began to listen at home to audio playback of her individual sessions. She said, "I can be frightening at times—hearing how I was breathing deeply and screaming while I'd been here and how I had to turn it off as it was so frightening—a feeling as if the whole world will blow up—as if my world will end if I let go of myself. At home alone I make connections that I hadn't while here with you. I can stop the tape and work through all the associations as I hadn't here in the office. I see how often I hadn't wanted to accept an interpretation you'd made while I was here. Then in going over it I see all the data to support the interpretation. It's irrefutable—it's there. With this second chance I can now accept it—or will go back again and again until I can understand and accept the interpretation. I often play way-back tapes as a kind of ego builder to see problems I had then which I have really worked through—or at least partially—like the tape on 'having to have my mother's consent to have sex,' or beating myself because I didn't do something I should have or did do something I shouldn't have. In the tapes I hear you repeatedly comment on my excessive expectations—and my inability to accept that I am where I am and am doing the best I can. I'm much better at that acceptance of myself now than before. I have less pressure from my 'should system' and that makes life much more feasible and livable. I still go through patches of uncomfortable living—like last week when I was beating myself all around—at work—socially—in my group—and privately, although privately I'm now more relaxed than any time

---

* D. E. Cameron, Psychic Driving, *American Journal of Psychiatry*, 112:502-509, 1956.

elsewhere. At work I've been treating supervisors less as fathers and more as friends. I feel less threatened with them now and can express my differing opinions with them instead of complying and later feeling angry or taking an immediate offensive, aggressive position and later regretting it."

It is important to keep in mind that confrontation with psychotic in-patients, with alcoholics, with couples, with marathon or sensitivity training groups or with patients in private practice has different as well as similar indications and may produce different as well as similar re-actions and long-term results.

I must state unequivocally my belief that confrontation alone is not enough to bring about the kind of characterological change and growth which is the usual goal of psychoanalytically-oriented psychotherapy. Al-most any confrontation can be accepted and assimilated to some degree if a patient is prepared for the work of psychotherapy, is in a state of positive transference to his therapist or group and there is enough mutuality, caring, regard, trust and intimacy present.

Whereas what is presented audiovisually to oneself in a videotape playback can be self-protectively denied if the patient is not ready to experience what is being presented to him "face-to-face," he may not be able to ward off direct confrontations in the kind of here-and-now en-counter group currently so popular in this country. Under the guise of "love," "caring," or "frankness," sadistic truths can be forced on par-ticipants in such groups if the leader is not trained, skillful or adept enough to prevent sadistic acting out or scapegoating. In such a group a young man already burdened with suicidal self-hate was told he looked like a freak, that he was ugly and unlikable. He was torn apart as though by lions in the Roman Coliseum. These confrontations further height-ened his feelings of inadequacy, impotency, unlovability and low self-esteem. He committed suicide after leaving the weekend group.*

There is a sense of unanimity amongst workers who utilize videotape confrontation that through this experience insight can be heightened; people can learn more of what is unknown about themselves but which is known to others; attitudes, roles and behavioral patterns can often be modified by increasing the variety and depth of information patients can obtain about themselves in relationship with their environment; and self-images and concepts can be clarified and frequently altered as individ-uals move toward a clearer sense of their own identity.

---

* Personal communication from a senior medical student at the College of Physicians and Surgeons.

REFERENCES

1. Carrère, J.: Le psycho-cinématographique. Principes et technique. Application au traitement des malades convalescents de delirium tremens. *Ann. Medicopsychol.,* 112:240-245, 1954.
2. Carrère, J., Craignou, C., and Miss Pochard: De quelques résultats du psycho-cinématographie dans la psychothérapie des delirium et sub-delirium tremens alcooliques. *Ann. Medicopsychol.,* 113:46-51, 1955.
3. Cornelison, F. S. and Arsenian, J.: A Study of the Response of Psychotic Patients to Photographing Self-image Experience. *Psychiat. Quart.,* 34:1-8, 1960.
4. Glover, Edward: *Psychoanalysis.* London: Staples Press, 1939.
5. Geertsma, R. H. and Reivich, R. S.: Repetitive Self Observation by Videotape Playback. *J. Ment. Nerv. Dis.,* 141:29-41, 1965.
6. Reivich, R. S. and Geertsma, R. H.: Experiences with Videotape Self-observation by Psychiatric In-patients. *J. of Kansas Medical Soc.,* LXIX:39-44, 1968.
7. Horney, K.: Alienation from Self, Chapter 6, 155-175 in *Neurosis and Human Growth.* New York: W. W. Norton & Co., 1950.
8. Berger, M. M., Sherman, B., Spalding J., and Westlake, R.: The Use of Videotape with Psychotherapy Groups in a Community Mental Health Service Program. *Inst. J. of Group Psychotherapy,* XVIII:504-14, 1968.
9. Winn, A.: The Laboratory Approach to Organization Development: A Tentative Model of Planned Change. *The J. of Group Psychoanalysis and Process,* II, 1969.
10. Paredes, A. and Cornelison, F. S.: Development of an Audiovisual Technique in the Rehabilitation of Alcoholics. Unpublished manuscript based in part on paper presented at the 19th Clinical Meeting of the A.M.A. in Philadelphia, Pa., Nov. 1965.
11. Sarbin, T. R.: Role Theory. In G. Lindsey, *Handbook of Social Psychology.* Cambridge, Mass.: Addison-Wesley, 1954.
12. La Barre, W.: Paralinguistics, Kinesics, and Cultural Anthropology, 191-220. In T. Sebeok, A. Hayes, and M. C. Bateson (Eds.), *Approaches to Semiotics.* London: Mouton, 1964.
13. Bernal, M. E.: Behavioral Feedback in the Modification of Brat Behaviors. *J. Nerv. Ment. Dis.,* 148:375-385, 1969.
14. Wilmer, H. A.: Use of the Television Monologue with Adolescent Psychiatric Patients. *Amer. J. Psychiat.* 126:1760-1766, 1970.

3
VIDEO FEEDBACK CONFRONTATION REVIEW

Milton M. Berger, M.D.

I. *Video feedback confrontation* can be accomplished:

1) via closed circuit television cameras and monitors presenting pictures and sound simultaneously with their being recorded at the site of the camera location and can also be viewed at other near or distant sites;

2) via videotaped recordings which can be seen

   a) immediately after part or the whole of a session or meeting is completed in what is referred to as instant playback.

   b) at a later time either at the same location as the taping or in other locations.

II. *Feedback of videotaped data* can be presented as:

1) general feedback of a whole session or meeting without any editing;

2) edited focused feedback of specific moments or segments of pre-taped interview in order to examine or highlight data for review, research, free-associations, awareness, enlightenment, or to promote interaction;

3) specific themes or subject material with titles, edited segments from one or more previously made tapes with and without narration, graphics or other audiovisual inputs to highlight, expedite or enhance achievement of the learning objectives for the tape.

Revision of material distributed at the Seventeenth Annual Frontiers of Psychotherapy Conference on *Feedback: A Royal Road to Adaptation and Change in Psychotherapy*, sponsored by the Temple University Health Sciences Center Department of Psychiatry and the Division of Psychiatry of Albert Einstein Medical Center, Philadelphia, Pa., in March, 1976.

III. *Video feedback offers:*

1) A sense of immediacy.

2) A sense of intimacy.

3) Magnification of all or part of a person during social interaction (face, hand, fingers, foot, etc.).

4) An opportunity to simultaneously see and experience oneself in one or more television monitors, through one or more different camera and positional views, as one is actually coming through to others verbally and nonverbally during social interaction in a psychotherapeutic or educational setting.

5) A "second chance" or repeated chances to experience oneself as one was coming through verbally and nonverbally, alone and/ or in interaction with others just previously or some time previously—that is, minutes, hours, days, weeks, months or years ago.

6) An opportunity to experience more objectively one's self, group, family members and therapist(s) with an expanded observing ego while not feeling the pressure of having to produce verbally during a psychotherapeutic session. There is a greater opportunity for "being" with the "self" one is experiencing.

7) An opportunity to witness, experience and react to how persons believe they are coming through to others and to how consonant or dissonant their inside picture is with the reality of how they really are coming through with their communications of self in relationship to other(s). This means that they now are confronted with how much of themselves has been observable and/or knowable to and by others

    a) which they thought they were successfully concealing and keeping secret and unknown to others;

    b) which was actually unknown to themselves but known to and being reacted to by others.

The data that are revealed at such moments primarily have to do with attitudes expressed through nonverbal behaviors as well as through tone, pitch, rhythm and other aspects of speech which may be in harmony with or contradictory to or otherwise implying something different from the actual words.

8) An opportunity to witness and gain awareness of our meta communications, i.e., how we "telegraph" to others messages

as to how they are to receive and react to our communications. If they are culturally at home with us, they will know whether to take our communication as playful, teasing or straight.

9) An opportunity to witness and experience how much of their mothers, fathers and other significant figures they have incorporated into themselves during their childhood.

10) An opportunity to become aware of
   a) how much of what we communicate is done to express and how much is done to impress in the service of our neurotic pride systems or idealized image of ourselves;
   b) how much of what we communicate is done to prove we really are what we believe we "should" be and how much to improve and express the persons we really are;
   c) how much of what goes on and influences and regulates interpersonal relationships between us and others comes from consciously intended sources and how much comes compulsively without our conscious intent from preconscious and/or unconscious sources.

11) A chance to resculpture or model by narrowing the physical space between people.

12) Alteration and accentuation of impact of contents and interaction by use of superimposed titles, narration, split screen and multiple images as well as other special effects.

13) Multiple simultaneous clear and distorted images of a person or part of a person to elicit free associations, anatomical, psychological and emotional connections to incorporated and/or repressed aspects of significant others in self and to aspects of self which have not yet been in awareness. (See Chapter 23.)

14) A chance to capture through the pause or freeze-frame potential of the video playback machine a look, a movement, a behavior which is characteristic, repetitive and has clear-cut impact on other persons but which has previously been elusive or unknown to the videotaped person experiencing the feedback. Such "looks" are highly significant in their capacity to serve as regulatory signals in family systems and relationships.

15) An opportunity to repeat and repeat the verbal and nonverbal context of human behaviors separately and together to reinforce experiencing, understanding and integration of new information.

SECTION II
Training

EDITOR'S INTRODUCTION

We have come a long way from the conclusion drawn at the conference on Psychiatric Education held at Ithaca, New York during the 1950s which stated that audiovisual media have little place in psychiatric education. Teaching with audiovisual adjuncts such as videotape reinforces what the student hears with what he sees. This reinforcement to learning goes far beyond the impact of one plus one equals two. Adding visual context, content, and process to what one hears amplifies and expands by geometric progression what is available to be perceived, reacted to and understood by those motivated to learn.

It is important that audiovisual adjuncts do not become an excuse for either lazy or inadequate teaching or treatment. It takes interest, enthusiasm, mental exercise, creative ingenuity and real knowledge of one's field of specialization as well as extra energy and time to review and edit, to utilize with "expertise" the manifest and latent content and process so profoundly communicated via videotape. Like certain pharmaceuticals which work well in small doses but not in larger ones, videotape playbacks used judiciously in psychiatric training and treatment programs can be of great value if not used for too long a period continuously. They must be interspersed in the ongoing training and treatment program and accompanied by preparatory, concurrent or later playback data and learning exercises to clarify and further validate what has just been presented.

Timing in the introduction and use of videotape is as important as appropriate timing in interpretations and other interventions in therapy or in the introduction of new material in teaching. Appropriate use and timing must depend not only on the availability of content on videotapes but also on whether the mechanical equipment for audio and visual playback is working efficiently. If the tracking head of a videotape playback machine is dirty or otherwise indisposed, the quality of the picture becomes so distorted and disruptive that students or patients not only cannot maintain continuous interest but also build up annoyance or anger and feel that their precious time is just being wasted. Proper timing includes a capacity to move the students from a passive observational

41

system to a more actively involved system of learning as developed by Barchilon.* He has focused his attention on such issues as learning blocks, pleasure in learning and its relationship to unconscious problems and conflicts of the learner and has found that "much of what has been observed in the doctor-patient relationship should and does apply more commonly and with greater frequency in the child-teacher interaction."

While noting that much learning is and should be essentially passive, Barchilon emphasizes that "the important step in education is to foster activity on the part of the student and hopefully to bring about or at least not hamper 'creative learning' as Joan Fleming** calls it." Barchilon has taught psychotherapy for many years by demonstrating treatment behind a one-way screen and later on through closed-circuit TV transmissions for the benefit of medical students or residents.*** He believes it to be the ideal medium for teaching technique, know-how and practical considerations almost impossible to learn elsewhere.****

> Nothing can match the actual looking at, without being immediately involved in the transaction, how to handle acted out hostility, how to interpret resistances, how to interact, smile, touch or not touch the patient, etc.

To undermine students' expectancy to passively observe and learn by osmosis, Barchilon developed a system in which: 1) students watch a televised session without a supervisor present; 2) students then act as supervisors of the observed therapist, formulating what happened and criticizing the therapist, a bit skeptical at first about this opportunity and therefore offering more praise than criticism; 3) if the therapist can maintain a relatively silent, non-defensive, accepting attitude and consider the truth in their remarks, students, gaining confidence rapidly, participate more actively, are happily outspoken and at times destructively critical of the therapist's blind spots and countertransference reactions which the TV lens has accurately reported. The teacher must maintain his

---

* Barchilon, J., "Some Conscious and Unconscious Factors in Teaching Psychotherapy with One-Way Screens, Closed Circuit TV or Movie Films," unpublished, 1964. (In a personal communication, Barchilon authorized me to quote at length from his paper, which I have done because of its imaginative nature.)

** Fleming, J. and Benedek, T., *Psychoanalytic Supervision*. New York: Grune and Stratton, 1966.

*** See article by Berger and Gallant on "The Use of Closed Circuit Television in the Teaching of Group Psychotherapy" in *Psychosomatics*, 6:16-18, 1965.

**** I was surprised to hear that such practical techniques and know-how learned through watching me demonstrate group psychotherapy via TV were referred to by my psychiatric residents as "Berger 'tid-bits.' "

"cool" without arguing or justifying himself despite the hostile, irrational transference reactions projected onto him. If he becomes defensive, students quickly revert to their usual passive attitude of: "Well you are the teacher so tell us." The excessive hostility of the students is due to the fact that for the first time in their learning experience the usual process of the student-teacher situation is reversed and their pent-up contained hostility and anger at having been subjected passively to so much teaching throughout their lives from pre-kindergarten on have a chance to finally be expressed against one of their teachers. This stage of hyper-criticism and transferential hostility lasts about three months, although it may end sooner if the patient involved in this exercise starts to improve and to overcome his or her resistances and to show signs of intrapsychic mobility and shifts. 4) The next stage is ushered in by a strong, partially unconscious identification with the therapist as students make slips of the tongue and may report their own associations to the material witnessed. They may say, "the patient told *me*, I mean told *you*, such and such. . . ." They may regard the patient as their own and as if the therapist was merely carrying out their instructions when treating the patient. At times, though, they revert to earlier patterns, conform and ask the teacher for his opinion. 5) Gradually their ambivalent identification is abandoned and students move into the stage in which a true realistic cooperation between equals becomes possible. Not being involved in the therapeutic transaction itself, their powers of observation are all focused on the process and they now become extremely perceptive supervisors.

Barchilon found that students ordinarily most refractory or insensitive or not psychologically minded in their previous residency experiences have surprisingly come forward in this type of exercise and demonstrated profound awareness, sensitivity and competency. His creative and courageous technique was successful in undermining passivity and reducing resistance or antagonism to learning.

In the actual conduct of psychotherapy, studies reveal that therapists tend to be more subjective and directive than formerly acknowledged. The nature of the therapist's directions or his way of directing is usually indirect. Videotape playbacks of sessions which he has conducted allow a therapist-in-training to see much more clearly that he in fact not only influences his patient in many ways, but influences him in ways that he the therapist had been unaware of previously.

He may realize more clearly the directive implications of many of his nonverbal mannerisms, particularly his facial movements including head cock, eyelid movements and verbal intonations as he asks simple questions such as "How do you feel about that?" This is a question that can be asked in a fashion which implies "You're serious about acting on that idea," or it can imply "Are you out of your mind? I can't really believe you'd go that far!"

It is not only for the psychotic or borderline psychotic patient or even for the extremely infantile or immature patient that the psychotherapist finds he sets limits. He finds on playback that limit setting is an influencing process involved in his psychotherapeutic approach with all patients.*

The subject of training has to include mention of the massive number of people who have had significant learning-training experiences on a variety of subjects while seated at home in front of their own television set either alone or with family or friends. Such subjects have been presented on talk shows at all hours and as regularly scheduled classes created and presented from university or commercial studios in cities of all sizes.

In 1952 W. J. McKeachie reviewed his experience teaching psychology on WWJ-TV in Detroit.** His weekly programs consisted of three 20-minute segments, with a viewing audience of many hundreds of students who registered for the telecourse and 150,000 people who viewed it because of its interest and value to them in living their daily life.

The title of McKeachie's first 15-week public telecourse was "Man in His World—Human Behavior." Preparation of his programs was accomplished through the following steps: 1) Three weeks before the program went on the air he outlined his lesson to two honor students in psychology who then wrote most of the supplementary reading materials for the registered students; 2) these written materials were edited by him a few days later; 3) six days before "show-time" he met with the television staff to outline the lesson and to discuss possible visual aids to enhance and clarify his material. Visual aids he found useful included posters, models, drawings, flip cards, photographs and concepts written on the blackboard in advance which could be turned to and underlined for emphasis during his presentation.*** On one occasion he used a film excerpt to "clearly

---

* Abroms, G. M., "Setting Limits," *Arch. Gen. Psychiat.*, 19:113-119, 1968.

** McKeachie, W. J. "Teaching Psychology on Television," *American Psychologist*, 7:503-506, 1952.

*** *Ed. Note*: This inexpensive technique of writing "headlines" or key points on the blackboard in advance means you can reinforce the learning experience by writing clearly and with enough heavy chalk so that the viewer doesn't get a distracting eyeful of illegible scribbles.

illustrate a given principle." 4) A rehearsal was held four days before "show-time" to check organization, clarity and rough timing; 5) a rehearsal was held two days before "show-time" to work on better timing and more clarity; 6) and then he appeared in the studio before show-time to rehearse camera movements, be available on the set for lighting adjustments and then two hours before producing his show "live" he went through a final rehearsal of his entire program with cameras and lights. All this was successfully done by McKeachie in 1951. His course content and sequence were as follows:

1. Determinants of Behavior
2. The Scientific Approach to Behavior
3. The Cultural Background of Personality
4. The Biological Background
5. Abilities
6. Perception
7. Thinking
8. Motives
9. Learning (Habits)
10. Conflict, Frustration, and Defense Mechanisms
11. Mental Illness and Mental Health
12. The Structure of Personality
13. The Development of Personality
14. Interpersonal Relations
15. The Individual in Society.*

Over the years we have seen sporadic attempts to introduce the daily work of psychiatrists and our colleagues in allied professions on commercial and public education TV. In the 1960s, "Road to Reality," a weekly series of analytic group psychotherapy sessions in which actors played the scripts taken from real sessions in the New York office of Dr. Richard Abell, was shown. Unfortunately it was received in the sense of "soap opera" rather than real preventive mental hygiene education by some, but many people did gain a great deal from it. Since then, actual encounter and marathon group sessions have been shown at times, but the distinction was not adequately made that these were "growth" groups rather than ongoing psychotherapy groups. In general the public

---

* *Ed. Note*: His content and format can still serve as an excellent basic course for professional and paraprofessional trainees in mental health and allied fields, as well as for the support services staff in all psychiatric and other health facilities.

reacted negatively to what they were seeing as if it were truly professionally conducted "group therapy."

On numerous occasions I have been approached by television program producers because of my long-term interest, identification and involvement with the field of group psychotherapy, as well as my identification with television in psychiatry, with a request for a program with actual patients instead of actors. I always refused to do such programs for public television because I believed that even if real patients gave their consent in writing to being shown it might be against their interests to reveal to such an unselected public audience what is usually considered confidential (see Section IV in this book).

In an overview of the field Lawrence Creshkoff, Director of Project Development, informs me that the Network for Continuing Medical Education (NCME), a pioneer in videopublishing, has produced and distributed videotaped programming for use in continuing medical education since 1963. In the field of psychiatry, more than 70 programs have been produced for use by internists, family and general practitioners, pediatricians, and other primary care physicians. In addition, a dozen titles have been developed for use specifically by psychiatrists.

The programs produced for general medical audiences are distributed to more than 700 hospitals and medical centers that subscribe to the NCME service.* Every year, 23 hour-long videocassettes (in color) are issued on a fortnightly basis; individual titles generally average between 15 and 25 minutes in length.

Among the psychiatric programs available through NCME are: "Body Language in Diagnosis" (G. H. Deckert); "Biogenic Amine Theories of Depression" (R. J. Baldessarini); "Differential Diagnosis of Depression" (F. T. Reid); "Drinkers in Crisis" (H. D. Abraham & J. A. Renner); "Managing the Depressed Patient" (G. L. Klerman); "Selye on Stress" (H. Selye); "What Goes on at Sex Therapy Clinics" (H. Lear); and a special 50-minute television workshop, "The National Sleep Disorders Update" (A. and J. Kales et al.).

Teaching techniques employed include actual clinical situations with real patients, simulated clinical situations with actors, televised self-assessment tests, panel discussions, and solo television lectures with film and animated graphics inserts.

Other programs specifically produced for and directed to psychiatric audiences have been developed in collaboration with the Video Subcommittee of the Scientific Program Committee of the American Psychiatric

---

* The service is supported in part by Roche Laboratories.

Association for presentation at APA annual meetings, beginning in 1972. These more specialized programs, which have been viewed by over 50,000 individuals, include: "Exploring and Exploding Myths about Hypnosis" (H. Spiegel); "Crisis Intervention" (L. Bellak); "The Use of Video in Psychiatric Treatment" (M. M. Berger); "Playroom Setting for Diagnostic Family Interview" (I. N. Orgun) ; "A Multi-Modality Approach to Ghetto Addiction" (G. Koz); "Psychodrama Sensitization for Crisis Intervention" (H. L. P. Resnik); "Psychiatry at Work in the Inner City" (E. Kovacs, I. Labourdette, et al.); "Diagnosis and Treatment of Sex Dysfunctions in Marriage" (H. S. Kaplan); "The Dynamics of a 'Normal' Family Over Time" (L. Wynne, C. Whitaker, et al.); "Three Families: Interactional Testing" (J. M. Lewis); "Impact of APA Decision Removing Homosexuality from Mental Illness List" (R. E. Gould, et al.); and "On Being the Child of a Psychiatrist" (M. A. Bartusis and D. Hays) .

Because of such factors as informed consent and the difficulties of achieving controlled sound and lighting in clinical situations, NCME prefers to produce simulated reconstructions in a studio setting. Scripts for such simulations are developed, where possible, from videotapes or audiocassettes made under conditions of actuality. It is felt that for teaching purposes, the production efficiencies and improved technical quality outweigh the possible loss of verisimilitude, and the dangers involved in invasion of privacy are averted (see Section IV).

Dr. Clarice J. Kestenbaum of New York City has written and directed a series of four child development videotape programs which present normal children from one month of age through 17.* In response to my question regarding any problems in creating these tapes, she stated:

> In thinking about our experience in videotaping school-aged children, my immediate reaction was that, in truth, we had no negative reactions at all. In taping several hundred children during the past years in a number of settings I could not think of a single instance when the children refused to cooperate. The anxious occasions encountered during an interview were in every instance contributed by the interviewing psychiatrist. In fact, children often spotted the examiner's nervousness and offered suggestions such as: "If you can't remember what to ask me next, why don't you ask me how I like baseball?"
>
> Most children are excited about the proposition of being on television, and the promise of seeing themselves following the taping

---

* Produced by Leonard Sussman and James H. Ryan, M.D. in the Department of Educational Research at New York State Psychiatric Institute. Dr. Ryan is the developer of the *Electronic Textbook of Psychiatry and Neurology* (a compilation of videotapes).

was incentive enough. I am speaking about working under various laboratory conditions where the camera was hidden, where the camera was in full view, and where the camera and technical crew were in the room with the child and interviewer.

We usually asked children under five if they would like to have their mother in the room with them during the taping. About half of the children ages three to five wanted mother to be present and all the children under three had a familiar adult with them during the interview. Even children with serious psychopathology were at ease during the taping, although I can envisage a situation where an overactive child might damage the equipment.

H. L. Muslin has pioneered in and written extensively about the use "of videotapes, audiotapes and films to train and evaluate learners in observing, collating (organizing clinical data in diagnostic categories), hypothesis formation, and management (use of therapeutic skills).* He states, "In the main, the audio visual media has not provided tests predictive of clinical performance." He points out that the development of reliable tests requires that the behaviors and processes to be measured be accurately determined and then examinations be painstakingly prepared according to what is to be measured. He says from a background of trial and error that "Learning and evaluation of the learning should be conceived in two phases, the first dealing with the processes of observation and the second dealing with clinical interaction with patients." He refers to the work of Stoller and Geertsma,** who as far back as 1958 were using filmed interviews to assess observing skills and clinical judgments in psychiatry by having their trainees evaluate 300 statements on the basis of their characteristicness in relation to the interview. Referring to his own work at the University of Illinois on the development of certifying examinations in psychiatry, Muslin's emphasis was on distinguishing between cognitive observations and inferences. The respondents were asked to choose from one of four categories and apply these choices to a series of statements related to segments of a videotaped clinical interview. He found that students "do indeed demonstrate increment in their scores over time. . . . The use of audiovisual mechanisms is valuable for assessment purposes since 1) it offers a standard stimulus and 2) the film or video can be reviewed repeatedly for purposes of consensual valida-

---

* Muslin, H. L.: "Overview: The Use of Recordings as Evaluation Mechanisms in Psychiatry," Chapter 5, pp. 77-85 in H. L. Muslin (Ed.), *Evaluative Methods in Psychiatric Education.* Wash., D.C.: American Psychiatric Association, 1974.
** Stoller, R. J. and Geertsma, R. H.: "Construction of a Final Examination to Assess Clinical Judgment in Psychiatry," *J. Med. Educ.,* 33:12:837-40, 1958; Geertsma, R. H. and Stoller, R. J.: "The Objective Assessment of Clinical Judgment in Psychiatry," *Arch. Gen. Psychiatry,* 2:278-85, 1960.

tion as to the observed data: what is or is not there. Thus problems of interobserver reliability can be resolved and provide for a fair assessment of the observed data for scoring purposes."

Two other Midwestern educators who have pioneered with the educative value of film and videotapes for medical students are John Schneider and Allen Enelow who worked at Michigan State University,* where they were also involved with Norman Kagan (see Chapter 6). Schneider and Enelow developed procedures to test cognitive objectives, behavior observation, interview skills and self-evaluation. They value audiovisual materials to evaluate attainment of skills because of such advantages as: "1) audiovideo exams offer a standard stimulus; 2) significant reliability can be attained by the faculty; and 3) the format lends itself to self-instruction."

Winslow Hunt, Roger MacKennon and Robert Michels used videotaped psychiatric interviews extensively in the clinical clerkship program in psychiatry they developed in the Department of Psychiatry at the College of Physicians and Surgeons of Columbia University. Their multi-level, multi objective basic clinical clerkship in psychiatry was aimed to fulfill the needs of (a) those medical students who plan to specialize in psychiatry, (b) those medical students considering psychiatry but who have not yet committed themselves and who thus found the program a testing ground helpful to vocational choice, (c) the great majority of students (those who will practice in other areas of medicine) for whom this "is often their only chance to acquire skills that they will later need in their daily work." They reported that their use of videotaped interviews were found to provide a valuable teaching format in that they "are effective in holding student interest, in avoiding the practical difficulties of live interviews, and in teaching active listening and interviewing technique as well as in demonstrating a variety of psychopathology."**

There is great diversity in the training programs which depend on video for detailed study and corrective feedback information among those

---

* Schneider, J. M. and Enelow, A. J.: "Assessment of Medical Students in Psychiatry: Applications of Film and Videotape," Chapter 6, pp. 87-100 in H. L. Muslin (Ed.), *Evaluative Methods in Psychiatric Education*. Wash., D.C.: American Psychiatric Association, 1974.

** Hunt, W., MacKennon, R., and Michels, R.: "A Clinical Clerkship in Psychiatry," *J. of Med. Education*, 50:1113-1119, 1975.

Ed. Note: These educators had the advantage of using the staff, equipment and electronic textbook videotapes prepared by the Educational Research Laboratory under the direction of Dr. James Ryan at the New York State Psychiatric Institute in New York City.

working in liaison with the efforts of mental health professionals. For a number of years Michael Carrera* has used the media to help trainees in the rapidly growing field of sex education. With collegiate students at the Hunter College Institute of Health Science and as administrator of a community sex information service which responds annually to thousands of cries for help and clarification coming in over the telephone, Carrera has found the incorporation of video feedback the best way to enhance and measure growth amongst trainees in the areas of comfort and sensitivity in communicating about sexual topics and practices. The trainees evaluate themselves as they discuss, present and openly communicate about sensitive topics previously "taboo" in open forums. Expressing and undermining nonverbal as well as verbal awkwardness are of particular importance in sex education, which requires presentations and discussions with young people, parent groups and school administrators regarding the actual content, nature and efficacy of sexuality programs.

The first chapter in this section on training presents some of the observations of Nancy Roeske of Indiana University School of Medicine on the potency of audiovisual material as an educational experience. She emphasizes the need for individualizing the use of videotaped educational materials in accordance with the teachers' concepts about the tape content and the principles of learning and theories respected by him or her. She outlines nine principles of learning to be considered if you are developing your own curriculum and she brings to us her experience as coordinator of medical education and director of the undergraduate curriculum of her Department of Psychiatry at Indianapolis.

The value of using simulations in training and in the creation of training videotapes seems to be increasingly clear and increasingly popular among experienced clinicians and teachers. The chapter by Dr. Robert Froelich offers a review of some key elements which are crucial for learning. He has successfully utilized simulations among medical students as a major tool for many years and gives us a step-by-step description of his method. The advantages of using simulations, as described by Froelich, were clearly outlined by Silverman and Fahy at their APA Video Continuing Education Session in 1975:

1. Primum non nocere:

   Simulation allows one to learn skills necessary to become proficient without subjecting a family to an inexperienced therapist.

---

* Personal communication from Dr. Michael Carrera, President of Community Sex Information, Inc. in New York City and Vice President of the American Association of Sex Educators, Counselors and Therapists.

2. Reducing the anxiety in a family:
   The anxiety occurring in a family that knows it is being utilized as a teaching object can often become an artifact that confuses the issues for a beginning therapist.
3. Reducing the anxiety in the trainee.
4. Repetitive exploration of family by trainee:
   The family can maintain a constancy that allows the student to perfect his skills until he or his teacher feels confident with his performance.
5. Models' responses can be altered to suit training situations.
   Problems and mode of interaction can be altered by simulators to expose trainee to graduated clinical settings.
6. Simulated family can be examined by many examiners, thus allowing comparison of techniques.
7. Simulated family participants can provide feedback to trainee about their experience as patients.
8. Simulator can feel through "role reversal" what a patient experiences in an interview.*

When I have created pre-scripted videotapes and films for pharmaceutical manufacturers and others I have found how important preparation is in producing a better end-result and how much aggravation and time are saved in editing by being clear as to what I want my simulators to express in their enactment. A two- to three-minute scenario can come out as a more natural production if you review in detail with the actor or actress the context and details of what actually happened with one or more patients involved in a similar situation or problem and then give them the liberty to free-associatively enact it in their own fashion as long as they present the same content and meaning as the patient(s) had expressed.

After Froelich's chapter comes Norman Kagan's report of his 15 years of experience with the training method called Interpersonal Process Recall (IPR). He presents a distillation of what he and his associates learned in refining this phenomenon to effect knowledge and improve human interaction, including when and how it could be useful as well as how other trainers could educate mental health trainees with the process called IPR. Working with class groups of 25 students it has become possible now for each IPR instructor at Michigan State University to offer

* S. M. Silverman, M.D. and R. Fahy, M.D. presented a videotape on "Simulated Families in Family Therapy Training" on May 7, 1975 at the 128th Annual Meeting of the American Psychiatric Association in Anaheim, California.

to 100 counseling students every 10 weeks the kind of individualized experiential learning which had previously been reserved for medical students or for graduate students pursuing mental health careers. He is doing what I have always dreamed of doing, namely, teaching what *really* goes on between people to all persons who will be working on a personal basis with other persons in human interaction.

The work of John Waldron has been placed after Norman Kagan's IPR because it is so closely related to it in the training of neophytes. This material is my version of the efforts by Waldron and his colleagues on the Psychiatric faculty at the Queens University in Kingston, Ontario. Just as Kagan's work is being utilized with people not directly involved in the "field of mental health" (actually we all are involved), Waldron's rating scales should be used not only with all professional and paraprofessional workers in our field but with all people engaged in working with other people. Communication is the key system in human interpersonal relationship and it's time that we recognize it as even more important than knowledge of the alphabet and begin to teach it and its implications in kindergraten.

There are many important points made by Douglas Weir in his chapter on "Evaluating Psychiatric Learning Through Videotaped Patient Interviews." He shares the skills necessary for the teacher planning to use edited, pre-taped video segments with psychiatric trainees at various stages of development to assess (a) knowledge possessed, (b) observational skills, (c) capacity for deductive reasoning and perceptive correlation, (d) diagnostic acumen, (e) appropriateness of therapeutic planning. He emphasizes the importance of appropriate selection of brief segments and, in view of the present state of the art, equipment and human video know-how available in most psychiatric settings, he makes a point I agree with wholeheartedly, namely, that black and white rather than color videotape is in general the recommended one to use. In general, anything which distracts viewer attention from patient(s) and patient-therapist interaction should be avoided. Videotapes which will be used for evaluating the viewer's sensitivity and knowledge should not direct the viewer's attention to a particular aspect of the patient's functioning, although videotapes which do are excellent for the basic teaching of new information. We once again see that the specific objectives for a tape should be kept in mind when it is produced and edited.

The spread of videotaped interviews of patients from the realm of individual medicine to the broader and more natural realm of family medicine is described in broad and then more detailed strokes by David Schmidt and Edward Messner in their chapter on the psyschiatric training of family physicians. The importance of this return to an awareness of family involvement and family systems in the development of individual illness, whether the more psychic or more somatic in original etiology, cannot be overemphasized. It is refreshing in this regard to learn that there are over 300 postgraduate training programs in family medicine as of 1977. The presentation by Schmidt and Nessner accentuates the significance of video in enhancing the ripple effect of psychiatric consultations so as to share significant knowledge sooner with non-psychiatrists and thus enhance their ability to recognize and more appropriately manage the emotional and psychic problems of their "somatically" ill patients.

In the next chapter Jim Lurie of Seattle shares his expertise in developing techniques and exercises utilizing video with trainees or actors and actresses. His approaches supplement the techniques offered by Froelich in Chapter 5, and Weir in Chapter 8. They are particularly valuable for general or family practitioners and come from Lurie's many years of experience in the experiential teaching of psychiatry to non-psychiatric physicians.

The next three chapters are concerned with the increasingly important subject of supervision. Most of those who became supervisors over the past 30 years were not trained specifically in the art or science of supervising others and approached their task with anxiety, confusion and a fragmented or partial approach. The chapters by Hirsh and Freed and by Gruenberg, Liston and Wayne deal directly with the how of supervision in working with trainees and cover many of the finer details of the experience. However, the chapter by Goin and Kline represents an important step forward in that it focuses on 10 years of study of the use of videotaped sessions of supervisors in the process of supervising their psychiatric trainees. This subject has received all too little study to date. Anxious trainees reporting non-objectively to supervisors who listened to "hearsay" about what happened describes what most of us experienced in our training in psychoanalytic institutes or other centers.

To my knowledge, the 1970 paper by Watters, Elder, Smith and Cleghorn entitled "Psychotherapy Supervision—A Videotape Technique"* was the first one which described the use of videotape to examine "the process of psychotherapy supervision, about which even less is known than about psychotherapy." The method they developed at the Master University in Hamilton, Ontario "consisted of putting together a composite videotape of both the psychotherapy session and the relevant super-

---

* Watters, W. W., Elder, P., Smith, S. K. and Cleghorn, J., "Psychotherapy Supervision—A Videotape Technique," *Canad. Psychiat. Ass. J.*, 16:367-368, 1971.

vision." The resident's therapeutic interview with the patient is videotaped. The resident and his supervisor then view this tape together, with
either of them interrupting at any point to discuss some aspect of the
therapy. Their discussion is also videotaped, and this record of supervision is then combined with the tape of the therapy session in such a
way that the viewer sees each successive segment of psychotherapy followed by that segment of supervision related to it. The final tape with its
alternating sequences of psychotherapy and supervision is then viewed
by members of a supervision workshop "consisting of other residents, the
therapist and faculty, including the supervisor. The main focus of the
meeting is on the particular supervisor's technique and upon the supervisory process itself. Supervisors are thus enabled to reconsider the effectiveness of their style and to make changes based on the valuable feedback given by the residents and faculty. The technique also helps residents to use supervision better than they had previously."

Earlier this year I learned of the efforts of George Zimmy, Thomas
Thale and Frank Muriel at St. Louis University Medical School to
develop a program of videotaping supervisors to help them develop their
supervisory skills. When they approached the supervisors with the idea
they found "the response was one of reluctant cognitive affirmation and
spontaneous affective ambivalence" as "receiving supervision of their
supervision via videotape seemed to be quite a different thing" than
supervising their trainees (personal communication). It took some months
for the idea inoculation to take and then they set up the following technique: In their recording studio with two cameras and split-screen the
television director decides when to record and thus records segments of
the supervisory sessions. Initially, critical comments by supervisors other
than the one who was taped for review were few. Interest was high and
the supervisor who was taped acknowledged how anxious he had been. In
the course of a year in which such review sessions have been held once
a month, questions have emerged as to goals of supervision, integrating
supervisory sessions with lecture courses on interviewing, and the amount
of time to be devoted to diagnosis and treatment of the patients problems rather than discussion of interviewing skills. Most important is the
fact that seeing themselves has led supervisors to change, to be more
direct and less protective. And learning that the supervisors are being
supervised has helped the trainees too!

The chapter by Goin and Kline presents significant findings to help
others better organize and conduct their supervisory programs. Most
significant have been the data they unearthed about supervisors' being
fearful of discussing countertransference problems because of blurring

between what is supervision and what is therapy and their feeling that therapy must be avoided when doing supervision. I personally don't see how it is possible to have absolutely crisp lines of separation between what is supervisory and what is psychotherapeutic in such a relationship experience. The three charts prepared by the authors should be most helpful as they reflect (a) an analysis of the content of the supervisors' statements, (b) the nature of the supervisors' activity, and (c) a questionnaire which can be used by supervisees to evaluate their supervisors.

While there is no separate chapter on video in group therapy training in this edition, the general principles and techniques in all the chapters are applicable. One videotaped group can serve to achieve many training and research purposes. The same tape can be used:

1. to teach individual psychodynamics;
2. to teach interpersonal psychodynamics;
3. to teach group dynamics;
4. to teach the nature of repetitive themes in the content of family or groups or individuals;
5. to teach the subtle nuances and regulatory mechanisms of conscious and unconscious nonverbal communications;
6. to teach therapeutic interventions made by the therapist and his or her functions as leader;
7. to teach the therapeutic impact of group members on and for one another;
8. to give an overview of what goes on in the beginning, middle and terminating phases of each session.

The different goals must be kept in mind when videotape is being used to teach first year medical students, fourth year students, first, second or third year psychiatric residents, paramedical personnel or older practicing psychiatrists who are developing an interest in learning about varied therapeutic group approaches.*

Video replay has become a major teaching instrument for trainees in family therapy. There is no better tool to teach the interplay and mutually influencing input of the varied multilevel systems operating within a family at any one moment. Family operations which can be assessed by trainees and instructor, or by trainees, instructor and the family together include but are not limited to:**

1. communications as to directness, truthfulness, completeness, frequency, clarity, etc.;

---

* See Rosenbaum, M. and Berger, M. M., *Group Psychotherapy and Group Function,* 2nd Edition. New York: Basic Books, 1975.
* See Chapter 9, "Optimal Family Functioning," in M. M. Berger, *Working with People Called Patients.* New York: Brunner/Mazel, 1977.

2. metacommunications as to ambiguity, contradictions, consistency, etc.;
3. atmosphere;
4. interest in one another;
5. capacity for, as well as ways and expressions of, caring;
6. frequency and mode of reaching out to and for one another;
7. degree of reality and objectivity in self-perception of family members and in their perception of other family members and the world-at-large;
8. emotional expression in terms of nature and impact, acknowledgment by others and what is permitted or forbidden;
9. evidence of operations supporting individuation-autonomy-separation or symbiosis-dependency-clinging;
10. power distribution and how it is used, expressed, and reacted to;
11. capacity of family members to be aware of problems and conflict, to identify them and to make efforts at solution;
12. degree and nature of initiative, spontaneity and assumption of leadership;
13. the nature and degree of role projection by the parents;
14. capacity of family members to share;
15. parental acceptance of each other and of the children;
16. family responses to pain, loss, failure and stress;
17. degree of curiosity and risk-taking;
18. frequency and nature of physical contact as well as its appropriateness and respect for the other person's physical boundaries;
19. sense of humor;
20. capacity for enthusiasm, optimism and joy in living;
21. the presence or absence of psychopathology;
22. the family's value-systems.

The varied approaches of the chapters in this section on training give ample testimony to the versatility of video as a tool and to the fact that the frontiers for new ways and new options to creatively exploit its potential are still open.

And finally I want to emphasize the value to video users of seeking basic training and experience with the equipment itself. Various professional groups intermittently conduct training workshops and institutes.*

---

* South Beach Psychiatric Center conducted two-day video institutes from 1973-1976; The American Group Psychotherapy Association has conducted two-day training workshops with video at its annual meetings; The American Psychiatric Association offered a course on using video for continuing education credit at its May 1978 meeting in Atlanta; South Beach Psychiatric Center has a 400-hour multimedia training program in clinical and community psychiatry.

4

VIDEOTAPES AS AN EDUCATIONAL EXPERIENCE

Nancy A. Roeske, M.D.

Audiovisual material can be a potent educational experience. However, the development and utilization of any video material must be considered within the context of the author's theories about learning. Every author will apply his or her concepts about the principles of learning to the production of this form of educational material. It is my belief that the content and methodological approach to curriculum should stimulate a learning process within the student, which eventually leads to the student's becoming his or her own teacher. Furthermore, the student, in the process of learning, comes to understand that learning is a lifelong process. Thus, the following principles of learning are considered when developing curriculum: 1) the ultimate responsibility for learning depends on the student; 2) students have great individuality in their needs and their capabilities for learning; 3) the course material should be both related to and relevant to the student as a person and as a professional; 4) application of course material by the student increases the possibility of remembering content and improving skills; 5) a problem-solving set increases the amount of learning; therefore, interesting questions and experiences can maintain and accelerate learning; 6) the time lag between learning and evaluation should be as brief as possible, since knowledge of the results of learning is an important condition for satisfactory learning; 7) material and skills are rapidly forgotten with non-usage; therefore, continuing practice and reexamination are necessary reinforcers for learning; and 8) the keystone of learning is aspiration. Thus, a major goal of the psychiatric teacher is to increase the student's aspiration level for psychiatric knowledge and skills. Audiovisual materials are particularly adept at fulfilling all of these principles of learning.

A major advantage in the use of audiovisual materials is the fact that students have had many years of learning from television. However, they have also learned to selectively tune out television materials. Therefore, audiovisual materials have a remarkably ambivalent position as a source of learning.

Nevertheless, audiovisual materials have a number of unique constructive attributes. These attributes include availability of material, focusing of attention, repetition of presentation, flexibility of presentation, and flexibility in the use of material. A frequent problem for an educator is to have the appropriate material available when it is required for the learning experience. Audiovisual material assures the availability of pertinent material for immediate use by the teacher and students and allows them to focus on a particular topic or aspect of a topic via the selection of content and the focus of the camera. This control over the content and methodology enhances the possibility for specific content and skills to be learned. The availability of the educational experience on an audiovisual tape allows for repeated presentation, thereby assuring reinforcement in learning. Further, the audiovisual tape increases the possibilities for flexible adaptation of the material to the demands of the group. For example, the picture may be larger than life-size, thus enabling students to see material more easily and completely. The videotape may be started, stopped, or repeated as necessary. The material may be used individually by students as a self-learning program. Or the material can be used by a teacher with varying numbers of students. Finally, audiovisual material can provide multiple stimuli. A given format can serve as a stimulus for a number of different types of learning experiences. For example, a three-minute presentation of a patient may serve as a stimulus for a discussion of the patient's mental state, interview questions and techniques, and the initial considerations for patient management.

On the other hand, there are special problems which are inherent in the use of audiovisual materials. Students have learned to tune out audiovisual materials through their lifelong experiences with presentations of commercials every three to four minutes. Students usually are unable to be intensely involved in learning from an audiovisual presentation for longer than 10 to 12 minutes. On the other hand, if the material is a lecture with interspersed diagrams or other material, the students' attention span is enhanced by taking notes and by being asked questions at the end of the program.

Presentation of psychiatric material presents very special problems for the student who is learning either on an individual basis or in a large group of students. Such material always evokes, at some point in time, an idiosyncratic emotional response in each student. The student's awareness of the effect of the material upon himself or herself, and his or her ability to comprehend and understand the meaning of the material are limited by the personal implications of the response. For example, the student may be unaware of the sexual stimulation of a videotape or his or her reaction to a person on the tape because of an association in the viewer's mind with a disliked person. Therefore, psychiatric material is most effectively taught if there is a skillful teacher present who is aware of the multiple ramifications of learning from this type of material.

All learning materials have limitations, some of which are inherent in the materials and some of which are inherent in the student and the educational system. The most valuable learning occurs when there is a combination of reading materials, learning from carefully edited and focused videotapes, and opportunities to apply the material, for example, by contact with patients. Reading a book and learning from audiovisual tapes are crucial aspects, usually prerequisites for contact with a patient. However, they can never replace the direct interaction between student and a patient.

The critical problem for the educator is to develop the most effectively stimulating and judicious blend of a variety of learning materials and experiences.

5

LEARNING VIA VIDEOTAPE SIMULATION

Robert E. Froelich, M.D.

"Are Medical Schools Neglecting Clinical Skills?" is the title of the lead editorial in a recent publication (1). "Physical Examination, Frequently Observed Errors" is the title of another recent article (2). The contention of these authors is that the technology of medicine is so seductive in luring the interests and attentions of the medical student and the clinical teacher that the learning of the clinical skills of interviewing, relating to patients, and performing the physical examination is being overlooked.

Videotape simulation is a teaching technique that focuses upon the skills of the student in a manner that facilitates effective learning. To understand how and why videotape simulation works, we will review the process of learning, clinical teaching goals, and some educational principles before describing the teaching technique.

PROCESS OF LEARNING

As Robert M. Gagne has pointed out, the learning of a skill requires a different process than the learning of facts, concepts, and problem solving (3). The learning of a skill requires the performance of the skill followed by accurate feedback, a change in the second performance of the skill with feedback from the second performance so that further perfection of the skill can take place. Experience without feedback and without the opportunity to review, critique, and correct leads to making the same mistake over and over on each practice of the skill.

Learning for a large percentage of medical students occurs with greater retention of the item learned when the following conditions are present: 1) The student is curious and/or interested in the item; 2) the student sees a need or relevance to the item in terms of his own personal future in medicine; and 3) the student discovers the item to be learned with the full impact of the cognitive understanding and the emotional charge

60

of the discovery process. To a questionnaire asking students how they most effectively learn, their responses were summarized by the following statements: 1) I learn best when I know what I am looking for; 2) I learn best when I dig it out for myself; and 3) I learn best when I set my own pace to find out what I am looking for (4).

Educational research indicates that the most effective learning occurs when the learning situation is similar to the actual situation in which the information is to be used. The material is then more readily transferred and will more likely be used in the real life situation for which the students are being trained (5). It sounds trite but it must be emphasized that students learn that which they themselves experience. Not only do they learn from that which they do but also from that which they see being done by others. In other words, they learn much by imitation of the role model.

Research into the learning process of students has shown that factual information which is acquired through the process of problem-solving considerably reduces the rate at which factual information is lost. The problem serves as the organizing framework for the bits and pieces of information (4). When we are able to teach factual information necessary for the practice of medicine in the context of a clinical problem, the students retain the information and are able to draw upon it with greater frequency and efficiency than when the information is not tied to a clinical problem.

Another aspect of student learning is that greater skill in attacking new problems develops when the student faces a large number of practice problems and less skill develops when he/she spends the same amount of time on fewer practice problems (6). Thus, the student's skill varies with the number and variety of practice problems with which he has worked and has received feedback.

TEACHING GOALS IN MEDICAL EDUCATION

The goal of medical education is for the student to learn 1) perceptual skills, 2) medical facts, 3) problem-solving skills, 4) professional attitudes, 5) professional values, 6) professional management skills, and 7) knowledge of behavior expectations.

When medical practice is reduced to its final endpoint, it rests upon interpersonal contact between the physician and a patient, a physician and another physician, a physician and a nurse, or a physician and an allied health professional; for these encounters, the physician must have expertise in communication skills in addition to medical facts. By way of illustration, I emphasize that it does the patient little good for the physician to successfully diagnose an early, life-threatening or disabling problem if he/she is unable through adequate communication to secure the patient's or the community's cooperation in efforts to arrest it.

If the student of today is to become a successful practicing physician, none of the seven goals listed above may be overlooked.

EDUCATIONAL PRINCIPLES

It is generally agreed that, in order to learn efficiently, the student must be motivated. Furthermore, learning occurs more readily if the student is rewarded for his/her efforts, and new information is acquired by the student more quickly if it is related to prior knowledge. Feedback in the learning cycle contributes to motivation, reward, and utilization of prior knowledge (7). This feedback creates motivation by acknowledging successes as well as failures. The learner is rewarded when he sees his own mastery develop by means of feedback. Feedback assists in the building of information upon prior knowledge and performance by providing awareness of and objectivity to the learner's behavior.

The goal of learning and of psychotherapy has the same quality. Each has a change in a behavior as the criterion of success. In treating patients in psychiatry, we have been confronted with the fact that learning on the intellectual level is only a part of the total learning process. Before behavior changes, there needs to be learning on the emotional level. The patient must be actively (emotionally) involved in the treatment-learning process. Similarly, the student must be actively involved in the learning exercise before meaningful learning occurs as judged by a change in behavior.

METHODS OF INSTRUCTION

We have reviewed characteristics of the process of learning, teaching goals in medical education, and educational principles. In light of this review, there are two instructional methods from which to choose when helping medical students develop interpersonal communicative skills, management skills, professional values, and problem-solving abilities. These are on-the-job training and simulation.

On-the-job training has the problem of giving the student responsibility for taking care of patients, directing nurses, and directing an allied health team with neither extensive experience nor legal backing. It is widely used as an instructional method in medicine and therefore does not need to be described. The value of on-the-job training as a learning method depends upon feedback given to the student. To insure that on-the-job training is really educational rather than experience without learning many feedback mechanisms have been developed. For example, special rooms with one-way mirrors, audiotape recorders, observers who have been carefully trained to take accurate notes on the interaction, motion picture film, and videotape to capture the audio dialogue as well as the nonverbal behavior of the situation have all been advocated. These techniques all involve some artificiality and distortion of the original scene by their intrusion.

The scene is unaltered only when recording is "double-blind" to the extent that a candid-camera technique is used and neither the student nor the interacting other is aware that the interaction is being recorded. Such recording involves such legal implications that I will not deal with it (see Chapter 25). The point is that even the on-the-job training situation is altered when it becomes a learning environment because of the intrusion of the third person, whether in the form of a machine or an individual.

The argument has been put forth that a simulation is not real, therefore it is not acceptable for learning. My answer is that the on-the-job training situation is no longer the same once it is made into a learning environment via recording.

Another argument for simulation has been the cost involved. In 1971 an hour of a student's time at the bedside of a patient in the University of Oklahoma teaching hospital cost the state $112.00. At the same time an hour of time spent by a student pilot on a 707 aircraft simulator at the Federal Aviation Administration center in Oklahoma City cost the government only $45.00. The cost of medical simulations developed in the last 15 years for learning various aspects of the physical examination, interviewing, and problem-solving, whether they involve computers, programmed patients, or paper-and-pencil problems have all (except for one anesthesia simulator) cost less than the $112.00 per student hour for a teaching bed. Even the anesthesia simulator cost per hour will decrease when its use increases and additional units are produced to overcome the initial research and development costs.

In dealing with the questions of the validity of a simulation, it has been our experience that some simulations bring out truer feelings than the on-the-job training method since there is less at risk. The real patient in the on-the-job training may have his/her life at stake. When there is less at risk, each can be freer in his/her expression of feelings and thoughts. In simulations, it is our experience that normally hidden aspects of the interactions and feelings become more easily evident.

Several techniques can simulate situations in which the students can apply the skills, values, and attitudes being learned. These include the case study method (8, 9), psychodrama (with variations of mirror techniques and role reversal), field problems, simulation games, and role-playing. The case study method, psychodrama, field problems, simulation games, and role-playing techniques have been used in management training (10), education of attorneys (moot court), officer training at the U.S. Army Command and General College, and other educational programs (11).

In the real life situations many of the psychomotor and affective elements of the organism remain unconscious and unavailable for discussion (12). Psychodrama, in particular, and the other methods of simulation as well, have all been devised to bring heretofore unrecognized aspects of interpersonal interaction into awareness for discussion and modification. Some of these interpersonal aspects may come from within oneself while some come from within the other.

Role reversal, mentioned earlier, is a technique in which a role player takes a role opposite to his own. For example, a husband may be asked to play the part of a wife, or a physician asked to play the part of a patient. Role-reversal techniques, in particular, are designed to bring out the feelings, attitudes, and values of another person.

Each technique has its own merits and limitations when applied to specific learning situations. The case study method is a technique wherein a real or fictitious case is presented from a printed record for discussion. The clinical pathologic conference is an example of the case study method. The case study method does not focus upon the interactional process, bring out the experiential background of the students, or define the roles of the participants as seen by the students. It usually deals with factual and concept learning rather than the learning of skills.

Psychodrama is a technique made popular by Dr. J. Moreno (9). In this method the patients are assigned roles and instructed as to some of the feelings they should portray. The roles are played as part of an unrehearsed dramatic production before an audience. Psychodrama brings the actors face to face with their audience as they play their part. Some inhibition of the actors as well as inhibition of the audience is fostered by this circumstance. Psychodrama or role-playing each relies upon notes, observations, and selective feedback by the participants on stage and in the audience. Thus, the feedback to the role-players is limited to notes and recall with all of the distortions inherent in this feedback process.

Problem-solving is a technique in which the class is presented a realistic problem. The class seeks the solution to the problem by analyzing the data and securing additional information from the teacher. Problem-solving focuses more upon the end results and decisions that were made than upon the interpersonal processes which take place in the communication networks. Again this technique lacks a recording process which focuses on the individual professional value system.

VIDEOTAPE SIMULATION TECHNIQUE

Videotape simulation is the combination of role-playing (with only the television camera and instructor as the audience) and videotape which records the dialogue and behavior of the role-players (13, 14). This combination is ideally suited for the learning of professional roles, professional values, behavior expectations, professional attitudes, and problem-solving skills. The teacher first selects a common clinical situation appropriate to his teaching goals (15). The situation has, as a part of it, role conflict and interpersonal disagreement, yet there should be no clearcut management procedure. The teacher defines very vaguely the role positions of the several persons normally involved in the problem (for example, patient, doctor, nurse, and spouse of the patient), and he/she describes the time and place the interaction is taking place. For example, one problem we have used to demonstrate latent feelings and content has involved a patient with a myocardial infarction. Other role-players are the young physician who sees the patient trying to direct his own treatment, the nurse who is following the doctor's orders but does not fully agree with him, and the patient's wife who knows that her husband is reluctant to admit to pain and fears that he will exert himself and die, leaving her with two young children.

Role-players are selected from the class that is being instructed. Each role-player is given the same brief statement of the problem which sets the stage and identifies each player by name and role position. This statement of the problem does not disclose the various points of view which are peculiar to the individuals involved. After noting the nature of the problem and the persons involved, each role-player is given a sealed envelope containing a statement which gives him/her, in one paragraph, information further defining his/her position, feelings and attitudes toward the problem. This paragraph is brief unless it is important to the problem that a role-player should portray a very specific viewpoint, feeling, or attitude. Frequently, as may happen in the real situation, the further information includes laboratory or social data applicable to that particular role-player and not known by the others. In general, the role-player is free to develop the role as he/she perceives it. No script or lines are provided and the role-players are discouraged from discussing the problem or their own role positions before the videotape recording is completed.

The teacher acts as director and calls into the room (on stage) those players who are in the first scene. Chairs are usually the only props that are necessary. Other role-players are kept in another room so they do not know what happens in the first scene. The instructor interrupts the scene when it has come to a natural conclusion, when a role-player requests that he/she be allowed to see another role-player (for example, the doctor asks to see the patient), or when the instructor feels that further interaction will not be instructive.

The videotape is restarted and scene two is recorded when appropriate role-players are assembled. Those who are not actively involved are waiting in the adjacent room. Similarly, in what would be a realistic progression of events, additional scenes are recorded. Usually the recorded material of all scenes runs from 20 to 30 minutes.

Ideally the videotape is stored for 12 hours or more before it is presented to the role-players and their peers in class. This delay between recording and class session allows the role-players time to detach themselves from the roles and to view the role enactments in the third person —"that was the way I played the role yesterday, that's not really me." This detachment allows the peer group greater freedom of expression in finding fault, commenting, and praising the performance they observe. Similarly, the role-players objectively comment on their own performance. The level of frankness and the honesty of comments approaches that in a "T group."

When the class session is opened, the students are given copies of the statement of the problem. They are asked what problems they see in the situation, how the different roles will be played, and what factors will be critical to the management of the patient. After some discussion, the videotape is started for all to view. The ground rules are that any student or teacher may interrupt the videotape at any time for a comment or question. The comment or question is discussed before the videotape is restarted, and before the related portion of the action is replayed. The discussion is the heart of the learning process. It is through the discussion that the insights become clear, the possible variations of playing each role become evident, and the latent content of the behavior becomes conscious. The value system of the role-player may be evident (for example, the physician felt that it was more important for the patient to follow his/her orders than to assume any responsibility for his/her own treatment). The teacher should set aside from one and a half to three hours for the class to work through a videotape simulation.

We have not found any teaching method that creates as much student participation or involvement as does videotape simulation. The reenactment of scenes is true to life because the role-players can be themselves without censoring their own behavior since they can hide behind the rationalization that they were just playing the role to please or to bring out a viewpoint as they were directed to do in their sealed envelope. In some respects, videotape simulation approaches reality more closely than does the recording of actual events because of the third person intrusion of the recording devices as discussed earlier in this chapter.

All of our videotape simulations have been filled with affect. The role-players have become involved in the situation and have expressed frustration, despair, anger, denial and other feelings common to the roles they were playing.

When we recall that the students learn best when they know what they are looking for, when they dig for themselves, and when they go at their own pace, we realize that videotape simulation provides a process which can fulfill all three requirements for efficient student learning.

Videotape simulation gives the student the opportunity to learn information in the way that he will use it in later life. In addition, he is learning information associated with a problem-solving situation which will act as an organizer of the information. As we learned earlier, this coupling of information to the problem-solving activity will lead to greater retention. As a class works through a number of videotape simulations, the members are rewarded by their peers as well as by viewing their own behavior. The information they gain is learned at the collective pace of the class discussion and is gradually built upon prior knowledge. As a side effect, one videotape simulation may have one set of teaching goals for first-year medical students and a second set of teaching goals for practicing physicians. Each audience's perceptions, background, and experience determine the direction of the discussion and the learning which occurs.

The obvious expression of affect associated with the solving of clinical problems facilitates learning on the affective level as well as the intellectual level. Videotape simulation solves the clinical teacher's problems by giving the students full responsibility for the situation, letting them learn by doing, giving them the freedom to proceed as they deem desirable, and letting them seek out the information they desire to manage the problem at hand both in the role-playing action and in the class discussion.

We have used videotape simulation successfully with groups of students ranging from 15 to 172 in number. We would prefer a small number in the class to a larger number, as it permits each student time for greater participation in the discussion. Our students have ranged from practicing physicians to first-year medical, dental and dental hygiene students. On several occasions the audience was made up of members of a Department of Psychiatry. The mixture of experienced physicians with young students seems to facilitate the discussion. Videotape simulation is also being used with other professional student groups with success.

The presentation of a videotape simulation to a class that did not participate in the recording of the problem has not been successful. The students did not have much interest in or involvement with the "foreign" tape recording.

THE FUTURE OF VIDEOTAPE IN TRAINING

When considering continuing education, an aspect of videotape simulation to be explored is the presentation of a recording of the classroom discussion of the videotape simulation to a "foreign" class or group. If the "foreign" class or group finds the recording acceptable and useful to learning, it presents a valuable tool to continuing education. In recent years recordings of grand rounds have been shared successfully between institutions. In a similar manner the sharing of videotapes of the classroom discussions may be useful.

Discussions of videotape simulations could be recorded and distributed to medical societies for self-study or small-group study and review. Videotape simulation may be a technical breakthrough for which we have searched so long to meet the needs of learning non-cognitive aspects of continuing and undergraduate education in medicine.

REFERENCES

1. Engel, George L.: Are Medical Schools Neglecting Clinical Skills? *J.A.M.A.*, 236: 861-863. 1976.
2. Weiner, Stanley, and Nathanson, Morton: Physical Examination, Frequently Observed Errors. *J.A.M.A.*, 236:852-855, 1976.
3. Gagne, Robert M.: *The Conditions of Learning.* New York: Holt, Rinehart and Winston, Inc., 1965.
4. Schorow, Mitchell: Problem-solving Theory and the Practice of Clinical Medicine. *Canad. Med. Assoc. J.*, 97:711-712, 1967.
5. Blair, Glenn: What the Psychology of Learning Says to the Teacher. University of Missouri Lecture, May 13, 1964.
6. Duncan, C. P.: Transfer After Training with Single Versus Multiple Tasks. In R. C. Anderson, *Readings in the Psychology of Cognition,* p. 641. New York: Holt, Rinehart and Winston, Inc., 1965.

7. Mosel, James N.: The Learning Process. *J. Med. Educ.,* 39, 1964.
8. Hunt, P.: The Case Method of Instruction. *Harvard Educ. Rev.,* 21:175-192, 1951.
9. Moreno, J.: *Psychodrama,* Vol. 1. New York: Beacon House, 1946.
10. Bavelas, Alex: Role Playing and Management Training. *Sociatry,* 1:183-191, 1947.
11. Boocock, Sarane S.: Simulation Games Today. *Educational Technology,* p. 7, April 30, 1968.
12. Moreno, J.: Psychodrama. *Amer. Handbook of Psychiat.,* Ch. 68, Vol. 2, p. 1375. New York: Basic Books, Inc., 1959.
13. Ramey, J. W., and Froelich, R. E.: Teaching Problem Solving by Videotape Simulation. *Council on Medical Television Health Science TV Source Book,* p. 70. Duke University Medical Center, 1968.
14. Froelich, R. E., and Bishop, F. M.: 1 + 1 = 3. *Medical and Biological Illustration,* 19, No. 1, January 1969.
15. Mager, Robert F.: *Preparing Instructional Objectives.* Palo Alto, Calif.: Fearon Publishers, 1962.

6

INTERPERSONAL PROCESS RECALL: MEDIA IN CLINICAL AND HUMAN INTERACTION SUPERVISION

Norman Kagan, Ph.D.

For all its apparent value in education and psychotherapy, media in general and the videotape recorder in particular offer us not one but many different tools, each best suited for accomplishing certain specific ends and not others.

In 1962 my colleagues and I first observed and later described (1) a phenomenon which seemed to have utility for effective knowledge and improvements in human interaction. We named the basic method Interpersonal Process Recall (IPR). It took five years of controlled studies (2) to discover when and how the phenomenon could be useful, and nine more years of research and development to produce and validate a film "package" (3) so that instructors in medicine and a variety of mental health programs could be trained to offer an IPR course to their students.

What we observed in 1962 was that if a person is videorecorded while he/she is relating to another and is then shown the recording immediately after the interaction, the person is able to recall thoughts and feelings in amazing detail and in depth. Usually there was some self-evaluation as well as a detailed narrative of the impact on the person of the "other" he/she had been relating with. If a remote control stop-start switch was given to the people so that they could stop and start the playback at will, usually a wealth of understanding about some of their underlying motives, thoughts and feelings during the interpersonal transaction could be verbalized by them. We also found, in these initial experiences, that the phenomenon could be counted on to work more reliably, and more information about underlying feelings could be elicited, if the person viewed the videotape separately from the original person with whom he interacted but in the presence of a third person who encouraged the viewer to verbalize and elaborate on that which is recalled.

We have found that the third person is most effective when he/she actively encourages the person, usually a student, to describe underlying thoughts and feelings. The third person's role requires that he/she ask such questions as, "Can you tell me what you felt at that point?" "Can you recall more of the details of your feelings . . . where did you feel these things, what parts of your body responded?" and, "What else do you think [the other] thought about you at that point?" The third person's role is that of an active, *inquiring colleague*. The term "inquirer" has been assigned to this third person in an IPR session.

IPR has proved to be a method by which mental health workers and a myriad of other professional and paraprofessional groups can learn and improve their ability to interview, communicate with, or help other people. It has also proved to be a useful vehicle for developing affective sensitivity scales (4, 5) for formulating theory about human interaction (6) and for the study of medical inquiry (7). Its potential for accelerating client growth in therapy is still under study (8, 9, 10, 11).

Until we came to understand better IPR as a tool and to learn something about what it could and could not accomplish, we met with some initial failures. Early in our experience with IPR we reasoned that the technique could be a powerful adjunct to or perhaps even a substitute for the usual supervisory process in counselor or teacher education. It seemed to us that the clients themselves could become the neophyte counselor's supervisor. We reasoned that this could be accomplished by videotaping the interaction between counselors and clients and by then replaying the tape for the clients and having the supervisor ask them about their thoughts, feelings and reactions to the counselors. By then giving the counselor an audiotape recording of the client's recall session or else arranging for the counselor to observe the recall session through a one-way mirror or on a TV monitor, a vehicle for learning about counselor impact on client would have been provided the counselor. The client's recall of the session is not only the most accurate available interpretation of the client's reaction to the moment-by-moment behavior of the counselor, but it is also immediate feedback for the counselor. Most important of all, we thought, the clients' statements of their own reactions to the counselors had greater credibility for the counselor than the supervisor's interpretations.

An experimental design was created to test this hypothesis. In the course of a master's level and again in a doctoral level counseling practicum the experimental procedures were compared with an equal amount of intensive traditional counselor supervision. The traditional supervision consisted of individual supervisory sessions between a counselor and a supervisor who had observed the counselor's session through a one-way mirror. Several such sessions were held. In the IPR treatment, the recall phenomenon seemed to be working well and consistently. Counselors heard their clients say such things as, "I wanted to talk about things which really bother me but the counselor didn't seem to want me to," "The counselor seemed scared and so I was trying to help him out," "I think she didn't like what I said but she wasn't going to say so directly," and an occasional, "I liked that, he really started me to thinking in new ways, there." It appeared to us that such client feedback would be highly instructive for the counselor, but it wasn't. The measured outcomes of the experimental procedures did not differ significantly from the outcomes of traditional supervision (12).

Why? We had simply failed to adequately analyze the nature of the learnings we hoped would emerge from the experience and then to fashion appropriate learning experiences to accomplish these. We had also failed to take into consideration the student's anxiety level and readiness for such powerful undeniable feedback *as a first experience* with the media. Analysis of what had happened led us to the development of the concept of interpersonal "developmental" tasks a neophyte would have to accomplish in order to obtain knowledge and skill in influencing human interaction. Subsequently the tasks of learning were ordered so they progressed from the least threatening to the most threatening phases.

The first phase in the revised model grew out of our early attempts to develop a behavioral counseling rating scale. We had developed the scale items by analyzing videotapes of counselors whose skills usually led to positive client comments on recall and comparing these with videotapes of counselors who seemed ineffective to their clients as well as to experts who reviewed the tapes. In addition we consulted the literature. Our conclusion was that, among other undefined characteristics, the successful counselors 1) focus much of their attention on client's affect; 2) listen carefully and try to understand fully the client's communication while conveying to the client that they are trying to understand; 3) could be extremely frank and honest (but gentle) rather than manipulative or evasive in responding to the client; and 4) respond so as to encourage the client to explore further and to assume an active role in the counseling process. These four behaviors were then used as a basis for rating of the trainee-client interviews. The first stage in the revised training system is to share these four concepts with the neophyte by means of a 52-minute color film in which a narrator presents examples and then simulation exercises for student practice.

The next phase of the emerging system was designed to help counselors overcome two dynamics which often interfere with the counselor's ability to understand the client or to communicate that understanding.* We had repeatedly observed in IPR sessions that people perceive and understand much more of their communication with each other than one would suspect as one observes the interaction. It appears that people "read" each other's most subtle communications fairly well, but as socialized beings often pretend that they read only the surface phenomena, the "official" message. Beginning counselors acted as if they did not perceive or understand the meaning behind many of their client's statements, but during recall indicated that indeed they did understand but were unable to act on their perceptions. In IPR sessions in which the counselor alone is the focus of the recall process, the "feigning of clinical naivete" becomes clear. "I knew she (the client) was very unhappy underneath that put-on smile, but—and I know this is stupid—I was afraid she might cry if I told her I knew she was 'hurting,' and then I would feel that I had made her cry," or "I knew (the client) was lying but I didn't 'call' him on it. . . . I was afraid he wouldn't come back for a next session if I was honest with him . . . he might even get up and walk right out of the room . . . I guess I would feel hurt if he did these things, and yet I know he probably wouldn't, but I couldn't risk it, I guess." The second dynamic which we hoped to influence in this phase of the system is the dynamic of "tuning out," of actually not seeing or hearing the other person for periods of time during the session. This usually occurred when the students were especially concerned about the impression they hoped to make on the client. For instance, during IPR sessions medical students often heard their patient for the first time say things of importance which they had not heard during the interview! The most frequent explanation by the medical students was, "I kept worrying about how to say things in such a way that I would appear to be older and more experienced than I am. I kept thinking about how I should look and how I should phrase my statements at those times. Even though I look as if I'm listening I really haven't heard a thing the patient said." Teachers often missed important cues about their students. The young teachers, not really comfortable with their subject matter, so often were "rehearsing" the material to themselves that they were simply not open to attending to external stimuli.

After recall sessions these two dynamics (feigning clinical naivete and

---

* *Ed. Note*: G. J. McMillan has condensed and altered Kagan's method in his approach as presented in "Video-Stimulated Recall in Pastoral Psychotherapy Training," *J. of Pastoral Care*, 28:262-266, 1974.

tuning out) were exhibited less often by students. The second phase in the revised supervisory system, then, was to set up a counseling session and do little or no recall with the client, but rather to conduct a recall session of the student. Typically, through this procedure, students learn to recognize where and how they failed to hear or to deal with client message. Students also usually became more sensitive to their own feelings in human interaction.

Awareness of and sensitivity to their own feelings and often inappropriate behaviors seemed to help students do a better job with their next clients or patients but awareness of self was often not enough. Typically the students still needed additional help to become more involved with their clients. It also seemed to us that by the time the second phase was completed the student was now also ready to learn more about client dynamics through feedback. An IPR tool was fashioned to both provide client feedback and afford the student additional experience using exploratory probes, the primary mode used in recall. In this phase, the students themselves are required to perform the function of inquirer with another student's client. Thus, the counselor has an opportunity to try out new behavior (the exploratory probes basic to the inquirer role) with the support of the videotape and the realization that they are working with their peer's client, not their own. When the students later switch roles, the counselor's partner then does recall with one of the counselor's clients. The students may agree to exchange notes later, to listen to audio recordings of their partner's recall or may even agree to observe the session through a one-way mirror and so learn about the client's recalled reaction to the session. Thus both students learn—the one in the counselor role and the one in the inquirer role. By this phase students are ready for such feedback and are not overwhelmed by it (especially since it is a peer, not the supervisor, who is the client's inquirer). The instructor or a staff member is available to be of assistance with any technical problems and to discuss with students their reactions to the role of inquirer and to the feedback they got from their clients.

In this phase students usually learn, often to their amazement, that they can be both confronting and supportive, that questions or comments raised by the interviewer which might be embarrassing or bold in most social settings are appropriate and productive in a counseling or medical interview when accompanied by communication of concern or interest. Students learn, too, how clients react to them and which of their behaviors clients found helpful and which they did not. Most often students are also amazed to learn of the extent to which clients are deeply concerned about the counselor's feelings about them. No matter how remote in space and time from the counselor-client interaction the content of the session appeared to be, they learn that a large part of the client's attention is focused on the here-and-now interaction between themselves and their counselor. This awareness creates in students a readiness for the fourth phase of the system.

It is one thing for students to learn experientially that an important part of client's concern involves the counselor and especially the client's anticipations but it is quite another thing for students to *learn to use the relationship itself* as a case in point to help clients understand their usual interpersonal behavior and feelings and to learn to relate in new ways. Again, with the developmental task defined and awareness of the probable readiness of the student for new learning, an IPR experience was fashioned to help achieve the goal.

Counselor and client are videotaped as before. During the recall session *both* counselor and client remain in the same room and are joined by an inquirer. During the recall session both counselor and client are encouraged to recall their thoughts, feelings and especially how they perceived each other and what meanings they ascribed to each other's behaviors. A situation is thus created in which two people, a client and a student, are helped to talk about each other to each other. Such *mutual recall* sessions typically enable students to better communicate with clients about the here-and-now of their interaction. Students become more involved, more concerned, more assertive, and more honest with their clients and use the ongoing counselor-client relationship as a case-in-point to help clients understand their relationships with others in their life.

Did the system which was developed to that point work? When neophyte counselor candidates were given only two sessions each of each phase of the above system (a total of eight sessions, each of approximately one and a half hours duration), they were rated as statistically significantly better than a comparable group of neophytes given intensive but traditional supervision of equal time. The counselors were so rated in a double-blind research design by Ph.D. level counselors as well as by their clients (2). Using even fewer sessions (hardly ideal!) Kingdon found that clients of counselors given IPR supervision made greater gains than clients of counselors supervised by other means (13).

Although originally designed for use with counselors, psychiatrists, and other mental health workers, the IPR model had an immediate appeal in undergraduate medical education. Most students enter medical school with an interest in human health and disease and because of the extensive knowledge they need before they can be of any help to patients they are usually not permitted to interview patients for some time. Certainly it would be helpful if they were able to have experience at interviewing early in medical school. IPR seemed to offer a solution, but modifications in the model were necessary. Under the direction of Jason (14) IPR was adapted for use with medical students. Amateur and professional actors and actresses were recruited. The actors were trained to play the part of patients in specified conditions of health or illness, friendly and unfriendly, communicative and uncommunicative, forthright and deceptive. The "concerns" which were to have brought each patient to seek medical care were always related to areas of study which the medical students had been through or else required no specific knowledge of disease entities, and so the students were potentially able to be of some help to the patient. It was hoped that talking with live people about their problems would help the students integrate their academic medical knowledge. After some pilot experiences it became apparent that the "tool" could help students to understand better their behavior with patients and to become more skillful at medical interviewing, both at eliciting information and at counseling patients. Often practicing physicians from the community could be recruited and, after themselves going through the various IPR formats, served as inquirers for the freshman medical students. Incidentally, these practicing physicians often volunteered that their own behavior with patients had improved in their practice.

The actors played their parts well. Although students were told their patients were actors, the interviews were considered to be very real and meaningful by the students. Evaluations of the program (15, 16) indicated that medical students made statistically significant gains in interviewing skills and in sensitivity to interpersonal messages. A very similar approach was later used in medical inquiry studies to demystify the diagnostic processes used by highly competent medical specialists (7).

Transfer-of-learning from the classroom or workshop setting, where students counsel with each other or with coached clients for practice, to the actual work setting with real patients and clients can be a very difficult process for some students. To aid in the transfer of skills to other settings students can be required later to use the various recall formats (counselor recall, client recall and mutual recall) in the clinic setting with real clients or patients. Where video recording is impractical (i.e., on rounds), simple audio cassette recorders have been used effectively.

To facilitate transfer-of-learning to the students' own personal "support system," IPR courses have been given for couples. The student and a significant other in his/her life take the course together. Several of the lab sessions are devoted to the couple's individually or mutually reviewing tapes of their interaction. For the past two years Joe and Fran Kertezs have offered such a couples IPR course at Michigan State University.

After the studies cited above validated the revised system, affect simulation or "stimulus" vignettes were added to the model (17, 18). The idea for such vignettes came from the experience of conducting hundreds of recall sessions. In numerous IPR sessions we observed that people often feared from each other behaviors which in all likelihood they would never be subjected to. Clients often feared, for instance, that if they told their counselor or psychotherapist "the truth" about themselves the counselor would walk out of the room in disgust, abandoning the client. Teachers often fantasized that if they gave up "too much" control in the classroom chaos and destruction would follow. Medical students often feared being discredited or even mocked by patients because of their age or fallibility. In general, the fears could be categorized under four general rubrics: fear of the other's hostility toward the student; the student's fear of loss of control of his/her own aggressive impulses; fear that the other would become too intimate, too seductive; and fear by the student of his/her own potential for seductiveness.

These "interpersonal nightmares" were often elicited and examined during recall sessions if the student was introspective enough and if the real or simulated encounter in the videotaped interview had stimulated the nightmare sufficiently, but it seemed to us that it might be possible to create a more reliable way of helping people face their interpersonal fears. It occurred to us that if we filmed actors looking directly at the camera lens (so that the resultant image then looks directly at the viewer) and if the content of the filmed sequence portrayed one or another of the more universal nightmares, then it might be possible to help students discuss and come to understand better their interpersonal behaviors. A series of filmed vignettes were made. These were meant to be used for a wide range of subjects and so actors were instructed to portray the various types of affect with varying degrees of intensity, but to avoid words which would ascribe a role to them or which would define too specific a story (e.g., in one vignette an actor looks at the viewer for a few seconds, tears appear in his eyes and between sobs he asks, "Why did you do that—I did nothing to you"). In another vignette a woman slowly licks her lips and tells the viewer that, "If you don't come over here and touch me I'm going to go out of my mind." Students are told to imagine that the actor is talking privately to them. Students are then asked such questions as, "Did the vignette have any impact on you? What did you feel? What did you think? Has anything close to that kind of situation ever actually happened to you? How do you usually respond? How do you wish you could bring yourself to respond? What did the person on the screen really want of you?" Most students have little difficulty in getting involved in the process.

After our initial experiences with the filmed simulation of general or universal interpersonal threat, we turned to creating vignettes of the kind of threat which might influence performance in a specific occupation. A series of films was made especially for teachers and instructors based on some of the fears teachers typically have. Similarly vignettes were made for physicians and medical students (e.g., "We've been to so many doctors who were just awful! But we're sure you'll be able to help us."). The vignettes are used with students in small groups. Other formats have also been used. In one, students and the image on the screen are videotaped using two cameras and a split-screen technique as the student watches the film. At the conclusion of the simulated experience students are then engaged in a video recall of the tape. In another format, each student's heart rate, skin conductance, respiration, and other physiological processes are also recorded and included on the videotape so that during the recall a student not only can see how he/she looked during the playing of each vignette but also how his or her physiological processes were responding.

Did the model which was now expanded to include affect simulation work? Controlled studies (19) indicated that the model reliably enables students to make significantly greater gains than control treatments. It was also found that the model was effective in other cultures (20). Especially exciting for mental health workers was the finding that the IPR model could be used to help paraprofessionals learn basic counseling skills. Dendy (21) provided a 50-hour program to undergraduate bachelor degree candidates. Among his findings were significant improvement in interviewing skills, significant growth on an affective sensitivity scale, and no loss of skills during a three-month no-training period. Most exciting of all, before the program was undertaken, independent judges rated the undergraduates' interview skills and also rated tapes of Ph.D. level supervising counselors employed at the university's counseling center. Both groups interviewed clients from the same client pool. Before the 50-hour program, there were large differences favoring the Ph.D.'s (fortunately!) but, after training, independent judges found no significant differences between the groups on scales of empathy and other basic communication skills.

Archer and Kagan (22) then found that these same undergraduates could, in turn, train other undergraduates so that the peer-instructed students scored significantly higher than other students who experienced an encounter group of similar duration. They also scored higher than a comparable no-treatment group, not only on measures of affective sensitivity and self-actualization, but also on scales given to roommates and other peers not in the study. When given lists of all participants, dormitory residents selected the IPR trained students as the ones they "would be willing to talk to about a personal problem" significantly more frequently than they rated either the encounter trained student or the control group member. Apparently, then, dormitory residents were able to identify the increased therapeutic skills of those peer instructed students in the IPR group.

Rowe (23) found that if, in addition to the experiential processes of the model, students were also exposed to relevant cognitive, theoretical constructs, their skill development was significantly augmented. Based on her findings, theoretical constructs about interpersonal communication were added to the IPR model.

Since our first publication reliable replication of the model by others has been a primary concern to us. The inquirer role so basic to the process is very difficult to communicate in writing. Even the filmed stimulus vignettes could easily be used in ways which would not encourage productive learning by students. This concern has led us to experiment with "packaging" the entire model so as to greatly simplify the task of the instructor and to make the model reliably replicable without the need for "outside" consultants. Our first attempt was limited to a black and white 16 mm film series containing illustrations, instructions, demonstration and didactic presentations but aimed primarily at mental health workers. The film package was obtained by more than 40 universities, schools, and social agencies, most of which reported satisfactory experiences. A controlled evaluation by one of them (New York University) indicated that counseling students taught by instructors using the package made significantly greater gains than a control group receiving an equivalent amount of other curriculum offerings (24). Recently, the package, entitled "Influencing Human Interaction," was revised and expanded so that it now consists of color films or color videotapes (3) and contains illustrations from a wide range of disciplines including medicine, teaching, and family therapy. An extensive instructor's manual and student handouts were also prepared. The new package is currently in use in medical, pharmacy, and law schools, hospitals, secondary schools, agencies, and prison personnel programs in the U.S., Canada, Australia, Sweden, Denmark, Norway, Germany, Puerto Rico, Israel and elsewhere.

The most recent modifications in the model grew out of an interest my colleagues and I have had for some time in the possibilities of influencing the productivity and happiness of entire communities of people by offering IPR training to large numbers of the people who would then be expected to use the skills and knowledge, not so much as counselors for others but as a way of relating more directly and being capable themselves of more intense involvement with those they live and work with. For instance, prison inmates who received IPR training at the prison reception center prior to assignment to the prison where they would serve their "time" were later rated by guards as more approachable than a control group of inmates (25). Teachers were rated by junior high school students as being more human and more likeable after the teachers received training (26).

In the IPR format described above the instructor or a trained cadre of instructor-aides had to conduct the first recall sessions for the students (prior to the students' learning the inquirer role and then conducting client and mutual recall sessions for each other). The number of students enrolled in such a course then would have to be limited to the number of inquirers the instructor could recruit or the number of recall sessions the instructor could reasonably conduct. Would it be possible to teach the inquirer role to students *prior* to the first IPR session so that their first interview is then followed by a recall session conducted not by the instructor or instructor-surrogate but by one of the student's peers? In other words, is it possible to teach students to supervise each other in this model right from the start? A controlled comparison (27) of the model using "outside" inquirers and a "self-contained" version indicated that very little was actually sacrificed for the increased efficiency.

It is therefore now possible for one or two people to have a positive influence on an entire school community (26). Based on class groups of 25, it has been possible, for instance, for each IPR instructor at Michigan State University to offer to 100 students every 10 weeks the kind of individualized experiential learning which had previously been reserved for medical students or for graduate students pursuing mental health careers. A typical ten-week course is presented in Figure 1.

Such courses are now also offered on a regular basis at MSU and elsewhere to nutritionists, nurses, prison personnel, and a wide range of students majoring in chemistry, business administration, and to persons who want to improve their ability to relate with others in professional or personal interactions.

These many years devoted to the development and validation of a single model have been exciting and, in my opinion, well spent. I won-

FIGURE 1

Basic Course Outline

Sessions*	Classroom Group	Lab
#1	Explain Background of IPR, development, uses and course objectives. *Class Structure*: Discuss how instruction is organized. *Class Requirements*: Explain the minimum expectations of the students; for example, the number of labs planned. *Collect Schedule Cards*: Explain the need for assigning lab sessions and, therefore, the need for knowing student availability for lab times throughout the term of the instruction. If the group is small this may not be necessary as students can assign themselves and choose lab partners. *Elements of Effective Communication*: Introduction to facilitating response modes: Exploratory Response and Listening Response.	None
#2	*Elements of Effective Communication* (continued): Affective/Cognitive Dimension, Honest Labeling; use exercises at the end of film for group practice. Explain what to expect from Lab Sessions; clarify roles of facilitator and "client." Discuss choosing *topics to share* in lab sessions.	Learn to operate VTR Individual (interviewer) Recalls Lab assignm. in pairs Outside (experienced) Inquirer
#3 and #4	Discuss lab experience with students. *Affect Simulation, The Process, Film #1.* *Affect Simulation, Vignettes.* *Affect Simulation, The Process, Film #2.* Individual Recall Film Example: e.g., a film from the "A" series. Conduct a classroom recall.	Individual (interviewer) Recalls Lab assignm. in pairs Outside (experienced) Inquirer
#5**	*Inquirer Training*: Inquirer Role and Function film. Relate students' experience of inquiring in their labs to a discussion of learning the role for themselves. Explain the functioning of the lab.	Inquirer Training Teams of 5-6 with a lab leader

* Allow approximately three hours, including breaks, for each session.
** In using a "self-contained" format session No. 5 precedes any Lab recall sessions, so that "outside (experienced) Inquirers" can be replaced by students serving as inquirers for each other.

FIGURE 1 *(continued)*

Sessions*	Classroom Group	Lab
#6	Discuss Inquirer lab experience. Complete Inquirer Training film. Individual Recall film example; e.g., a film from the "A" series.	Inquirer Training Teams of 5-6 with a lab leader
#7	*Individual Recall (Client)* Discuss lab experience in small groups. Filmed examples; e.g., a film from "B" series.	Client Recalls Teams of 3 Students acting as inquirers for each other
#8	*Discussion Film* Encourage student reaction in small groups. Suggest possibility that some questions may lend themselves as themes for subsequent lab sessions.	Mutual Recalls Teams of 3 Student Inquirers
#9	Mutual Recall Discussion Discuss lab experience in small groups. Filmed examples; e.g., films from "C" series.	Mutual Recalls Teams of 3 Student Inquirers
#10	Mutual Recall Discussion Filmed examples; e.g., films from "C" series.	Recalls with Significant Other Student Inquirers Teams of 2 plus invited outside person

der, too, if those who would develop models based on media might learn from our initial errors. Let me conclude by repeating my introductory statement that ". . . media in general and the videotape recorder in particular offer us not one but many different tools, each best suited for accomplishing certain specific ends and not others."

REFERENCES

1. Kagan, N., Krathwohl, D. R., and Miller, R.: Stimulated Recall in Therapy Using Videotape—A Case Study. *Journal of Counseling Psychology,* 10:237-243, 1963.
2. Kagan, N., and Krathwohl, D. R.: *Studies in Human Interaction: Interpersonal Process Recall Stimulated by Videotape.* Educational Publications Services, Col-

lege of Education, East Lansing, Michigan: Michigan State University, 1967. Currently available on microfisch through the ERIC system.

3. Influencing Human Interaction. Distributed by Mason Media, Inc., Box C, Mason, Michigan 48854.
4. Campbell, R. J., Kagan, N., and Krathwohl, D. R.: The Development and Validation of a Scale to Measure Affective Sensitivity (Empathy). *Journal of Counseling Psychology*, 18:407-412, 1971.
5. Danish, S. J., and Kagan, N.: Measurement of Affective Sensitivity: Toward a Valid Measure of Interpersonal Perception. *Journal of Counseling Psychology*, 18:51-54, 1971.
6. Kagan, N.: Influencing Human Interaction—Eleven Years with IPR. *The Canadian Counselor*, 9:74-97, 1975.
7. Elstein, A. S., Kagan, N., Shulman, L., Jason, H., and Loupe, M. J.: Methods and Theory in the Study of Medical Inquiry. *Journal of Medical Education*, 47:85-92, 1972.
8. Schauble, P. G.: The Acceleration of Client Progress in Counseling and Psychotherapy through Interpersonal Process Recall (IPR). Unpublished doctoral dissertation, Michigan State University, 1970.
9. Hartson, D. J., and Kunce, J. T.: Videotape Replay and Recall in Group Work. *Journal of Counseling Psychology*, 20:437-441, 1973.
10. Van Noord, R. W., and Kagan, W.: Stimulated Recall and Affect Simulation in Counseling: Client Growth Reexamined. *Journal of Counseling Psychology*, 23:28-33, 1976.
11. Tomory, R. E.: The Acceleration and Continuation of Client Growth in Counseling and Psychotherapy: A Comparison of Interpersonal Process Recall (IPR) with Traditional Counseling Methods. In progress.
12. Ward, R. G., Kagan, N., and Krathwohl, D. R.: An Attempt to Measure and Facilitate Counselor Effectiveness. *Counselor Education and Supervision*, 11:179-186, 1972.
13. Kingdon, M. A.: A Cost/Benefit Analysis of the Interpersonal Process Recall Technique. *Journal of Counseling Psychology*, 22:353-357, 1975.
14. Jason, H., Kagan, N., Werner, A., Elstein, A., and Thomas, J. B.: New Approaches to Teaching Basic Interview Skills to Medical Students. *American Journal of Psychiatry*, 127:1404-1407, 1971.
15. Resnikoff, A.: The Relationship of Counselor Behavior to Client Response and an Analysis of a Medical Interview Training Procedure Involving Simulated Patients. Unpublished doctoral dissertation, Michigan State University, 1968.
16. Werner, A., and Schneider, J. M. Teaching Medical Students Interactional Skills. *New England Journal of Medicine*, 290:1232-1237, 1974.
17. Kagan, W., and Schauble, P. G.: Affect Simulation in Interpersonal Process Recall. *Journal of Counseling Psychology*, 16:309-313, 1969.
18. Danish, S. J., and Brodsky, S. L. Training of Policemen in Emotional Control and Awareness. *Psychology in Action*, 25:368-369, 1970.
19. Spivack, J. D., and Kagan, N.: Laboratory to Classroom—The Practical Application of IPR in a Masters Level Pre-practicum Counselor Education Program. *Counselor Education and Supervision*, 3-15, Sept. 1972.
20. IPR Workshops Conducted for the United Nations World Health Organization in New Guinea and Australia. See "Assignment Reports," Kagan, N., and Byers, J., 1973 and 1975, WHO, Manila, Phillipines.
21. Dendy, R. F.: A Model for the Training of Undergraduate Residence Hall Assistants as Paraprofessional Counselors Using Videotape Techniques and Interpersonal Process Recall (IPR). Unpublished doctoral dissertation, Michigan State University, East Lansing, Michigan, 1971.
22. Archer, J., Jr., and Kagan, N.: Teaching Interpersonal Relationship Skills on

84		*Videotape in Psychiatric Training, Treatment*

Campus: A Pyramid Approach. *Journal of Counseling Psychology,* 20:535-541, 1973.
23. Rowe, K. K.: A 50-Hour Intensified IPR Training Program for Counselors. Unpublished doctoral dissertation, Michigan State University, 1972.
24. Boltuch, B. S.: The Effects of a Pre-practicum Skill Training Program, *Influencing Human Interaction,* On Developing Counselor Effectiveness in a Master's Level Practicum. Unpublished doctoral dissertation, New York University, 1975.
25. Singleton, N.: Training Incarcerated Felons in Communication Skills Using An Integrated IPR (Interpersonal Process Recall) Videotape Feedback/Affect Simulation Training Model. Unpublished doctoral dissertation, Michigan State University, East Lansing, Michigan, 1976.
26. Burke, J. B., and Kagan, N.: Influencing Human Interaction in Urban Schools, NIMH Grant #1+21MH13526-02, 1976, Final Report.
27. Bedell, P.: A Comparison of Two Approaches to Peer Supervision in the Training of Communication Skills Using a Videotape Recall Model. Unpublished doctoral dissertation, Michigan State University, East Lansing, Michigan, 1976.

7

A COMMUNICATION SKILLS ASSESSMENT RATING SCALE

John Waldron, M.D.

Over a period of years at the Psychiatry Faculty of Queens University in Kingston, Ontario, we have developed a glossary and interview rating scale useful in assessing the communication skills of third-year medical students.* The technique we have found useful (1) is to demonstrate interviewing styles to medical students in their second year and "to inform them about some of the basic maneuvers in talking with patients." Third-year students twice conduct 40-minute videotaped diagnostic interviews with patients, which are simultaneously monitored by the tutor and the two or three peers in his small group. The student has been instructed to so conduct the interview that by the end of it he can "make a tentative diagnosis, discuss the prognosis and report on the patient's mental status. During the actual taping of the interview the tutor uses the experience being observed to teach the other students with him." After the interview the student rejoins his group and "when it is deemed suitable, the tutor may ask the patient to join the first part of the discussion to give his impressions of the student's performance." Then peer teaching is emphasized as the tutor joins the discussion which centers on the data and reactions to the videotape playback. Afterwards the student interviewer returns to the studio to again review the tape, either alone or with his peers, and is guided by a written critique of the interview which has been prepared by the tutor.

It is through the following interview rating scale that the tutor's assessment is passed on to the students. It shares valid information in a succinct and relevant manner while underscoring and repeating the essentials of the interviewing process.

Ed. Note: In my opinion the rating scale should be used in the very first year of training not only for medical students but also for psychologists, social workers, nurses and all others involved with patients on paraprofessional as well as professional levels.

Our experience "is that the experience of viewing oneself in replay is probably the single most important learning experience for the student. Students have repeatedly told us that the tutor's written and spoken comments were hardly necessary to point up their errors since they were painfully evident when viewed on the television screen" (1).

The Queens University Interview Rating Scale is presented here in two parts as it is actually used with students. Part I is composed of six sections and indicates the meaning of the scores rated on a scale varying from 1) very poor to 5) very good. Part II is a succinct glossary for the use of the rater.*

PART I

QUEEENS UNIVERSITY INTERVIEW RATING SCALE

DATE: _____

STUDENT: _____

RATER: _____

PATIENT: _____

TAPE NO.:_____

SCORES

SECTION I	_____	1 — VERY POOR
SECTION II	_____	2 — POOR
SECTION III	_____	3 — AVERAGE
SECTION IV	_____	4 — GOOD
TOTAL	_____	5 — VERY GOOD
SECTION V	$\times 23 =$	
SECTION VI	_____	

SECTION I — INTERVIEW STRUCTURE:

1. Establishes terms of reference   1 2 3 4 5
2. Maintains appropriate control   1 2 3 4 5
3. Follows leads   1 2 3 4 5
4. Pays attention   1 2 3 4 5

----

* *Ed. Note:* I believe the student should know the contents of this glossary.

SECTION II — INTERVIEWER ROLE:

1. Maintains control over own feelings	1	2	3	4	5
2. Reassures patient appropriately	1	2	3	4	5
3. Is appropriately congenial	1	2	3	4	5
4. Is appropriately self-assured	1	2	3	4	5

SECTION III — COMMUNICATION IN THE INTERVIEW:

1. Question structure	1	2	3	4	5
2. Language/concept choice	1	2	3	4	5
3. Allows appropriate flow	1	2	3	4	5
4. Clarification techniques	1	2	3	4	5
5. Listening posture	1	2	3	4	5
6. Handling emotionally-loaded material	1	2	3	4	5

SECTION IV — HISTORICAL CONTENT IN INTERVIEW:

1. Elicited chief complaints	1	2	3	4	5
2. Established time of onset	1	2	3	4	5
3. Characterized course	1	2	3	4	5
4. Delineated activity limits	1	2	3	4	5
5. Explored etiological factors	1	2	3	4	5
6. Elicited sufficient data to establish mental status	1	2	3	4	5
7. Explored suicidal intent	1	2	3	4	5
8. Explored previous history	1	2	3	4	5
9. Explored physical symptoms	1	2	3	4	5

SECTION V — GLOBAL ASSESSMENT OF INTERVIEW:

1   2   3   4   5

SECTION VI — DIFFICULTY OF PATIENT:

Easy   Difficult

1   2   3   4   5

PART II

REVISED GLOSSARY FOR USE WITH QUEENS UNIVERSITY INTERVIEW RATING SCALE

The following is to be used by the rater for consultation at the time he is completing the rating scale on the interview he has just observed. It contains:

(1) The questions he should ask himself in reference to rating each item on the scale;

(2) Special scoring instructions where appropriate.

SECTION I—INTERVIEW STRUCTURE

Item 1—Establishes terms of reference:
Did the patient know *whom* he was talking to, and *why?*

Item 2—Maintains appropriate control:
Does the examiner *persistently pursue the main purpose of the interview* (gathering data relative to a diagnosis) *without allowing himself to be frustrated by the patient* on the one hand, or *cutting off the patient excessively* on the other hand?

Item 3—Follows leads:
Does the examiner *reject offerings* and, if so, is this because of *rigid adherence* to a system, or because of the unacceptability (because he finds them emotionally charged or irrelevant) of these offerings? Does he *overlook significant statements?*

Item 4—Pays attention:
Does the examiner overlook what the patient has already told him?

SECTION II—INTERVIEWER ROLE

Item 1—Maintains control over own feelings:
Does the examiner betray emotional responses which significantly interfere with communication? Does the examiner maintain emotional control of such rigidity that it significantly interferes with interest and concern coming through?

Item 2—Reassures patient appropriately:
Does the examiner (a) *recognize* and (b) *respond* to appeals for reassurance?
Note: The rater will encounter interviews in which the patient neither overtly nor covertly seeks reassurance. In this event, a score will be assigned on this item equivalent to that awarded under Section V (Global Assessment of Interview).

Item 3—Is appropriately congenial:
Is the examiner's behavior in terms of congeniality essentially that appropriate to a professional rather than social encounter?

Item 4—Is appropriately self-assured:
The question applying to this item is similar to that under Item 3.

SECTION III—COMMUNICATION IN THE INTERVIEW

Item 1—Question structure:
Is there sufficient flexibility with regard to open versus closed questions? Does the wording of the questions minimize or maximize the amount of useful information to be obtained from the patient?

Item 2—Language/Concept choice:
Does the patient know what the examiner is getting at? Is the examiner's use of language acceptable or offensive to the patient?

Item 3—Allows appropriate flow:
Is the examiner intolerant of silences? Does he interrupt excessively? Does he *not* interrupt when appropriate?

Item 4—Clarification techniques:
Does the examiner make adequate use of summary statements? Does he attempt to resolve ambiguities in the patient's statements? Does he give adequate explanations of changes of direction during the interview?

Item 5—Listening posture:
Is the examiner's *postural/motor behavior* such as is appropriate to a professional encounter facilitating trust and empathy?

Item 6—Handling emotionally-loaded material:
Does the examiner show excessive avoidance or insistence on emotionally laden material? Is his timing appropriate in dealing with this? Is he made unduly anxious by it?

SECTION IV—HISTORICAL CONTENT IN INTERVIEW

Item 1—Elicited chief complaints:
Do I, having listened to this interview, know what this patient is complaining of and *the reasons* for admission?

Item 2—Established time of onset:
Do I, having listened to the interview, know for how long the patient has had his complaints?

Item 3—Characterized course:
Do I, having listened to this interview, know what has been the sequence of events in this patient's complaints?

Item 4—Delineated activity limits:
Do I know what the patient's average day is like at the present time?

Item 5—Explored etiological factors:
Did the examiner make inquiries about the patient's life situation at the time of onset of symptoms? Did the examiner make

inquiries into etiological factors more distantly removed in time from onset of symptoms? More emphasis on present breakdown.

Item 6—Elicited sufficient data to establish mental status:
Could I, having listened to this interview, give an adequate account of the patient's mental status?

Item 7—Explored suicidal intent:
Was this area explored and could I, having listened to the interview, make a meaningful statement about the risk of suicide in this case?

Item 8—Explored previous psychiatric history:
Did the examiner inquire about previous psychiatric symptoms or breakdown? Did the examiner make an attempt to assess the patient's premorbid personality?

Item 9—Explored physical symptoms:
Was specific inquiry made with regard to physical symptoms? If such symptoms were mentioned by the patient, was further inquiry made about their nature and their relation to other symptoms?

REFERENCE

1. Waldron, J.: Teaching Communication Skills in Medical School. *Am. J. Psychiatry,* 130:579-581, 1973.

8

EVALUATING PSYCHIATRIC LEARNING THROUGH VIDEOTAPED PATIENT INTERVIEWS

W. Douglas Weir, M.D.

The advent of simplified and economical video recording equipment has allowed for a new dimension in psychiatric education. Creative use of this medium has resulted in the introduction of a level of immediacy and realism in psychiatric teaching unheard of a decade ago. In many centers, the retrospective technique of psychotherapy supervision has been replaced either by the use of closed circuit equipment (1) or videotape recording (2). Numerous stratagems have been devised for using television in teaching clinical psychiatry in medical schools across the country (3, 4, 5). Little, however, is found in the literature regarding the use of television for evaluating psychiatric learning.

The evaluation of clinical psychiatric acumen and skill is vital at all levels of training, as well as in the sphere of continuing education. Whether one is a medical student, board candidate, or graduate physician, it is the ability to apply one's knowledge in the solution of actual clinical problems which is of central importance. Written and oral examination techniques, no matter how ingeniously devised, suffer significantly from the absence of actual patient material. At the clinical level, it is the ability of the examinee to apply his factual knowledge to the patient as he presents himself which should be the focus of evaluation. By using the actual clinical problem as the test material, it is possible to measure not only the cognitive material possessed by the student, but his ability for perceptive correlation. This, in turn, reflects his observational skill and ability to reason deductively with regard to accurate diagnosis and appropriate therapeutic planning. Further, the introduction of actual patient material into the test situation brings with it the element of interpersonal stress, of recognized or unrecognized countertransference. While difficult to quantitate, these elements can have significant impact on both the diagnostic and therapeutic outcome of the doctor-patient interaction. Thus, insofar as possible they should be a part of every examination at the clinical level.

With these considerations in mind, the optimum clinical examination would allow for the student to examine several different patients under faculty observation and subsequently to discuss the case in whatever depth was deemed appropriate for his level of training. Such a format has been used widely and there is little doubt that given our present state of knowledge in psychiatry it represents, perhaps, the best approach. There are, however, serious practical limitations associated with such an evaluative design. First, suitable patient material is frequently not readily available at the time of the examination, especially in the large volume necessary for individual interviews. Reports regarding the use of actors to simulate patients have been published (6). This technique appears, however, to have numerous limitations not the least of which concerns the fact that the examinee, more likely than not, is aware of the simulation, thus obviating its purpose.

Realistically, as the number of medical school students, annual board candidates, and other potential examinees increases, the direct patient technique requires an increasingly large expenditure of time. Typically the direct technique requires approximately two hours per examinee, per patient. Given a group of 30 examinees, this would total at least 60 hours of faculty time, which does not take into account the preparation of grading reports. Even then, the examination would be limited to only one patient, allowing the student to demonstrate his knowledge in a limited diagnostic-therapeutic field. Such an examination would not only be inadequate but patently unfair.

Faced with this dilemma, the decision most frequently made is to give a purely written examination in clinical psychiatry. This is a poor solution since it fails to test the most fundamental aspect of clinical psychiatric practice, namely, the examinee's observational skill and subsequent ability to deduce a diagnostic impression based on actual clinical material.

THE VIDEOTEST

The use of videotaped patient interview material offers a means of obviating many of these difficulties. Carefully selected patient interview material, coupled with an appropriately designed examination instrument, allows for a clearer delineation of the student's ability to apply his cognitive knowledge in a more realistic and meaningful way. Having used such a technique, termed a videotest, over the past three years, we have found a high degree of acceptance on the part of clinical level medical students, at times bordering on enthusiasm—a rare phenomenon, indeed, for medical students confronted with any examination.

Consistently we have found that this examination format introduces an element of immediacy which captures the imagination of the students. This, combined with its obvious relevance, has led the majority of students to remain after the examination to go over the material with the examiner. And, since the patient interview material is prepared on tape, this requires no more effort than reversing the machine for review. Discussion is generally lively and it is clear that a great deal of additional learning occurs at these post mortems.

For the videotest which we are currently using, tapes have been prepared which contain three carefully selected five-minute sections of previously recorded patient interview material. The aim of this examination, which is given to third-year-level medical students who have just completed their clinical clerkship, is as follows:

1. to determine whether the student is cognizant of normal and abnormal behavior and mental status and is able to record his observations using the proper terminology;

2. to determine whether, on the basis of the behavioral and mental status material recorded, he is able to arrive at a reasonable diagnostic impression and/or differential;

3. to determine whether, on the basis of the diagnosis he has arrived at, the examinee can formulate, in broad outline, a therapeutic program for the patient.

The examinees are shown the first patient one time only, since among other things we are interested in assessing the acuteness of their perception. They are then given 20 minutes to complete their write-up on this patient. The same procedure is followed with the remaining two segments on the tape. A sample of the answer sheet used by the examinees is shown.

Using this protocol, the entire examination requires one hour and 15 minutes to administer. Further, it could obviously be administered to as large a group as desired simultaneously given adequate equipment. As noted previously, while not originally planned, the students' interest in reviewing the material after the examination has made us extend the total period by 15-30 minutes. Though some of the students remain simply to find out "the right answer," most participate actively in the observational and diagnostic process as the material is reviewed.

Name _____

Score _____

CLINICAL EXAMINATION
JUNIOR PSYCHIATRY

Patient Number _____

A. List behavioral and mental status features demonstrated by the patient. Include positive and negative features, as appropriate, *using proper terminology.*

_____   _____
_____   _____
_____   _____
_____   _____
_____   _____

B. Differential Diagnosis: Given the behavioral and mental status material noted in "A," make a diagnostic differential using proper terminology. Be as specific as possible. Circle the single most likely diagnosis in your opinion.

_____   _____
_____   _____
_____   _____
_____   _____

C. Case Management: Write a brief paragraph: What type of therapy might be indicated *on the basis of your primary diagnostic impression?* Be specific; if drugs, what drug, what dosage—if psychotherapy, what type; should the patient be hospitalized, for what reason? Are further studies indicated; if so, what studies and for what purpose? Be brief and specific.

_____
_____
_____
_____
_____
_____

FIGURE 1

In essence, this examination results in an evaluation not only of the student's factual knowledge in the areas of mental status, diagnostics and therapeutics, but also of his ability to perceive and discriminate significant behavioral and mental status features as manifested by an actual patient. Next, his ability to integrate this observational material into a reasonable diagnostic framework is demonstrated. While the procedure does not permit evaluation of a student's performance with a live patient—a particularly stressful situation for the inexperienced clinician —as contrasted with a written examination, a more complete assessment of the examinee's ability to perceive, discriminate and integrate patient material into a clinically meaningful configuration has been achieved.

The examination described is currently used with clerkship level medical students. It could easily be adopted for use with residents, and even board candidates. Considered from the standpoint of utilizing identical taped material, the basic difference would be in the scoring. One might not anticipate that junior medical students would pick up a subtle seductiveness on the part of a patient, whereas residents might well be held accountable for this feature. Diagnostically, more precision, reflected perhaps by a less diffuse differential, would be anticipated on the part of the resident. A markedly more sophisticated treatise on therapeutics would certainly be expected from the resident or candidate level examinee.

While the question of selection of patient material for use in an examination will be discussed in the next section, it seems relevant to remark that the degree of symptomatic subtlety demonstrated by a patient should be correlated to the level of student to be examined. Resident and medical student alike would be expected to recognize frank delusional thinking characterized by marked grandiosity and religiosity. This, accompanied by pervasive hostility and associational difficulties, should result in a strong presumptive diagnosis of paranoid schizophrenia by both. On the other hand, while the detached manner and shallow affect of the simple schizophrenic should be recognized by the resident, it is perhaps unrealistic to expect this of a junior clerkship medical student.

SELECTION OF TEST MATERIAL

The central consideration in preparing a clinical videotest is the selection or production of suitable test material. This is a multifaceted problem which must be approached from two varying perspectives. The first might be termed the clinical-academic viewpoint, the second the technical aspect. While a successful synthesis of these two parameters can often easily be effected if one is producing videotaped material specifically for testing purposes, much excellent material can also be derived from careful review of previously videotaped interviews.

Clinical-Academic Considerations

Prior to the review or production of videotaped material there is one paramount question which must be answered. What is the clinical level of the student to be examined? How much clinical experience does he possess? Based on knowledge of this parameter, what degree of symptomatic subtlety should he be able to appreciate?

It is vital for the examiner to confront and clearly define in his own mind the level of diagnostic and therapeutic acumen it is reasonable to expect of a student at a given level of training. This must be based on a consideration of total basic course content and the length and type of clinical experience that precede the examination. For example, the examination format outlined earlier is given at the conclusion of the third-year clinical clerkship in psychiatry at our institution. The student has had direct patient contact with both inpatients and outpatients, working under the preceptorship of faculty and residents. All students have been exposed to a variety of psychotic, neurotic and characterologic entities. In addition, they have been given free access to our catalogue of self-instructional videotaped patient material during their clerkship. Level specific seminars on diagnosis and therapeutics have been given regularly during the six weeks of this clinical rotation. Prior to the clerkship they have experienced a two-year course in basic psychiatry including growth and development, psychodynamics, interviewing techniques and mental status examination, psychopathology (utilizing extensive videotaped patient material) and elemental psychotherapeutics. It is reasonable, therefore, to anticipate that they should be able to recognize and properly report the features of a depressive reaction and to determine whether it is of neurotic or psychotic proportions. Similarly, they should be able to delineate the organic brain syndrome from the schizophrenic. Based on their training background our expectations with regard to their therapeutic knowledge are much less. We could expect, however, that they would prescribe a major tranquilizer for an acutely psychotic patient in an appropriate dose, rather than a drug from the minor group. And, on the basis of their training we would also anticipate that they would recognize the appropriate use of psychoanalytic therapy as contrasted with supportive techniques.

A judgment must be made as to how obvious symptomatic material must be in order that it is reasonably apparent to the level of student being examined. Parallel to this is the question of how much symptomatic material must be presented before it is reasonable for the student to be able to arrive at an appropriate differential diagnosis. Both of these considerations obviously rest on an accurate appreciation of the student's clinical level. As an example, one segment which we are currently using at the junior clerkship level demonstrates the following features in a late teen to early twenties Caucasian male: disheveled appearance, total lack of eye contact, pervasive hostility, marked guardedness, repeated associational difficulties, loosely organized delusional thinking, prominent tendency toward grandiosity and ambivalence. It is reasonable to expect that, having recognized this symptomatic constellation, the student will arrive at a strong presumptive diagnosis of schizophrenia, paranoid type. The student would be given extra credit for recognizing that a similar picture might also arise secondary to the ingestion of an hallucinogenic drug, particularly given the patient's age group.

The segment cited above contains frankly psychotic material with a clear paranoid trend. A segment containing much more subtle paranoid material and less direct hostility would be more appropriate for residency level examinees. In general, as regards selection of material the degree of symptomatic subtlety should increase as the level of training.

As a general principle, using this test format, the inclusion of historical material within the test segment takes second place as contrasted with the behavioral and mental status features demonstrated. This is dictated principally by the fact that only brief segments of tape are used. It should be pointed out, however, that careful editing of material will often result in finding interview segments which not only illustrate excellent mental status material, but also include highly relevant historical material. For example, another segment we have used shows a middle-aged, tearful female manifesting psychomotor retardation, difficulty with memory, and depressed mood. During the course of the tape run, she also reports progressive inability to function at home and on the job, anhedonia, early waking insomnia, anorexia and weight loss and the occurrence of a mastectomy three months previously. Such material is clearly diagnostically relevant, thus leading to our selection of this particular segment for examination purposes.

The length of the tape run selected for testing depends upon the aim of the examination and the level of student being tested. The aim of the examination scheme outlined previously is to determine whether the examinee can recognize abnormal behavioral and mental status features. It is entirely possible to select segments lasting as little as five minutes or less which contain a wealth of such material. The two examples noted illustrate this admirably. One is a full five minutes in length, while the other lasts only slightly longer than four minutes. Little would have been gained by lengthening either of these pieces since, as they stand, they represent a succinct and highly characteristic picture.

Technical Considerations

Surely it goes without saying that the technical quality of videotapes used for examination purposes must be very high. This is particularly true when only brief segments of tape are used in the testing situation. The examinee can hardly be held accountable for material which he cannot hear and see clearly. Careful quality control must be exercised in the selection (from pre-recorded material) or production of videotest tapes from a technical as well as clinical viewpoint.

Picture quality should be characterized by well defined images in clear focus which possess sufficient contrast for good definition. Audio levels should be appropriate to the content of the material, reflecting as closely as possible the reality of the situation. For example, the low pitched, waning voice of the depressive should not be boosted artificially in order to attain audio balance between patient and interviewer. The audio signal should be as free as possible of ambient noise. In this respect a comment regarding automatic level microphones is in order. This type of microphonic system is best avoided since its use often results in a highly distracting signal between verbal interchanges.

As regards the use of color versus black and white recording, it appears that while an argument might be made for the added realism of and increased viewer attention to color tapes, the use of color can introduce complications. When using color much greater care must be exercised in set design in producing tapes for testing purposes, since color can be highly distracting when inappropriately used. Brightly colored furnishings and accessories add interest to the picture but they also tend to divert the attention of the viewer. Thus, careful control must be exercised in this respect in the production of patient interview tapes destined to be used for examination purposes. On the whole, no appreciable advantage is realized with the use of color, whereas considerable added expense is incurred for the equipment and supporting technical personnel needed to produce high quality color videotapes.

As a defining principle in the selection or production of patient interview videotapes to be used for testing purposes, the following guidelines are given: Anything that distracts viewer attention from the patient should be avoided. By the same token, anything that directs viewer attention to a particular aspect of the patient should also be avoided. The purpose in using the videotaped patient interview is to determine how perceptive the examinee is of those features demonstrated by the patient. It is, therefore, unacceptable to utilize any technique which alters the clinical realism of the interview situation. On the other hand, manipulation of the camera in such a way as to emphasize particular portions of the patient's anatomy with close-up shots obviates the assessment of observational skill. While such techniques are highly valuable in the production of teaching tapes, a different perspective is necessary when considering videotapes for test purposes.

Set design should be kept as simple as possible. An arrangement utilizing two arm chairs of equal height, angled toward one another at approximately 45 degrees, provides an excellent set. Additional furniture and ornaments, which can be distracting, should be avoided. Microphones of the lavalier or slip-on type are the least obtrusive and provide the best sound pick-up, if they are of good quality.

Two basic camera shots are all that is necessary. The first should include a head to foot view of both therapist and patient. The second should be a full head to foot view of the patient alone, preferably a full frontal shot. Even given this limited range of shots, there should be no more than one change of view within a five-minute segment. The eye of the observer will divide the picture in front of him. The more skillful he is the more relevant will be his division.

Figure 2 illustrates both set design and camera angles.

As compared to film, the video image is of lower quality. Thus, the two camera angles recommended above should hone in as closely as possible on patient and therapist in order to derive the greatest detail. However, focusing on particular aspects should be left to the examinee. Another limitation of the video camera, as contrasted with film, is its intolerance to extremes of light. Care must therefore be taken to light sets properly if good picture quality is to be attained. Both patient and therapist should avoid white or light colored clothing, particularly if either of the participants has a dark complexion. The video camera cannot reconcile such marked contrasts leading to poor image definition, particularly of facial features.

It is apparently based on the considerations outlined above that neither great technical skill nor extensive personnel are required to produce excellent videotaped interviews for testing purposes. A wide range of expensive video hardware is not required, although it will be found that a machine capable of producing crisp tape edits is a sine qua non. Recently, modestly priced machines with this capability have become available, thus simplifying the work of assembling a videotest tape

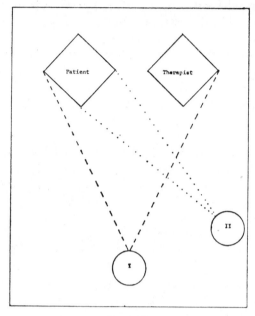

FIGURE 2

containing three or more consecutive interview segments. Finally, a comment relative to software is important. The modest added expense of the newer high density tapes is more than justified in terms of picture quality. This is particularly true if the plan is to use a given tape frequently or over a long period of time.

TEST VALIDATION

Emphasis has already been placed on the need for an acute awareness of the clinical level of the students to be examined when selecting material for this type of examination. Experience has shown, however, that it is wise to seek validation of each taped segment used for testing purposes. After a segment thought to be suitable is selected, it should be reviewed for appropriateness by several faculty clinicians who are active in the teaching program. If this review results in a lack of observational and diagnostic consensus, the segment should be eliminated. In effect, the reviewing faculty takes the examination, utilizing the same form illustrated in Figure 1. A conscious effort is made to confine the scope of the answers to the clinical level of the students for whom the test is proposed. This process, aside from resulting in a judgment as to the level appropriateness of a given segment, also allows for the generation of a scoring profile for each segment used. This procedure tends to lend greater objectivity in scoring.

Over the past decade and a half, videotape recording has been used widely for clinical psychiatric instruction. It seems clear that it has much to offer as a medium for the assessment of clinical skill and knowledge, awaiting only imaginative application.

REFERENCES

1. Kornfeld, D. S., and Kolb, L. C.: The Use of Closed-Circuit Television in the Teaching of Psychiatry. *Journal of Nervous and Mental Diseases*, 138:452, 1964.
2. Gruenberg, P. B., Liston, E. H., and Wayne, G. J.: Intensive Supervision of Psychotherapy with Videotape Recording. *American Journal of Psychiatry*, 23:98, 1969.
3. Suess, J. F.: Teaching Clinical Psychiatry with Closed-Circuit Television and Videotape. *Journal of Medical Education*, 41:483, 1966.
4. Benschoter, R. A., et al.: Use of Videotape to Provide Individual Instruction in Techniques of Psychotherapy. *Journal of Medical Education*, 40:1159, 1965.
5. Ryan, J.: Teaching by Videotape. *Mental Hospital*, 16:101, 1965.
6. Froelich, R. E.: Teaching Psychotherapy to Medical Students Through Videotape Simulation. In Milton M. Berger, M.D. (Ed.), *Videotape Techniques in Psychiatric Training and Treatment*. New York: Brunner/Mazel, 1970, pp. 55-64.

9

THE USE OF VIDEOTAPE TECHNIQUES IN THE PSYCHIATRIC TRAINING OF FAMILY PHYSICIANS

David D. Schmidt, M.D.
and
Edward Messner, M.D.

INTRODUCTION

Since the establishment of the American Board of Family Practice in 1969, over 300 postgraduate training programs have been developed in family medicine. More than 50% of the medical schools in the U.S. have undergraduate programs in family medicine. The latter are predominantly preceptorships with practicing physicians.

Considerable attention has been given to the appropriate psychiatric curriculum for these programs (1, 2, 3). Several general goals have evolved: 1) The family medicine trainee should increase his self-awareness. He must gain an appreciation for his effect on patients, and his personal reactions to patient demands. Furthermore, he should learn to use himself as a therapeutic agent. 2) The family medicine trainee should become a master at patient interviewing and develop new skills in the area of counseling and short-term psychotherapy. 3) The family medicine trainee should demonstrate cognitive knowledge of the common psychiatric syndromes that are catalogued in Table 1. He should know that the organic psychosis may require emergency management and should understand the complex physiologic disturbances involved in these syndromes. 4) The family medicine trainee should demonstrate both cognitive knowledge and management skills for the common emotional problems that are seen in family practice (Table 2).

General agreement exists that one of the major tasks of the future family physician is to help his patient cope with emotional problems and that the educational goals listed above are desirable. Still there is

TABLE 1

A. *Organic psychosis*

1. Organic brain syndrome
2. Alcoholic psychosis
   a. Delirium Tremens
   b. Korsakoff's psychoses
3. Psychosis with acute poison and intoxication

B. *Non-organic psychosis*

1. The schizophrenias
2. Manic depressive illnesses
3. Involutional melancholia
4. Psychotic depressive reactions

C. *Neuroses*

1. Anxiety neurosis
2. Hysterical neurosis
3. Phobic neurosis
4. Obsessive-compulsive neurosis
5. Hypochondriacal neurosis
6. Depressive neurosis

D. *Personality disorders*

1. Hysterical personality
2. Antisocial personality
3. Passive-aggressive personality
4. Inadequate personality

TABLE 2

A. *Psychophysiologic disorders*

1. Musculoskeletal (low back pain, tension headache)
2. Respiratory (asthma)
3. Cardiovascular (cardiac neurosis)
4. Gastrointestinal (peptic ulcer disease, spastic colon)

B. *Behavioral disorders of childhood and adolescence*

1. Hyperkinetic reaction of childhood
2. Learning difficulties
3. Adjustment reaction of adolescence

C. *Depression*

D. *Anxiety states*

E. *Sexual malfunction*

F. *Disturbed family relationships (and family counseling)*

G. *Alcoholism and Drug Abuse*

H. *The emotional problems that accompany acute and chronic illness or death*

I. *Geriatric problems and the emotional needs of the elderly*

considerable difficulty translating these objectives into successful methods of instruction. The principles involved in the management of emotional problems are often difficult to teach by such traditional methods as lectures and readings. In addition, the supervision of the trainee's care of emotionally disturbed patients is extremely time consuming, and the clinical material available during a given rotation may be limited. The widespread availability of video recording has greatly enhanced the ability of family practice educators to implement the teaching of the psychiatric aspects of this discipline. The methods described here include:

1. developing a library of video recordings which contains illustrative examples of the psychiatric syndromes catalogued in Table 1 and the family practice management problems that are listed in Table 2; and

2. recording of trainees during routine medical encounters and during counseling sessions for later review with supervising faculty.

DEVELOPMENT OF VIDEOTAPE LIBRARY

Academic exercises specifically created for the purpose of combining the behavioral and medical sciences have been video recorded (4). They form the heart of such a library. The family physician, a psychiatrist, and student(s) gather together for a conference designed to exemplify psychiatric problems which are common and/or particularly difficult in family practice. The family physician selects from the patient population individuals and/or families around which the conference is centered. Two general criteria for selection are 1) the family physician believes that study of their problems contributes meaningfully to the teaching program, and 2) treatment of the patient(s) would be enhanced by psychiatric consultation.

The family physician explains to the patient(s) in advance that he will be interviewed by a psychiatrist in the presence of student(s) and that the entire proceedings will be recorded on videotape. Informed consent forms are signed by the patient(s) and are witnessed. There should be an explanation of the future use of these tapes, and the patient should be given a genuine option to refuse.

Prior to the interview of the patient(s), the videotape recording begins as the family physician presents a relevant history and his involvement with the management of the patient to the student(s) and psychiatrist. This is followed by questions and discussion among all participants. The psychiatrist then makes some statements about his preliminary impression of the situation, theoretical or therapeutic principles which might be involved, thoughts about how the interview might further clarify the problem, or other ideas which he believes might be useful to the student(s), the family physician, and the future audience of the videotape.

The patient(s) is then invited to join them and is introduced, usually for the first time, to the consultant and to the student(s). He then is reminded of the videotape and his attention is called to the camera, which is in plain view. The videotape equipment is operated and monitored by a technician in another room, an arrangement which has been explained to the patient in advance. This technical assistance improves the quality of the recordings with respect to lighting, contrast, sound, and continuity. The 45-minute interview is conducted mainly by the psychiatrist, with participation by others as the situation permits, in a relatively informal atmosphere.

Following the interview, the student(s), family physician and psychiatrist discuss the patient's situation further. The psychiatrist attempts to draw inferences from the interview, make therapeutic recommendations, comment on the preliminary discussion, and explain how features of the patient's condition can be generalized to other patients' situations.

The videotape recording enables the participants to review, in detail, the conference in which they participated. Other physicians or medical students can use it to reexamine details of technique or history, or participants can refresh their memories of significant parts of the conference.

Each participant has access to the tapes and may replay them at his convenience to review the conference in which he took part. More important, one can gradually develop a library of such tapes. This permits trainees to view conferences on problems which have not emerged in their own clinical experience. By drawing from this library, the family practice educator is able to cover a wide range of subjects with each trainee. Each time a student views a past tape, the family physician is able to discuss with him any new issues that were not covered in the original conference. In our experience, the student's interest in and empathy with the patient recorded on the tapes appear to equal that of the student(s) who took part in the original recording session.

RECORDING OF TRAINEE-PATIENT ENCOUNTER

In the current American medical educational system, there are few if any opportunities for a student or resident physician to observe an experienced clinician obtaining a history and performing a physical examination. Furthermore, few instructors take the time to watch a trainee while he performs a patient evaluation. Most instruction centers around what was done or should be done, with little direct observation. The technique of video recording patient-physician encounters offers an opportunity to correct this situation. Many family practice residency programs have begun recording these encounters on videotape. The subsequent review of these by the trainee and faculty becomes a potentially powerful learning experience. The objectivity of this technique provides the trainee with considerable insight. Often the resident himself is most critical of his behavior. Below are examples of what one looks for during a review of a recorded routine physical examination.

In the opening moments of the encounter, particularly with a new patient, one is looking for a warm natural introduction. The trainee is encouraged to show a respectful concern about the patient's complaints no matter how trivial they may appear. Although the interview should begin with open-ended questions, the resident is encouraged to probe gently for underlying fears that may accompany the complaint. It is stressed that if the physician can help the patient to be explicit about his concerns, the physician can be more effective in utilizing the physical examination, laboratory evaluation, and finally the summarizing conclusion of the encounter to alleviate these fears.

The resident is asked to examine the quality of the communication between himself and his patient. Does he use medical jargon or a language the patient fully understands? Does the physician make every effort to release tension? Does the patient feel comfortable? Is the physician sensitive to the patient's emotional response to the interview and physical examination? Is the physician warm and gentle, non-judgmental, and accepting, or is he distant, harsh, judgmental and patronizing? Is the physician efficient without appearing hurried? Does the patient have the opportunity to express himself fully? Does the physician pick up and adequately pursue symptoms or feelings casually mentioned by the patient? Does the physician give false reassurances? Is the physician abstract and non-specific in his explanations? Is the closure of the encounter timed appropriately? In the concluding moments of the encounter, has the physician made an effort to deal with each problem that was identified by the patient or doctor? Were the plans for follow-up or the regime for care carefully explained to the patient by the physician? Are there any hints on the recording that would suggest the patient's emotional response to this encounter?

The video recorded interview is most meaningful when the patient, himself, joins the resident and faculty member during the review session. This arrangement has been described in detail by Kagan (5, see

Chapter 6). It is an educational experience that provides for the resident insight into his effect on patients, his response to patients, and his ability to use himself as a therapeutic agent.

Reviewing videotaped interviews is a very effective means for sharpening the psychotherapeutic skills of family practice residents. When a trainee becomes involved in short-term psychotherapy usually centered around problems that are commonly seen in family practice (Table 2), he is encouraged to videotape all or selected sessions. The later review of these sessions with a supervising faculty member can be most helpful. We would like to cite a few specific examples.

Every physician who finds himself dealing with death, and in particular the family physician to whom the bereaved family members frequently turn for help, will be considerably more effective in alleviating his patients' pain and suffering if he has a working knowledge of certain principles for the management of grief that have developed since Lindemann's classic article in 1944 (6). Experience through videotape will better prepare him to help patients "work through the grief." A review of a tape session may show that the patient is talking in general terms by saying "Oh, Doctor, I am so unhappy!" or "Doctor, life simply is not the same." This protects the patient from experiencing the pain that would result from a detailed description of a particular event or situation involving the lost loved one. The supervising physician reviewing the tape with the training family physician might suggest to the resident that he ask the bereaved to describe a particular time or event in some detail. The patient might be encouraged to describe their last evening together: Where did you go? What did you wear? What did your lost loved one wear? What did you have for dinner? One should encourage the bereaved to talk about his relationship with the deceased until words flow without inhibition and carry with them the full expression of emotion. This mental effort required to face the pain of the loss is what we have come to call the work of grieving. The resident can be guided by these suggestions during the next session with the patient. He and his supervisor can evaluate the effect of his attempt to get the patient to work through his grief by reviewing the video recording of that second session.

A second example is an encounter between a male resident and a female with a hysterical personality disorder. The management of such a patient requires considerable skill even when one does not attempt formal psychotherapy. In order to help the patient shift emphasis from control of others to control of self, the resident himself must learn to be a model of self-control. This means that the resident must not allow himself to be manipulated emotionally at one extreme; nor at the opposite extreme should he totally reject the patient because of the discomforts that result from her seductive behavior. Review of serial tapes can demonstrate that a closeness develops in the doctor-patient relationship, the patient may feel uncomfortable and try to provoke the doctor into rejecting her. Provocations may well produce anger in the resident. This can be captured on the videotape. The resident physician must be helped through replays to understand the origins of his anger, realize that the patient is trying to get him to reject her, and remain steadfast in his willingness to maintain a mature doctor-patient relationship.

Armed with the insight that comes from viewing the videotape, the resident may be successful in his effort to demonstrate for the first time to the patient that she can participate in a non-threatening relationship with a man. When the resident recognizes that the patient is trying to arouse emotion in him, he can be encouraged to invite the patient to examine the interaction. The supervising faculty member can suggest that at the next session he might initiate this process by saying to the patient "It might be well to look at what is happening here," or "Let's try to understand what's going on," or, "Perhaps we can find out what this might lead to." The main idea is to present an attitude of observation in which both patient and clinician cooperate. This sort of cooperative effort is known as the therapeutic alliance. As the resident attempts to develop such a therapeutic alliance during the next few encounters a review of the videotapes can assess the effectiveness of this effort.

DISCUSSION

It is extremely rare for a patient to refuse the request for videotaping. It is always emphasized that this academic exercise will contribute to the development of new physicians. When approached in these terms, most patients are willing to make a personal contribution to the training program. Although the residents who are being videotaped demonstrate some initial anxiety, this decreases, without exception, after one or two experiences. The family practice residents readily appreciate what a powerful learning experience the videotapes provide.

Medical students utilize the one-to-two-hour taped conferences from the library even more than the residents. Frequently these tapes represent the first exposure for the student to this emotionally laden content material. In addition, medical students are more accustomed to playing a passive role in the learning process.

Resident physicians, on the other hand, have heavy patient service commitments and may become impatient with prolonged conferences. Their resistant attitude has been met by presenting to the resident physician group an edited and shortened version of the patient interview. An instructor then facilitates a group discussion centered around this interview which provides active participation for the residents. The value of the videotape technique in the education of residents persists. Over a period of years, illustrative case interviews can be collected and shown to each new class of residents. Each group is thus assured exposure to the designed curriculum.

The active collaboration between family physician and psychiatrist has been rewarding. The psychiatrist has come to realize that the family physician deals with emotional problems earlier and on a different level than the consulting psychotherapist. The traditional modes of psychotherapy can be altered to become more appropriate for the family physician. Through this collaboration, the family physician has accumulated a body of knowledge and skills that has supplemented his strong desire to help the patient at a time of emotional crisis. To his compassion has been added some additional competence. This has contributed to our effort to combine medical and behavioral sciences. During the review of routine medical encounters, the consulting psychiatrist often joins the family physician and the two together supervise the family practice resident. Again, this collaborative effort brings together the expertise of the behaviorist and the credibility of the experienced family physician. This collaboration and the use of videotape techniques have proven to be a most effective teaching method.

CONCLUSION

We now have six years of experience using videotape techniques in the training of medical students and resident physicians in the psychiatric aspects of family medicine. This experience includes a student preceptorship in a private practice (4) and a family practice residency program which is university based. Several conclusions can be drawn from this experience: 1) The uses of videotape as described above have proven to be a most effective means of accomplishing the stated goals. 2) The ability to capture on tape graphic examples of psychiatric disorders makes the learning process far more efficient than simply relying on utilizing live clinical examples that happen to be available during any given rotation. 3) The objectivity and faculty feedback during reviews of trainee-patient encounters are powerful means of gaining increased self-awareness for the resident.

REFERENCES

1. Fisher, V. F., Mason, R. L., and Fisher, J. C.: Emotional Illness and the Family Physician. *Psychosomatics,* 16:107-11 and 171-177, 1975.
2. Stephens, G. G.: Should the Primary Physician Do Psychotherapy? *Psychiatric Opinion,* Vol. 13, No. 3, July 1976.
3. Smith, C. K., Anderson, J. C., and Masuda, M.: A Survey of Psychiatric Care in Family Practice. *J. Family Practice,* 1:39-43, 1974.
4. Messner, E., and Schmidt, D.: Videotape in the Training of Medical Students in Psychiatric Aspects of Family Medicine. *Int. J. Psychiatry and Medicine,* 5:269-273, 1974.
5. Kagan, N., et al.: *Studies in Human Interaction: Interpersonal Process Recall Stimulated by Video Tape.* East Lansing: Mich. State Un. Ed. Pull. Services, 1967.
6. Lindemann, E.: Symptomatology and Management of Acute Grief. *Am. J. Psychiatry,* 101-141, 1948.

10

VIDEOTAPE DEMONSTRATIONS AND EXERCISES IN THE PSYCHOLOGICAL TRAINING OF FAMILY PHYSICIANS

Hugh James Lurie, M.D.

Videotape can offer effective additions to the usual teaching armamentarium used in training family physicians. This chapter will briefly outline various kinds of video usage which the author has found particularly useful in the undergraduate, postgraduate, and continuing education training of primary care physicians.

DEMONSTRATION OF A CLINICAL STATE

The signs and symptoms of a clinical state can be clearly demonstrated on video, using either live patient material or dramatized vignettes produced with actors. For example, the instructor may illustrate the manifestations of depression with videotaped examples which show an individual's decreased motor activity, sullen facial expression, handwringing and agitation, or slowness of speech. Particularly when the "freeze-frame" technique is used (where the tape is stopped to examine a particular scene), the precise visual images diagnostic of a clinical process have a marked and lasting impact on physicians viewing the tape. Such audiovisual usage may be incorporated into a lecture or demonstration, or may be used as a focus of small and large group discussion to increase, for example, the abilities of the viewers to diagnose a clinical condition based on nonverbal behavior.

TEACHING INTERVIEWING INCORPORATING VIDEOTAPE PLAYBACK

Live and (ideally) immediate videotape replay after a clinical interview between the student and a real or simulated patient can be used at all levels of training for feedback and self-scrutiny about the success of a particular interview technique or strategy, for a closer inspection of patient behavior in an interview, or for illustration of some nonverbal aspects of therapist behavior such as distracting gestures, restlessness, or excessive nodding. Video playback is also unique as a teaching device to demonstrate the communication of affect between patient and therapist, e.g., the therapist who becomes progressively slower and more detached in his speech in response to the depressed patient's slow speech, or the therapist who responds to a patient's seductive gestures with reciprocal seductive behavior and/or embarrassment.

In the author's experience, the process of being videotaped must first be demonstrated by the instructor, in order for the physician-student to be willing to consider a similar process himself. Confronting one's own image is often a rather traumatic experience even for the experienced interviewer, and it is important that the teacher share his own feelings of discomfort and be open about the shortcomings of his own interviewing strategies or nonverbal behavior as he sees it on the television monitor. Because physicians, particularly, are often defensive about whether they will be ridiculed or criticized in front of their peers, video playback must be introduced gradually and gently, with a clear explanation of the objectives of the experience, as well as a description of the discomfort that viewers often experience in response to their own images.

Several adaptations of usual videotaping and critique are useful for a defensive physician group: one is Kagan's Interpersonal Process Recall (IPR) in which one member of each group of three persons becomes trained to be a neutral inquirer and facilitator to ask about feelings, looks, and the meaning of specific nonverbal behavior. With IPR, the participating trainee can view the interviewing process rather more objectively and experience "criticism" from a single designated peer rather than through a public critique (1, Chapter 6). Another way to reduce the anxiety of the physician-trainee group is to use actors to portray the patients who are to be interviewed on video. This method allows the physician to be less guarded in the interviewing process as he does not have to fear that any mistake will be potentially harmful to the real patient. Actors who are to be objective about interviewing techniques and effectiveness can also provide feedback to the student while not being seen as threatening to the teacher. The teacher who wishes to use actors as credible patients and objective observers of an interview must establish clear teaching objectives which the actors will fulfill, as well as have some knowledge of how to train actors for these roles (2). Finally, the experience of being criticized personally can be diffused by the instructor's showing small segments of a number of different interviews that have been made with trainees, and asking the group as a whole about their reactions to the different interviews. This technique focuses on the process of the interview and successful and unsuccessful strategies, rather than on the specific participants involved.

ATTITUDE CLARIFICATION

Unconscious prejudices and biases (such as sexual or racial attitudes) can strongly influence medical and mental health judgment and decisions. A heightened awareness of such attitudes must be included in the training experience of each physician. Videotaped stimulus materials can be used in a variety of structured exercises to help the physician personally confront his own attitudes. Stimulus materials are often constructed using actors in a short and dramatic vignette; maximal psychological impact is most often achieved if the vignette is taped "subjective camera" (with the actor speaking directly into the camera as if talking directly to the viewer).

Exercise 1:

Video: A hostile black patient speaking: ". . . Listen, you honky, why don't you just shut up and leave us blacks alone . . . you can't possibly understand me and why I get uptight at work. . . ."

Instructor: "How does it make you feel?" or "What would you say next?" This strategy of asking for a behavioral response is often more effective in eliciting attitudes than is a direct inquiry about attitudes.

or

"How would you advise your office nurse to handle the situation?" Looking at attitudes through a consultation model is not so personally revealing or threatening.

SKILL DEVELOPMENT

Video can be extremely valuable in the rapid acquisition of a variety of clinical skills. Although immediate video playback is one way to achieve this goal, another alternative is to use dramatized video vignettes to project the physician rapidly into the interviewing role. Particularly in a workshop setting, the vignette may set the stage for the interview, briefly develop the role, and then facilitate the viewer continuing the role play.

Exercise 2:

Video: The vignette is staged subjective camera, with closeup views of a disheveled and clearly hostile man wearing dirty work clothes. The monologue is approximately the following: "... All right, give me the lecture: that's what my wife wanted you to do, right? I mean, you're the doctor. You know all there is to know about drinking problems. Do you know what my life is like at the shop ... the way the foreman looks at me. ... So I drink to get away from it a bit ... and all my wife does is nag. So if you want to give me a lecture about my drinking, go ahead ..."
(Slow fade with extreme closeup of man's hostile face.)

Instructor gives one of the following instructions:

Instruction A: At the conclusion of the vignette take one minute to decide what you'd say next. (The instructor then compares responses in the large group discussion.)

Instruction B: At the conclusion of the vignette, decide what you would say next. We'll videotape each of your responses as you sit in front of the monitor and react to the vignette as if to a patient with whom you are speaking. The responses will then be criticized individually and in a group. (This method requires two videotape recorders: one for playing of the prerecorded vignette, and one for recording the responses.)

Instruction C: Divide into groups of two (or three, if an observer is desired). Number yourselves one and two. At the conclusion of the vignette, number one continues in the role of the patient depicted on the monitor; number two responds as the doctor with whom the patient is talking would respond. After ten minutes of role playing, each group spends five minutes giving feedback about the intervention, what kinds of statements helped the patient to feel "understood" and less angry, and which statements seemed to increase the patient's anger or level of discomfort.
    At the close of this time, the facilitator may either call on several of the small groups to share their successful and unsuccessful strategies with other participants or allow time for each group to retry the interventions. This latter method is a particularly useful technique for those interventions which have been unsuccessful, as it permits the participants to have a greater opportunity to experience success.

Exercise 3:

Video: An interview between a real physician and a real or simulated patient. Just as the physician starts to tell the patient about the need for surgery the tape is stopped.

Instructor asks the small groups to play the tape from where the video ended. After role-playing, feedback, and discussion time, the rest of the original interview can be shown to reveal what the doctor actually did. This, in turn, should provoke further discussion.

A different kind of clinical skill development can be facilitated by video through the use of a vignette which depicts a particular clinical state and which requires either a diagnostic scheme, a treatment regime, or both (Exercises 4-7).

Exercise 4:

> *Video:* A dramatized vignette portrays a withdrawn, depressed elderly woman in a nursing home. She is complaining about the arthritis in her hands; she is obviously somewhat disoriented for place and time, and she becomes quite paranoid as she describes her daughter's visits to her (". . . who is that girl who comes to see me? She says she's my daughter, but she couldn't be my daughter. I think she's after my money. . . .").
>
> *Instructor* asks the participants (in groups of six or so) to make a comprehensive diagnosis and treatment plan for social, psychological, and physical rehabilitation. The participants may also be asked to develop an appropriate team to implement this plan; such an exercise allows the physician to become more aware of all of the different primary care needs of such a patient which the physician alone cannot meet.

Exercise 5:

> *Video:* A stimulus tape showing a family crisis which might confront a family physician—for example, a family with a suicidal family member, or a family where one family member is still missing in a flood.
>
> *Instructor* may ask the group to develop a crisis plan, role play the plan, critique it, and then try it again following the critique. The different strategies may then be compared.

Exercise 6:

> *Video:* A vignette of a couple with a sexual problem.
> *Instructor* asks the viewers to become a sexual therapy team which is hearing about the sexual problem for the first time and needs to develop and try out an interviewing approach to explore further the dimensions of the problem.

Exercise 7:

> *Video:* A monologue by a rape victim, including some of the details surrounding the attack (all described in a subjective camera vignette by a very hysterical and agitated young woman).

Instructor assigns the group to form a rape crisis team at the hospital where the victim presents (emergency room physician, emergency room nurse, psychiatrist, police officer). Every member of the team must sort out his personal response to the plight presented by the rape victim on video, as well as what his particular role would be to best help the victim.

CONCLUSION

Teaching family physicians on an undergraduate or graduate level about their attitudes and helping them develop new skills for psychological intervention may be considerably enhanced by the use of videotape. Video may be used in various ways to actively involve the learner in his own educational process and to promote self-scrutiny about skills, attitudes, and deficits. Depending on the educational objectives of the instructor, an educational experience for training family physicians might use many of the techniques described above in different combinations (3). Video as a part of a teaching program helps facilitate peer feedback and peer learning, as opposed to overreliance on the "expert" for the major psychological outcomes. Optimally, video may be used to provide the possibility for the best adult learning experience for the participating physicians (5).

REFERENCES

1. Kagan, N., and Schauble, P. G.: Affect Simulation in Interpersonal Process Recall. *J. Couns. Psychol.*, 16:309-313, 1969.
2. Lurie, H. J.: The Actress as a Mental Health Teacher. *Psychiatry in Medicine*, 4:2, 1973.
3. Lurie, H. J., and Gallagher, J. M.: Innovative Techniques for Teaching Psychiatric Principles to General Practitioners. *J.A.M.A.*, 221:7, 1972.
4. Lurie, H. J., Callen, W., and DeMurs, J. L.: Teaching Behavioral Science Skills Using Experiential Methodology. *The P. A. Journal*, 6:3, 1976.
5. Barber, W. H., and Lurie, H. J.: Designing An Experientially Based Continuing Education Program. *Am. J. Psychiatry*, 130:10, 1973.

11

PATTERN SENSITIZATION IN PSYCHOTHERAPY SUPERVISION BY MEANS OF VIDEOTAPE RECORDING

Herman Hirsh, M.D.
and
Herbert Freed, M.D.

We have been using closed-circuit television (CCTV) with videotape recordings (VTR) for the supervision of psychiatric residents in psychotherapy for the past two years. In brief, our procedure is as follows: Two residents are assigned to one supervisor. The patients are seen on a once-per-week basis but alternate sessions are held in the CCTV setting so that the interview can be observed and recorded. In this way, each resident makes a recording on alternate weeks of the psychotherapeutic sessions with his patient. One pair of residents has been permitted to make their own recordings without immediately being observed by the supervisor. The other pair of residents has been observed by their supervisor who concurrently makes the videotape and at times during the course of the interview may make telephone contact with the resident if he feels that his comments may be of immediate value.

Let us discuss the rationale for using this technique for the sensitization of residents to effects and patterns of response. We hope particularly to focus upon the process of sensitizing the resident in his own pattern of behavior. The term includes attitude, mood content of verbalization as well as motor activity. Today it is popular to talk of and develop models to better understand behavior. Indeed we are told that no theory of behavior will be of value unless we can formulate a model of it which we can program in a computer. Too many of us fail to realize that we start after birth to develop and store our own models of the world in our own super brain. To develop these models we act as 'three channel' individuals in our learning activities. The very young child learns the language without books more effectively than the adults who read, memorize and even rush to Berlitz. This is the action motor channel with the learning residing in the musculature as it is in the pianist. The second channel is the image channel utilizing visual and the other sensory organizations. The third channel is the symbolic in which there is the translation of experience into language and the internalization of language for thought and for model formation.

If we go a step further we realize that the relationship of the host of internalized models makes for patterns—for sets of relationships which allow for predictability. These are the basis for the formulation of Grey Walter: "Science is pattern finding; Art is pattern making." During supervision of residents the relevance of videotaping and replay to patterns now becomes obvious since we are all three channel individuals. The patterns may be character traits which are crystallized in mannerisms, posture and gesture or even in tone of voice where affects become evident. The patterns of transaction between patient and resident remind us of our prime interest in the transference-countertransference phenomena.

We would like to return to the comment about our three channel learning and emphasize a conviction: It is that the second channel—the image channel, utilizing visual and the other sensory organizations—is the major force in the development of empathy in the resident. McLuhan says that watching TV is a tactile rather than a visual experience; he says it energizes involvement. We would put the emphasis on its empathic value. That is, an empathic perceptiveness is cultivated and helps in the establishment of the therapeutic alliance. Even more we have found our visualization of the tapes of superior value in establishing the supervisor's empathic perceptiveness and thereby useful in establishing and maintaining the learning alliance between the supervisor and the resident. This concept the "learning alliance" has been stressed in the writings of Fleming and Benedek.

Of course, the other channels are also contributing to bringing us the multiple meanings in the patient's communication. We supervisors are challenged to demonstrate and simplify to the residents the complexities of the patterns rather than to be compulsive in our emphasis on content.

We anticipate the criticism that the use of videotaping may result in a serious contamination of the therapeutic process. This can occur. It probably is most likely with certain patients and most frequently in the early phase of a course of treatment. We have the impression that the resistance to the use of recordings is lessening. An indirect indication of this is the statement by Fleming and Benedek from their book on supervision of analysands (1), doing psychoanalysis. Transcriptions of the supervisory hours, and "vitality of the supervisory process could be emphatically tasted by the reader."

You will recall that we utilize the pattern of the developing transference neurosis to encourage both insight and conviction in the patient. We found that the resident's observation of his image carrying out some nonverbal action is most convincing and cogent evidence of either adaptation or defense on the part of the resident to the interview situation. One rather cocksure resident denied feeling much anxiety in the interview situation, but on replay of his videotape saw himself light several cigarettes and eagerly puff away at them during several tense moments throughout the hour. In the discussion of his behavior he was able to recall the tension and consider the possibilities of its origin. Another resident was observed to become caught up in irrelevant discussions about the patient's husband each time the patient made seductive gestures and become coy with the resident. Almost half of the interview thus became sidetracked into a subject which the patient was unwilling to follow. The resident was finally informed by telephone that the patient wanted to talk about herself and was evidencing some transference manifestation towards him. His resistant pattern thus became broken and he finally permitted the patient to go on in the direction she chose. Upon replay of this tape, the meaning of the telephoned interpretation of the resident's resistance to the transference was so much in evidence throughout the part of the interview prior to the telephone call that the resident easily recognized his own pattern. He then commented favorably and appreciatively about our interpretation to him. Many clues to the affect of the resident and patient can be revivified on playback and many times affective components of the interview which were missed by both the interviewer and the observers are detected in the relatively neutral atmosphere of the playback session.

We found it expedient to develop the resident team of two, the resident as therapist and his colleague who would act as "engineer" and determine when he would alternate in recording the doctor or the patient. The lack of a split screen monitor was probably serendipitous we felt. It encouraged the resident's sensitivity to hints of a rhythm in the doctor-patient transactions. It should be noted that it was the residents themselves who noted what might be called kinetic (nonverbal) markers. We used such observations to spur consideration of content, e.g. transference-countertransference. Another incidental observation we found of value was the observation of the pattern of movement and sound which can be noted in the fast forward movement of the tape.

The sensitization to effects would seem a "natural" to many of us. Videotaping gives us a second look, a chance to overcome the resistance to observing ourselves present in all of us and especially in the novice in psychotherapy. In addition this opportunity to integrate the multi-level messages—verbal and nonverbal—can help the resident integrate these observations to determine discrepancies such as flattening of effect as well as the sorting out of effects and their relationship to the psychodynamics of the patient.

One of the benefits emphasized by the residents involved in the training program thus far was the diminution of free floating anxiety which they had previously experienced as therapists. The repeated statement was: "When I observed that A had anxiety and frustration just like I had, I could relax." It would seem that the television image of the colleague could do as much as, if not more than, any degree of reassurance from the supervisor. Although we do not recommend self-teaching or supervision of one resident by the other, we have found it useful to allow the residents to make a critique of their own tape or of the tape of the partner who is working with him. It has long been our feeling that residents and students can learn from each other once they have an idea of what is to be learned.

SUMMARY

CCTV with VTR and replay is probably the most effective form of psychotherapy supervision available at this time. We focus on patterns of behavior as revealed in the replay of the therapeutic session and attempt to sensitize the resident pairs to these patterns. We find this technique useful in establishing a learning alliance between resident and supervisor. It recalls a statement about learning once read which we will attempt to quote. To read is not as effective as to be told. To be told is not as effective as to be shown. But to see for ourselves is perhaps the most insightful method of learning. VTR and replay lend themselves to this best way of learning.

REFERENCE

1. Fleming, J. and Benedek, L.: *Psychoanalytic Supervision*. New York: Grune and Stratton, 1966.

12
INTENSIVE SUPERVISION OF PSYCHOTHERAPY WITH VIDEOTAPE RECORDING

Peter B. Gruenberg, M.D.
Edward H. Liston, Jr., M.D.
and
George J. Wayne, M.D.

PHYSICAL SETUP AND FORMAT (METHOD)

The Department of Psychiatry at the UCLA School of Medicine operates a television facility which is located in the Outpatient Department of The Neuropsychiatric Institute. It consists of two contiguous rooms —an interview room and a control room. The interview room is comfortably furnished with chairs, tables, and a sofa. It has drapes along two walls and is carpeted. A microphone is suspended from the ceiling near the participants. The control room contains the camera, videotape recorder, monitors, and auxiliary equipment. The two rooms are divided by a wall in which are two camera ports. Affixed to this wall is a bookshelf, the back of which is made of clear glass. This bookshelf is situated directly in front of the camera ports so that the camera in the control room sees through a port and through the partially filed bookshelf. In the control room each camera port is covered by a piece of black cloth through which the camera lens protrudes. Little effort is made to hide the camera completely, but it is unobtrusive. All patients know of the camera and all sign consents to be videotaped. We have a videotape recorder and several monitors. Our vidicon camera is equipped with a

Ed. Note: The historical section which appeared in the first edition of this chapter has been omitted, since it would be redundant at this time. The authors noted particularly the importance of immediacy with video recording and playbacks. The authors continue with their discussion of the program at UCLA School of Medicine.

12-120 mm zoom lens. Thus, the camera operator can establish wide shots, medium shots, and close-ups of one or both participants.

The resident sees his patient for a 50-minute session twice weekly. On one of the days he reviews the recording immediately after the session. On the other day the supervisor observes the session on the monitor while it is being recorded. Afterwards, the supervisor and the resident can review portions or the whole of one or both tapes of that week. Their discussion includes the content and meaning of the transactions, suggestions for appropriate interventions, nonverbal communications. and a general critical evaluation of the therapy session. Of special value, the resident can observe his own nonverbal communications about which he may have been unaware during the session. Each week the supervisor and resident spend two to three hours together in viewing and discussing. The resident spends up to an additional three hours weekly reviewing the tapes by himself.

Once each month a continuous case conference is held for all members of the outpatient staff. One patient is presented for the entire year. Rather than having the resident read from notes, segments of representative sessions are shown by videotape. The conferences are conducted by the resident's supervisor and by visiting consultants. During these two-hour conferences the consultants, members of the full-time staff, residents, psychologists, and social workers discuss their reactions to the patient, to the resident, and to the treatment. The result is an additional dimension in supervision. There is a free exchange of ideas among all staff members, irrespective of their level in the professional hierarchy. Thus, the resident is afforded the opportunity to profit from the ideas of diverse professionals, as well as of his colleague-peers.

DISCUSSION

Supervision with videotape recording is a revolutionary change which brings the teaching of psychotherapy very close to the traditional teaching techniques of subjects like surgery, medicine, and obstetrics. A strong feeling of teamwork and personal participation has existed since the introduction of this technique. Except for rare occasions, in the past the supervisor did not ordinarily see the patient. He had contact with him primarily through the subjective reports of the resident. The supervisor felt no genuine sense of encounter with the patient. Videotape has changed this. There is an additional "plus." With this technique we find that the supervisor is, in effect, a co-therapist—the resident's ally in assuring a therapeutic result.

Too often the patient can become the "forgotten man" as a result of our concern with and focus upon the teaching-learning experience. We may lose sight of the patient's need for help. With the greater sense of engagement with the patient provided by videotape, the experienced supervisor can protect him against possible antitherapeutic maneuvers by the resident. The supervisor is better able to make transient identifications with the patient and the resident, enhancing his grasp of the entire transaction. It is easier with videotape for the supervisor to maintain a good, usable, reality-oriented working relationship with the resident. The supervisor is not so much in the dark—he can see what is going on. Although the supervisor does not see every recorded session, just being able to see one session a week gives him sufficient familiarity so that a verbal presentation from the resident for the unseen session is enough to grasp the whole picture. A supervisor more in touch makes for a more comfortable and honest relationship between himself and the resident. Supervisors are aware of certain residents' needs to impress them by presenting fabrications. With videotape all that can be removed. Making process notes may also create learning difficulties for the resident. Attention that ought to be invested in the patient is drained off in note taking. The resident worries whether his notes are complete, and the patient worries whether the resident is more interested in notes than in him. This, too, is eliminated by videotape.

There are times when the resident engages in certain forms of nonverbal behavior which introduce artifacts into therapy and which he could not possibly believe himself. With the one-way mirror the supervisor may observe something which he feels is detrimental. Telling the resident about it often results in his denial of it. Such acts can be seen and repeated on videotape and short shrift made of them. The resident no longer has the defense: "You are just reading something into my behavior." The data are there for both resident and supervisor to observe. Vital nonverbal communications are now easy to deal with. Heretofore, they were generally overlooked.

Residents often do not recognize opportunities for appropriate therapeutic interventions. Formerly, they had no accurate way of examining and questioning their techniques. Similarly, the supervisor under traditional circumstances was unaware of what had been missed. With videotape, the supervisor can see missed opportunities and point them out. Additionally, the resident reviews by himself every recorded session. Even without comments by the supervisor, he is able to see elements in his technique which were not apparent to him during the session. Thus, the videotape allows him to observe and, in a sense, to supervise himself.

The continuous case conference series provides an additional level of supervision. Visiting consultants who come once a month discuss special subjects germane to therapy in general, such as transference, counter-transference, working through, insight, interpretations, and so forth. Several times over the past year visiting consultants focused upon aspects of treatment that had been underemphasized or interpreted somewhat differently by the resident and his supervisor. A fresh and perhaps more objective view was thus introduced, facilitated by the videotape. We have also seen visiting consultants viewing small, edited pieces of tape out of context and making marked misinterpretations. For the consultant to be of maximal value he must grasp the continuity and the main trends. More than just a few edited strips here and there are necessary for him. In the continuous case conference everyone tends to get into the "supervisor-act." Too many supervisors may complicate the therapy. Moreover, this process is sometimes traumatic for the resident. This is unfortunate but unavoidable. The uneasiness felt by the resident is due to this unique type of "public exposure" of his work.

When we began this project, we used a room where the camera was obviously present. In this situation the resident was always aware that his performance was under observation. The following episode is noteworthy. Some time after therapy had begun the facilities for videotaping were interrupted for nearly two months; and the resident had to see the patient in his own office. During this period a notable change occurred in treatment. Both resident and patient expressed the opinion that therapy seemed to be slowing down.

At the end of this two-month period the patient and resident moved into new facilities which were more spacious and comfortable. Moving into the improved quarters seemed to result in an increase in the tempo of therapy. This indicates that the cessation and subsequent resumption of videotaping were clearly related to the effectiveness of therapeutic activity. Succinctly stated, when one is under intense scrutiny, whether he is doing psychotherapy or surgery, it is reasonable to expect a more intense investment of attention to the problem at hand.

SUMMARY

The use of the new technique of videotape recording to provide long-term, intensive supervision of psychiatric residents doing outpatient psychotherapy is described and the advantages of this method over the classical method of supervision are discussed. The method and format are outlined as well as some of the effects that this technique has upon the therapist, the supervisor, and the patient. The videotapes are used as part of a continuous case conference and this entails rewards and problems. The authors conclude that this technique offers unique advantages over the classical method of supervision. Supervision becomes more complete and honest and provides the resident and supervisor the necessary feedback with which to determine the progress of the patient and the resident. Residents who have used this technique feel that, while they may not have learned faster how to do psychotherapy, they have learned it better.

13
THE USE OF VIDEOTAPE IN STUDYING AND TEACHING SUPERVISION

Marcia Kraft Goin, M.D.
and
Frank Kline, M.D.

INTRODUCTION

Ten years ago when we started to study the process of supervision we began by talking with residents. We asked, what was a good supervisor? This seemed like a simple enough question. But the residents could not clearly say *why* certain supervisors were highly valued. In contrast, the residents were definite on *who* the good supervisors were.

We decided to videotape supervision. With the event preserved, participants could look at it, say what they thought was going on, and explain when and why it was good. Researchers could also study the tapes, analyze the content and look for differences between good and bad sessions.

Videotaping supervision had another value besides preserving the moment for future study and allowing the participants to see themselves. It also permitted supervisors to learn from observing one another, just as surgeons can learn from watching each other operate. In this way, looking at videotapes of supervisors at work is an active and exciting method of teaching supervision.

VIDEOTAPE STUDIES OF SUPERVISION

We studied first videotaped sessions of five supervisors (1) and later videotapes of 24 supervisors (2). These videotaped meetings between second year psychiatric residents and their supervisors provided an opportunity to look at and analyze what actually transpired between supervisor and supervisee. Previous publications about supervision had not

126

contained reports of actual observation. Typically, our conclusions about how supervision should and should not be taught have been derived from personal experience or discussion with others, rather than from actual observation of the interaction (3, 4, 5, 6, 7, 8).

In an analysis of the sessions the supervisors' comments were noted and their teaching styles categorized and graded (Table 1). The data which emerged showed there were distinct differences between the outstanding supervisors and those considered by residents to be average (see Tables 2 and 3). The valued supervisors showed a high incidence of specific, definable, teachable behaviors. They were active and aggressive in their teaching. They encouraged the resident to formulate conceptions about the patients and to consider new ways in which to arrange the observed data. They pushed the residents towards clearer formulations and were not satisfied with incomplete ideas. The supervisors' comments were unambiguous and clear. They focused on specifics such as transference, patients' dynamics, and understanding the process going on between the patient and the therapist. They also extrapolated from the data presented and predicted the future behavior of the patients.

We also concluded that the good supervisors remained in touch with the central therapeutic problems. The supervisors conveyed a feeling of enthusiastic emotional involvement in the supervisory process, the residents, and the patients discussed.

The outstanding supervisors rarely talked about themselves or their experience with patients.* They rarely discussed general psychiatric principles unless they related to the specific case presented and were not afraid to redirect the resident's attention.

The supervisor who was passive, afraid to take a clear-cut position on the material presented, and who failed to focus on the specific material presented was not as highly valued by the resident. A neutral stance and free-floating attention may be useful in psychotherapy, but are deadly in supervision.

We were also interested in how the 24 supervisors dealt with countertransference. It turned out to be surprisingly neglected (8). Analysis of the sessions showed that only four of the 24 observed supervisors talked about countertransference a great deal. Twelve avoided the subject completely, and several talked about it only indirectly. This lack of consideration of the subject took place in the face of many obvious countertransference problems and opportunities for discussion.

---

* Undoubtedly appropriate clinical examples are helpful. Unfortunately, supervisors who like to use their own patients as examples tend to do this too much and to disrupt the supervisory process.

TABLE 1

Content Analysis

Focus of the Supervisor's Statement is Directed Towards:

Item   *PATIENT*

1. Understanding his dynamics or the content.
2. Understanding the process between the patient and therapist.
3. Discussing the transference.

THERAPIST

4. Provide support in therapy situation.
5. Consideration of countertransference.
6. Improve rapport between therapist and supervisor.
7. Encourage discussion.
8. Express approval or agreement with the resident.
9. Express disapproval or disagreement with the resident.
10. Redirect attention.
11. Further information requested.

SUPERVISOR

12. Empathetic with patient.
13. Talk about his experience with patients.
14. Talk about his personal life.

INFORMATION GIVING

15. Techniques.
16. Principles of psychotherapy.
17. General psychiatric knowledge.
18. Uses extrapolation.
19. Analyzes large units as opposed to isolated segments.

OVERALL IMPRESSIONS

20. Stimulate to conceptualize.	1 — 2 — 3 — 4 — 5
21. Push to limits of capacity.	1 — 2 — 3 — 4 — 5
22. Unambiguous communication.	1 — 2 — 3 — 4 — 5
23. In touch with therapeutic problem.	1 — 2 — 3 — 4 — 5
24. Communicates emotional involvement.	1 — 2 — 3 — 4 — 5

TABLE 2

Behaviors of Supervisor

Factor I		Supervisor Activity	
Item	20	Supervisor stimulates resident to conceptualize a theoretical understanding	.91
	21	Supervisor pushes resident to limits of capacity	.89
	22	Supervisor shows unambiguous communication	.82
	23	Supervisor is in touch with therapeutic problem	.77
	24	Supervisor communicates emotional involvement	.74
	25	High resident evaluation	.67
	10	Redirects attention	.51

Factor II		Information Giving and Integration	
Item	16	Principles of psychotherapy	.89
	11	Further information requested	—.69
	18	Uses extrapolation	.50
	17	General psychiatric knowledge	.44

Factor III		Correctional	
Item	9	Express disapproval or disagreement with the resident	.86
	6	Improve rapport between therapist and supervisor	.75
	5	Consideration of countertransference	.70
	15	Techniques	.44

Factor IV		Information Giving, General and Personal	
Item	17	General psychiatric knowledge	.76
	19	Analyzes large units as opposed to isolated segments	.68
	13	Talk about his experience with patients	.63
	14	Talk about his personal life	.49

Factor V		Patient Focus	
Item	3	Discussing the transference	.73
	1	Understanding his dynamics or the content	.63
	2	Understanding the process between the patient and therapist	.62
	18	Uses extrapolation	.53
	25	High resident evaluation	.51

In the literature, discussing countertransference seems to be equated with doing therapy. It is usually concluded that therapy has no place in supervision. The videotaped supervisors may have purposely avoided countertransference in an attempt to avoid the temptation of becoming involved as therapists. In so doing they betrayed their educational responsibility to help residents learn about important countertransference issues. Supervisors, working in isolation from their peers, do not realize that they need to find an identity as supervisor that is separate from that of therapist, while still incorporating many of the same techniques

TABLE 3

Supervisor Assessment Form Used by Residents

My Supervisor:

1. helps me synthesize (make a coherent whole of) data about my patient.
2. directs my attention to areas I had not considered before.
3. helps me understand the dynamics of my patient.
4. discusses principles of psychotherapy with me.
5. directs most of his comments to the therapeutic problems of my patient.
6. talks a great deal during our sessions.
7. makes me feel relaxed and comfortable.
8. provides a therapeutic model.
9. stimulates me to conceptualize a theoretical understanding of the patient.
10. talks very little during our session.
11. is aware and works with my current interests and needs.
12. talks about my countertransference.
13. points out my mistakes.
14. seems really interested in what I present.
15. increases my understanding of the technique of psychotherapy (the how to do it aspect).

and material as a therapist. Probably a clearer understanding that discussion of a therapist's feelings (and their effect on his therapeutic interactions) does not necessitate investigation of the origins of these feelings would free more supervisors to talk about countertransference.

The ease with which a few of the supervisors could directly approach discussion of countertransference was illuminating. Their frank and open approach did not lead to deeper probing of the therapists' intrapsychic conflicts. The valued supervisors did not use discussion of countertransference as a weapon. The work between these supervisors and residents continually focused on the latter's work with their patients. The openness did not appear to elicit anxiety, and this impression was later confirmed by discussions with the residents apart from their supervisors.

VIDEOTAPE USE IN TEACHING SUPERVISION

Having learned that valued supervisors exhibit definite and apparently teachable behaviors, the authors arranged a teaching program for 15 supervisors (9). Psychiatric supervisors were invited to watch and discuss videotapes showing the work of supervisors rated by the residents (in their annual assessment) as excellent teachers of psychotherapy. This proved to be an effective method to increase the observing supervisors' teaching skills—effective as demonstrated by both the residents' subsequent assessment of their supervisors and the supervisors' reported reactions to observing the videotapes.

Supervisors who attended the meetings looked at and talked about the videotapes of six highly valued supervisors. In an evaluation by these supervisors' residents, the trained supervisors increased their focus on the patient, therapy, and theory. The supervisors talked more about the patient's dynamics, the technique of therapy and provided a theoretical understanding for the problems. Those attending the meetings also became aggressive teachers about patient-oriented matters. These changes were not seen in a control group of 15 supervisors who did not attend the meetings.

Those seeking to learn more about supervision have usually been directed to study groups where supervisors discuss case material which has been presented to them by their students (5, 6, 10); it also has been suggested that supervisors educate themselves by returning for supervision of their own cases (3, 10). These approaches both focus on the patient and handling of the patient material, but do not look at the supervisor-supervisee interaction. Observation of actual supervision could focus on that vital interaction.

Since our previous study showed that most supervisors avoid a discussion of countertransference, we were especially interested in seeing if the teaching sessions altered this behavior. Two of the supervisors in the teaching film were quite free in allowing and encouraging discussion of the residents' reactions and we wondered if the observing supervisors would identify with this behavior. They apparently did. Their evaluations showed increased talk about countertransference, and increased pointing out of residents' mistakes. Countertransference, which had been a neglected and probably forbidden subject, was no longer so avoided.

The supervisors' reports on the teaching program emphasized two areas: 1) personal emotional gains and 2) practical ideas about the teaching process. They said the meetings helped to strengthen their identity as supervisors and decreased their anxiety about teaching. They felt freer not to be liked and were relieved to see their feelings and reactions were not unique but shared by others. They also said they recognized the residents' needs for structure, the importance of long-range teaching goals and the need to attend to the material presented by the residents.

132   *Videotape in Psychiatric Training, Treatment*

Psychiatrists' needs in assuming their role as educators have long been neglected. With the advent of videotape we have a method with which to begin the observation and teaching of supervision.

REFERENCES

1. Goin, M. K., and Kline, F. M.: Supervision Observed. *Journal of Nervous and Mental Disease*, 158:208-213, 1974.
2. Kline, F. M., Goin, M. K., and Zimmerman, W.: You Can Be a Better Supervisor. *The Journal of Psychiatric Education*, Vol. 2, Fall/Winter 1977.
3. Grotjohn, M.: Problems and Techniques of Supervision. *Psychiatry*, 18:9-15, 1955.
4. Kubie, L.: Research in the Process of Supervision in Psychoanalysis. *Psychoanalytic Quarterly*, 27:226-36, 1958.
5. Ekstein, R., and Wallerstein, R. L.: *The Teaching and Learning of Psychotherapy.* New York: Basic Books, 1963.
6. Fleming, J., and Benedek, L.: *Psychoanalytic Supervision.* New York: Grune and Stratton, 1966.
7. Semrad, E. J., and Buskard, V.: *Teaching Psychotherapy of Psychotic Patients.* New York: Grune and Stratton, 1969.
8. Goin, M. K., and Kline, F. M.: Countertransference: A Neglected Subject in Clinical Supervision. *American Journal of Psychiatry*, 133:1, January 1976, 41-44.
9. Goin, M. K., Kline, F., and Zimmerman, W.: The Use of Videotape in Teaching Supervision. Accepted for publication in *The Journal of Psychiatric Education.*
10. Moulton, R.: Views on the Supervisory Situation: Multiple Dimensions in Supervision, My Memories of Being Supervised. *Contemporary Psychiatry*, 5:146-157, 1969.

SECTION III

Treatment

EDITOR'S INTRODUCTION

My current working definition of psychotherapy is that: Psychotherapy is the active process of a trained psychotherapist meeting over a period of time with a self-acknowledged patient, while participating in an "I-Thou" dialogue, for the purpose of expressing, eliciting, diagnosing, accepting, and working through one's conscious and unconscious bio-socio-psychological intrapsychic and interpersonal functioning while developing one's healthier potentials during an experience of communing, communicating, relating, and working with others (individuals or groups) in an intimate, corrective, interactional, exploratory, re-educative, emotional and attitudinal encounter focusing on individual and group dynamics in a spirit of trust, sharing, mutuality and confidentiality.

Many, if not most, patients come to the psychiatrist to get relief from symptoms, pain or misery, not wanting to have their basic neurotic character structure touched or influenced. In deep psychotherapy the therapist is usually far ahead of the patients as far as goals are concerned and usually the therapist has to modify his more perfectionistic goals for his patient and settle for less. Video playback allows the patient to obtain a clearer picture of what in his personality was thought by him to be private but actually is visible to the public-at-large and influences them in their ways of reacting to him. It may also allow him to learn much about himself which was formerly secret to himself. It is of great import to the patient when he learns that what was secret to himself about himself was in fact known and overt to others.

In every kind of analytically oriented psychotherapeutic approach, with every patient, there is an uncovering process, a process of bringing into awareness and clearer focus that which is vague, elusive, subliminal, preconscious or unconscious.

In reviewing the aims and conduct of psychotherapy Jules Coleman has succinctly stated, "Whatever form of psychotherapy one practices, it must be based on being able to hear what the patient has to say, to be

133

able to understand what he means, and to be able to respond to what he offers with appropriate sympathy, discretion and discrimination; appropriate in the sense of being therapeutic, directed at the clarification and working through of unexpressed feelings and fears at whatever level or in whatever context they are offered."* Video closed circuit and particularly playbacks allow the cooperating, motivated patient as well as the therapist a chance to repeatedly observe and listen to the patient's overt or manifest productions while they mutually work towards perceiving and understanding his latent, covert, double-binding or multi-channeled other messages which may or may not be in harmony with his overt statements about himself and others. Such cognition and understanding may lead to emotional as well as intellectual insight which can be the forerunner of change in image, self-concept, attitude, emotional reactions or behavior.

The crossing over of creative or practical uses of technological advances can be no better illustrated than in the area of security. Banks, stores and buildings use closed circuit television circuits to keep an "eye" on what is going on in unguarded or unobserved places. Hopefully the time will come when all patients in so called "seclusion" or "isolation" rooms in mental hospitals will be observed continuously through an audiovisual closed circuit television unit transmitting to the nurses' or attendants' station. In September, 1969, a patient in such a room was set on fire and suffered serious burns following some act of her own doing while unobserved and unheard by the nurse on duty in her station.

I have witnessed one modern psychiatric unit with a closed circuit monitor system transmitting from the private room of each patient in a costly, most-up-to-date facility. Although the monitors were on in the nurses' station the nurses and attendants rarely looked at them and the psychiatric residents rarely used the opportunity to observe the patients' behavior when alone.

In 1954 Parloff, Kelman and Frank** focused on an increase in self-awareness as a major criterion for improvement in psychotherapy. To this day universally applicable ways of determining improvement in psychotherapy are still something to be desired. However, it is generally accepted that to know oneself is to have a greater opportunity to grow in a self-fulfilling manner than to be ignorant or unaware of who one is.

---

* Coleman, J. V.: Aims and Conduct of Psychotherapy. *Arch. Gen. Psychiat.*, 18:1-16, 1968.

** Parloff, M. D., Kelman, H. C., and Frank, J. D.: Comfort, Effectiveness and Self-Awareness, Criteria of Improvement in Psychotherapy. *Amer. J. Psychiat.*, 3:343-352, 1954.

In the last 20 years many patients have come to psychotherapists, not with any one specific bodily symptom or complaint, but simply with the massive statement, "Doctor, I come to you because I don't know who I am." So then, movement towards accuracy and completeness of self-awareness may very well be among the most significant goals of psychotherapy. To this end the use of videotape can be a major help in bringing about just the aforementioned self-awareness.

Videotape playbacks and closed circuit television allow a patient to more totally see and hear and sense what and how he is in the here and now. He can experience himself as a subjective-objective-participating person while relating to and with his therapist, spouse, family or peer group members. While becoming increasingly aware of himself as he is in the here and now he is able to compare and evaluate the similarities or differences between this knowledge of himself now and the knowledge he has of what and how and who he was in the past when alone or relating with others.

Through a videotape confrontation of self alone and with others, one can become more familiar with his own anatomical, psychic, emotional and attitudinal identity and become clearer about the impact of this self on others as well as about the impact of others on self. Heightened self-awareness can lead to deeper knowledge of self, including one's transferential transactions. This increased scope of knowledge can serve as an enlarged basis for wholeheartedly working through what needs to be given up because of the crippling consequences of such neurotic distortions and thus allow a patient a chance to function more realistically and with greater authenticity.

Parloff and his co-authors also focused on the processes of comfort and effectiveness as bases for noting improvement in psychotherapy. Here too videotape has high value in helping both the patient and his therapist to assess his degree of comfort as reflected nonverbally and not just verbally and also the degree of his effectiveness as a communicator and as a person who relates with and to others.

The majority of reports concerning the results of videotape self-confrontation written by clinical psychiatrists, psychologists, social workers and nurses have in general indicated the positive values of video feedback techniques in psychiatric treatment (see selected references on videotape, p. 000). These papers were based in general on work with patients by highly trained and seasoned practitioners who did not use the video equipment in any rigid or set pattern. The clinical experiences reported on were for the most part evaluated subjectively by the therapist and patients reported on. On the other hand, a number of papers have come from the field of research psychology based on an attempt to research the impact of video self-confrontation with a control group compared to the experimental group being researched. For the most part I have found that the researchers were too narrow in their concept and structure, lacking in clinical skills and experience, used college students instead of patients for their experimental and control groups and conducted their research over too short a period to bring about positive effects attributable to the video experience.*

To attempt to assess the results of video self-confrontation alone may be of interest scientifically but it is not the intent of skilled psychotherapists who integrate video self-confrontation with their other psychotherapeutic approaches to insist on defining the values of video self-confrontation as a separate entity. The authors, including myself, who have repeatedly supported its use are capable of and usually advocate integrating its use with a multiplicity of simultaneous or alternating techniques and theoretical approaches used in psychotherapy with a patient, a couple, a family or a group. It is not simply a single video self-confrontation replay which is used in clinical practice; at times segments are played repeatedly with discussion guided by the therapist to enable the patient to comprehend the impact of what is experienced during replay. This is what makes the video self-confrontation a valuable and positive experience for the patient. Researchers almost always report their use of a one-time replay of previously taped interviews. The positive results found by experienced clinicians lie in the fact that repeated replays increase awareness, lead to deeper understanding or insight and may heighten the patient's motivation to work towards change.

It is not my intent to foster a form of treatment to be called "videotherapy" although writers and editors love to label this aspect of our work in that dramatic fashion. The *Time* magazine article in 1973 on some aspects of my work with video in psychiatry resulted in the editor's insisting on captioning the article "Videotherapy" despite my plea against that and despite the strong views of the writer of the article, Virginia Adams, who supported my position.* I take a very strong position against the use of video self-confrontation with patients which is not guided by and integrated with their therapeutic work in its context at the time of the replay as known to the therapist and patient. Therefore to research the impact on patients of video self-confrontation alone would seem to

---

* *Ed. Note*: See papers and their review by Fred Stoller and M. M. Berger in *J. Comparat. Group Studies*, pp. 177-190, May, 1970.

* *Time*: Feb. 26, 1973, p. 58, Behavior section, "Videotherapy."

me to be producing artifact-data which are not in fact consonant with the best interest and treatment of the patient.

"The word is not the thing." That is the motto of semanticists starting with Korzybyski and Hayakawa and continuing into the present. From my point of view, the trend to label as "media therapy" some educational and therapeutic approaches to the prevention and treatment of psychiatric disorders which use video is indeed a mistake. The therapy is not rendered by the media. The media is a tool in the therapeutic armamentarium available to the eclectic psychotherapist. I loudly protest that labeling educational approaches and the use of that electronic recording and communication conduct called video by the name "media therapy" just doesn't make the media into what we call therapy.

I hope to influence, if not convince, proponents of this and equivalent terms to question its use and hopefully to give it up. Ivey, in an article entitled "Media Therapy,"* states in his opening paragraph "Media therapy had been proposed as an educational or preventative supplement to the psychotherapeutic program. This article discusses the mode of operation and potential effectiveness of a frankly educational, as opposed to therapeutic program, in the treatment of the hospitalized psychiatric patient." And then in the fifth paragraph of his introduction Ivey clearly states, "The objective of this article is to describe the combination of behavioral intervention, the video feedback learning system, and a systematic educational approach as a new treatment method for psychiatric patients."

So Ivey clearly proclaims his advocacy of video as an important component in an educational and feedback learning system and my work and writings support his position from my experience as an educator and psychoanalytic psychotherapist. Psychotherapy at times functions largely as an educative process as the patient is freer to learn new modes of experiencing being and becoming. As crippling, restrictive, maladaptive ways of functioning can be given up with the guidance and aid of a trained therapist, energies which formerly served to sustain neurotic systems are freed for learning new concepts and new ways of functioning and to fuel the patient in his attempts to risk new behaviors which he is learning may be more adaptive, satisfying and fulfilling intrapsychically and interpersonally. *The video has served as a tool to facilitate* the learning and awareness of new information, the clarification of behavior to be changed, to feedback to the patient and therapist data for ongoing evalua-

---

* Ivey, A. E.: Media Therapy: Educational Change Planning for Psychiatric Patients. *J. of Counseling Psychology*, 20:338-343, 1973.

tion as to whether or not change which is desired has yet occurred so that the therapist with the cooperation of a motivated patient can truly serve as a change-agent or facilitator in his or her task of being therapist. *The media is not the therapy or the psychotherapist* but rather a facilitative electronic tool similar to what a microscope is to a physician who can better and more appropriately diagnose, prescribe and function as a healer after integrating the data obtained through the medium of the microscope.

Another advocate of video enthusiastically but erroneously labels her "use of videotape feedback to enhance group process" as "TELETHER-APY."* Brooks reveals little knowledge of the large literature on the use of videotape in psychiatric facilities when she states that the usefulness of videotape feedback "for self-evaluation by group members and as an enhancer of group process is just being realized." (See Chapters 15-19 in this section). Her use of TELETHERAPY is equivalent to media therapy and videotherapy, and all are inaccurate, inappropriate and contextually incomplete concepts even in their inventor's writings. In concluding my remarks on this subject, I repeat that the use of videotapes for playback in the course of psychiatric treatment may indeed be therapeutic if it is not used as a technique by itself but as a part of a total treatment program conducted by a therapist with a theoretical and clinical understanding of the human personality and an awareness of the profound impact video feedback almost always has on patients or clients exposed to it.

In the broad realm of treatment we have seen a rapid proliferation of the use of videotape playbacks to reach almost every group of patients treated or counseled by members of the psychiatric or allied professions. A number of these approaches will be touched on in this introductory section to the use of videotape techniques in psychiatric treatment to convey the spirit of this creative growth in the conceptualizations for the use of videotape.

In 1973, Resnik and his colleagues reported on the use of videotape confrontation after attempted suicide.* In the emergency room of the National Naval Medical Center in Bethesda, they recorded on videotape the patient as he was brought in to show his condition, the measures being taken to save his or her life and the reactions of the family. After the patient was rescued and available for psychotherapy the videotape

---

* Brooks, D. D.: "Teletherapy," or How to Use Videotape Feedback to Enhance Group Process. *Perspectives in Psychiatric Care*, 14:83-7, 1976.

* Resnik, H. L. P., Davison, W. T., Schuyler, D., and Christopher, P.: Videotape Confrontation After Attempted Suicide. *Am. J. Psychiatry*, 130:460-463, 1973.

made in the emergency room situation was played back. The method is useful in challenging the patient's denial of despair and suicidal intent by confronting him with the consequences of his suicidal behavior. Seeing themselves receiving gastric lavage, tracheotomy, being sutured and receiving intravenous punctures and emergency oxygen motivated patients to accept responsibility for their own self-destructive behavior and their ambivalence about living. They engaged in a therapeutic alliance more rapidly than many suicide attempters do and quickly gave up their rationalizations, denials and projections. Resnik emphasized the impact of replay of closeups which had captured "the patient's facial expression (confusion, disorientation, agitation or lethargy) as well as those of his family (concern or indifference)." It was hypothesized that this technique is "relevant to the treatment of a broad spectrum of self-destructive patients who have traditionally been viewed as problems in medical and psychiatric management."

In a brief clinical note written in 1974 of his videotape feedback technique to successfully treat six couples with sexual dysfunction, Serber emphasized clearly the protective precautionary measures he utilized as well as the significant improvement direct visualization led to during the treatment period.* His untimely death removes a courageous innovator with a high sense of professionalism from our contemporary work. He had previously used videotape as a component in behavioral therapy to produce aversion to deviant acts such as exhibitionism with the technique of "shame aversion therapy."**

In Serber's treatment of sexual disorders couples signed clearly stipulated consent forms agreeing to be videotaped while alone in an attractive room resembling a bedroom and engaging in "live" sexual activity. The contract stated that the patients would own and have the videotape in their possession at all times both during and after the taping. No live closed-circuit immediate feedback through a TV monitor was used in order to reduce the anxiety and factors of unnaturalness. Serber used a wide-angle camera lens placed about 12 feet away from the double bed and placed a microphone on the floor near the bed to record the verbal interchanges between the couple. The lens recorded the couple sitting up as well as in a horizontal position. The couple were instructed how to start and stop the recording equipment. The videotape was reviewed by the therapist and it was often found that the behavior seen on videotape

---

* Serber, M.: Videotape Feedback in the Treatment of Couples with Sexual Dysfunction. *Arch. of Sexual Behavior*, 3:377-380, 1974.

** Serber, M.: Shame Aversion Therapy. *J. of Behavioral Therapy and Experimental Psychiatry*, 1:213-215, 1970.

had little in common with what the couple had previously reported. Couples were motivated by the video playback and discussion to complete their assigned homework in a more systematized fashion and also experienced a desensitization to formerly anxiety-producing behavior. His preliminary report offers hope to couples and therapists that they can more clearly delineate their actual problem and be helped to resolve it through the use of the videotape playback.

In the addiction rehabilitation program at the Donwood Foundation Hospital in Toronto extensive use is made of videotapes recorded in the hospital as lectures given by Dr. Bell and his colleagues in the second phase of rehabilitation.* After the initial phase of hospitalization which consists of a complete study of the physical and psychological effects of the patient's addiction, together with medical treatment when required, the patient enters the second phase which lasts for three weeks and consists of daily lectures and group therapy sessions designed to enable the patient to understand the reasons for his addiction, to clearly realize the effects of it, and to remove the underlying cause of the addiction. Videotaped lectures are also used in the third or outpatient phase which lasts up to two years. The videotaped lectures are successfully used to stimulate discussions with family members as well as alcoholic and drug-addicted patients.

Over a period of five years we successfully used serial video closed-circuit self-image confrontations with hard-core drug addicted females in our one-year residential rehabilitation program at the Quaker Committee on Social Rehabilitation Baird House in New York City. Later review of videotapes of how they had appeared physically, emotionally, and attitudinally upon admission was a source of great amusement and heightened motivation to our residents three, six and nine months later.

The positive effect of peer confrontation in psychotherapy and encounter groups with delinquent and addicted adolescents has led to the addition of videotape playback to the overall treatment method in some centers. Pascal, Cottrell and Baugh** reported in 1967 that they used videotape as a self-confrontation device with adolescent boys referred by the juvenile court. Their objectives were not only to use it to provide a corrective experience but also to condition an avoidance reaction to the deviant behavior seen on the television replay monitor. They felt that the

---

*VTR Plays a Key Role in Rehabilitating Addicts. *Canadian Hospital*, 46:36-37, 1969.

**Pascal, G. R., Cottrell, T. B., Baugh, J. R.: A Methodological Note on the Use of Videotape in Group Psychotherapy with Juvenile Delinquents. *Int. J. Group Psychother.*, 17:248-251, 1967.

videotape could act as a positive reinforcer for desirable behavior as it enabled the boys to recapitulate the lesson with time and thereby benefit from hindsight.

In 1974 Marvit, Lind and McLaughlin* created a project involving 44 delinquent adolescents being treated by four different agencies, staffs and programs in Hawaii. Their goal was to induce attitude change through the use of videotape. Agency 1 has a guided group interaction program and places a major emphasis on group responsibility. The boys treated here are referred by the court, have long histories of deviant social behavior, and may have been committed to youth correctional facilities previously. Agency 2 is a runaway shelter for girls which has no structured treatment; its major emphasis is on crisis intervention and referral to other helping facilities. Agency 3 is for girls with histories of law violations who are involved with the family court. A reward behavior modification approach is used with an emphasis on both a token economy and goal setting. Agency 4 is a residential treatment center for boys and girls which provides a family-type living arrangement for children with intolerable home situations and for those who cannot return home following their participation in court proceedings. Thus, the sample population included youths with short and long histories of trouble with the law who came from varied socioeconomic levels, some high and others from welfare families.

In this study 23 youths were in the experimental group and 21 in the control group. All of them completed a pre- and post-project questionnaire to assess their attitudes about themselves and other people and their perception of the attitudes of others as they related to themselves. The experimental group was videotaped during its next four group psychotherapy sessions and after each taping they viewed the tapes together as a group and discussed the content, including their feelings and other reactions to seeing themselves. In this group they compared their self-image with the video playback of their appearance and behavior in the dynamic interaction of the group.

The results of comparing the analysis of the attitude questionnaires revealed significant changes in the responses of the experimental group. Confronted with their self-defeating behaviors and images they became more upset initially, more sensitive to feedback from others, more critical of themselves and more defensive about their behavior. Their feeling of being "on top of the world" was diminished as they used less denial

---

* Marvit, R. C., Lind, J., McLaughlin, D. G.: Use of Videotape to Induce Attitude Change in Delinquent Adolescents. *Am. J. Psychiatry*, 131:996-999, 1974.

regarding their behavior and circumstances. Reality made an impact on their distorted self-perception and alienation from self. The false façade of self-confidence common to delinquents diminished as they saw the reality of themselves as others saw them and a more genuine confidence based on reality was formed. They became more willing to discuss problems with others rather than keeping things to themselves. Initially their participation in community affairs became less active as they developed a more reflective attitude, became more aware of their shortcomings, felt less confident, and put less energy into social activities as a way to avoid painful affects.

In the area of self-concept Marvit and his colleagues noted that the videotaped group became more aware of how they appeared to others and experienced an increased fear of others as a reflection of reduced denial and an increased fear of rejection due to their behavior. They saw how other people actually saw them and why others did not take them seriously or treat them with respect or serious consideration. The initial negative responses to self shifted during the four weeks of the project and the videotaped delinquents began to see themselves as better looking at the end of the series. They were better able to select both positive and negative feedback from the videotape and group discussions and more realistically work through negative feelings with the support of their peer group. As has been noted in other work with televised groups (see Chapter 15 by Stoller in this section) the concern with appearance led the group members to improve their appearance as they changed the way they dressed and behaved. I have seen this occur in a number of adolescent groups when I have used videotape playbacks in psychiatric and drug-treatment settings. As unrealistic expectations of others they were involved with interpersonally were reduced, a more realistic appraisal and experiencing of themselves and the world around them occurred so that hostility, resentment and rebelliousness could be kept to a minimum.

In summary, the authors noted the lack of resistance to such a therapeutic approach with videotape, even in a population of delinquents, probably because they were reared with television. The videotaping experience was positive in that for the first time these youths were exposed to themselves and their behavior in a unique and fascinating way.

I want to emphasize that although Marvit's groups initially reacted with great anxiety and initial disappointment they gradually recouped positive feelings and found more of themselves to be pleased about. This reaction of initial social self-criticism is pointed out elsewhere in this book (p. 000) and is a frequent finding in my work with patients. The psychotherapeutic prognosis can be made on the basis of how soon and how positively patients move from that degree of social self-criticism to social self-restitution which allows them to be more comfortable and at times even pleased with the feedback image they experience. The video experience reported on by Marvit et al. led to improvement in posture and general health care as well as to improvement in dress.

The chapter by Philip C. Morse in this section reports on an innovative use of videotape feedback with emotionally disturbed children in a summer camp setting. The research compares a control and an experimental group and reports on the usefulness of feedback in treating children with problems related to impulse control, reality testing and low self-esteem. In relation to my earlier comments about the drawbacks associated with rigid time and frequency of videotape playback we see here the positive results associated with an individually scheduled timing for frequency and length of the playback experience. The chapter also includes a review of the literature on video usage with anorexic children, borderline schizophrenic children and others with varying degrees of immaturity and psychopathology. The capacity of video to expedite the decentering process and help children gain a more realistic perception of themselves in relationship to others is a major contribution.

Harry Wilmer expanded our clinical use of video with his report of a "television monologue"* with 100 adolescent psychiatric patients. He developed this technique while he was directing the youth drug study unit at the Langley Porter Neuropsychiatric Institute. He developed a method of soliloquy which involves a patient sitting alone in a room talking to a television camera for a short period of time. It is thus possible to give the patient a tool to externalize his inner speech and to make it available to himself and others, and to experience this free of the contamination of human interaction. This type of self-encounter or self-confrontation is not familiar to the patient from any previous experience and provides a new dimension for the study of personal and individual social perception. The method developed by Wilmer was to inform new patients on their admission to the ward that they would be asked to make such a television monologue within two or three days. Instructions were minimal. The patient was told that

. . . he is to do his own thing for 15 minutes before a camera alone and that after watching the replay alone he may have the tape erased if he wishes. Any further explanation is strictly in response to the

---

* Wilmer, H. A.: Use of the Television Monologue with Adolescent Psychiatric Patients. *Amer. J. Psychiat.*, 126:102-108, 1970.

patient's questions. . . . The setting is informal. . . . The camera is placed before a comfortable chair in which the patient sits and it is focused on the upper half of his body. . . . We prefer to use an over-head microphone on a boom so that the patient's movements are not restricted and he is not physically attached to the machinery. The technician, having arranged the setting, leaves the patient, tell-ing him he will be back in 15 minutes. He goes into the adjoining room and starts the videotape recorder. At the end, the technician returns to the room and, with minimal conversation, turns off the camera, turns on the monitor, then rewinds the videotape and plays it to the patient, again alone in the room sitting on the same chair. If the patient requests that the tape be erased, this is done with no attempt to persuade him otherwise.

The patient and his psychiatrist almost always review the mono-logue together within a day or two. The patient may elect to show the monologue to other patients or to the community. His monologue is also used for supervision and in formal case presentations to con-sultants. The patient is also told that he may make subsequent monologues if he wishes, but he is not urged to do so. . . . Recent modifications of the technique include reducing the monologue time to 10 minutes and to videotape the patient again after the replay, talking about the monologue or continuing it for another five min-utes and then replaying that five-minute segment to the patient.

In his overview of the patient monologues Wilmer (a) referred to their uniqueness as a clinical record for later review or for later therapists, (b) saw them as a fascinating revelation of the patient's inner speech, (c) noted how some tapes are remarkable examples of free association and others of regressive behavior. In some tapes the patient is willing and able to talk freely about painful, personal, intimate or historical material that as yet can't be discussed with the therapist or group. The patient has the stage all to himself with no human parental surrogate facing him. Wilmer also (d) noted how some patients use it as a panto-mime experience or kind of psychodrama. One patient used the mono-logue as a means of loosening her "uptight straight" psychiatrist by tak-ing off her clothes and doing a topless dance. He further (e) commented on the fact that the few patients who verbalized nothing in their mono-logues revealed a great deal through their physical behavior. Most often it was a defiant and rejecting act toward the doctor and the community, but sometimes it exemplified an overwhelming sense of inhibition and phobic reaction. Such patients generally did poorly in the community, so pervasive was their withdrawal and their commitment to deviant, non-revealing behavior. In one such patient, this was clearly a reenactment of his dominant childhood behavior, when he dared reveal nothing in-timate for fear of being hurt, rejected, or given the silent treatment by his parents. Others, in their silence, act like little children reverting to a kind of sign language, using playful self-distortion as they once did before mirrors. Wilmer (f) noted how some patients talked excessively to avoid self-revelation; (g) commented on those patients who relied on objects and clinging to objects such as books and musical instruments to establish relationships; (h) reported that some read prepared auto-biographies or from books and one withdrawn schizophrenic patient read poetic essays from a book in Joyce-like fashion, reading only one line from each page.

Wilmer states:

> The monologues present the patient in ways that, for practical purposes, may be classified as follows: 1) predictive, diagnostic; 2) informational, historical; 3) behavioral representation of self; 4) psychotherapeutic effect; and 5) record of the patient at a given time and place.
> This technique lends itself to objective measurement. Time of eye contact with camera, speech non-fluencies, repetitive gestures or metaphors, specific references to time, persons, places, events, speed and volume of speech, silences, and opening phrases, body touching, etc. can be tallied.

The developer of the monologue approach described it as "a new form of metaphorical experience. . . . The monologue opens new vistas for self-observation in often poetic and creative ways. In it, each in his own way is exploring his own version of the most famous monologue of all: 'To be or not to be: that is the question.' "

Clause Bahnson, a pioneer in the use of video self-image confrontation, has continued his work with video self-image confrontation in long-term treatment of two patients diagnosed as multiple personality.* Over the three-year period of therapy with these patients he has learned that the strong resistance to its use with such patients is to be expected because their very symptoms are tenaciously held defenses against seeing and experiencing a unified self. In affirming the dictum we have learned regarding the use of video equipment, namely, that the equipment should be in the service of the patient and not vice versa, Bahnson states he does not use the video replay on any fixed schedule with such patients but uses it when the clinical picture warrants or clearly calls for it. He tapes a whole session and reviews material between that and the next regularly scheduled psychotherapy session. He then selects passages of from four to six minutes for focused feedback at the next session. He

---

* Personal communication.

recommends that it be used with great caution and consideration with such patients and that the therapist may find the effects of replay to be quite dramatic, e.g., equivalent to the uncovering of particularly traumatic and usually violent early memories.

In 1972 Silk reported on the use of a variety of video methods to assist the therapist in brief joint marital treatment for marital adjustment difficulties.* Silk's goal is to utilize the limited therapy time available by maximizing its use with video; he recommends 1) reviewing the videotape made of the couple in their initial interview at the start of the second session, and 2) having the couple in the third or fourth session review the videotape made of each one separately at the time of the first interview. In this manner the couple is given something quite tangible to work with, e.g., such data as the clear fact that they do not look at each other when they talk, that their words carry double meanings, and they quickly stop efforts to prove what's happening as "the other person's fault." Major areas of marital conflict can be more fully and rapidly assessed to decide on some tentative treatment measures. The second session video replay sets the stage for illustrating the degree of patient responsibility involved in successful treatment. The videotape stresses "that the couple is being dealt with as a unit with videotape expected to help them experience each other more fully." By the third session the couple is helped to make emotional contact with each other by creation of a problem-solving situation to be discussed and solved in a specific amount of time. Communication styles, distortions and problems can be focused on as partners assume greater responsibility for the contribution of each to their marital problems and realize the need to learn how to compromise and move towards conflict resolution. The brief therapy can be terminated as the couple learns to cope with each other more effectively.

The chapter in this section by Ian Alger** on his use of freeze-frame video in psychotherapy details his theoretical views on and practical experiences with this technique of stopping the action on the monitor at crucial moments in the therapy session with families and couples. Stopping the movement allows for the dissection of complex behavioral interactions as they are reviewed in the light of context, frequency, and

---

* Silk, S.: The Use of Videotape in Brief Joint Marital Therapy. *Am. J. Psychotherapy*, 26:417-424, 1972.

** *Ed. Note*: This chapter was written for this edition by Alger to replace the chapter in the 1970 edition entitled "The Use of Videotape Feedback in Conjoint Marital Therapy" which was co-authored by his long time associate, Peter Hogan. Peter Hogan met with an untimely death during the early summer of 1977. We will miss his warmth and creativity.

regulatory impact on the family system. He emphasizes the retentive impact of such visual images which become milestones in awareness and insight. Such illuminating moments can lead to increased motivation to change as well as to change itself. Freeze-framed moments of images are seen by Alger as powerful metaphors whose symbolic quality serves as a kind of shorthand to communicate a wealth of emotional ideational and behavioral material.

The first chapter in this section presents the now classic 1964 paper by Moore, Chernell and West reporting on television as a therapeutic tool. This report is quoted more often than any other by those writing on aspects of videotape usage in treatment of psychiatric patients. The authors reported the results of the first experimentally designed controlled study with 80 psychiatric inpatients to evaluate whether or not seeing themselves on videotape would have a marked and beneficial effect on their improvement.

Stoller's report on televised group psychotherapy with hospitalized patients in Chapter 15 received much attention as an innovation when reported initially in the *American Psychologist* in 1967. Its potential for the hundreds of thousands of patients in our mental hospitals has hardly been realized, but I am still hopeful that video will have great impact on the lives and therapeutic outcome of these patients. Stoller's premise was that a successful series of performances could contribute to a dramatic alteration of the self-image held by regressed individuals with histories of repeated failures.

In his afterthoughts, written in 1968 at my suggestion, Stoller more clearly delineates and vigorously attacks the self-perpetuating systems involved in fostering chronic institutionalization. His strong position against traditional concepts of privacy, secrecy and confidentiality as being due more to the anxiety of therapists about being open than to the real interest of patients is continued in his later chapter on videotape in marathon and encounter groups (see editor's introduction to Section IV on legal, moral and ethical considerations).

In the next chapter I have brought together my experiences in using videotape with flexibly integrated treatment of individuals, couples, families and groups in private practice. The scope of the chapter runs a wide gamut: from ways of introducing its use to patients to emphasis on humanistic concerns being even more important than legalistic concerns; from examples of initial self-confrontation reactions to examples of how video helps in demonstrating to family members the system of unconscious arrangements which perpetuate their hang-ups; from clarifying neurotic claims and externalizations to pinpointing the roles and games and self-

148   *Videotape in Psychiatric Training, Treatment*

defeating arrangements people make; from examples of the values for the therapist of really seeing himself as he is rather than as he thinks he is to clarifying the nonverbalized impact people have on one another; from utilizing a patient's videotaped group session in his later individual psychotherapeutic hour to utilizing a videotaped couple session during a later group session; from the use of four live monitors during sessions to watching playbacks without sound.

In Chapter 17 Mayadas and O'Brien present a comprehensive overview of the experiences of various authors with videotape in group psychotherapy. They emphasize the self-corrective dimension of instant replay when added to the consensual validation found in the group. They note especially how denial and resistance to change are considerably reduced with video feedback. They note how the combination of videotape playback and the group therapy experience allows members to test out hypotheses about self in a structured simulation of the social environment so that discrepancies between cognitively perceived self-images and socially projected images can be experienced and confronted. Their review encompasses the work of leading figures, including Alger, Hogan, Benschoter, Berger, Czajkoski, Danet, Miller and Stoller in the use of video in group therapy. They repeat my own observation that, the more open are the presence and use of video cameras, the easier is the acceptance by the group and the less is the use of video a hindrance to the group process.

Clelia Goodyear,* a New York social worker whose specialty is working with terminal patients, has been using video replay with 25 individual and group patients during the past five years. These are all patients who are aware that they have a terminal illness, although of course many of them still use a great deal of denial in relationship to that reality. She has never used the video equipment in the first session, but only after a relationship of trust and positive transference has been established and the patient has a sense of her being there, as a real person, for him or her. This is sound clinical practice with all patients, not only with those who are terminally ill.

My own concern about using video with the aged and terminal patient had originally been that the self-image confrontation might increase self-hate. Goodyear hypothesized that her patients would in fact be very interested in seeing how they actually appear physically and emotionally since they are so terribly concerned both about their physical appearance and their psychological bearing. Most terminal patients are greatly

* Personal communication from C. Goodyear who is in private practice.

concerned about their depressed emotional status and how their depression affects others, especially family members. She did not screen patients out of the experience even though they showed physical evidence of the effect of the disease if she felt their ego was intact enough to handle it. She reports most patients said, "I am concerned about what I'm going to see. . . . I'm afraid to look at myself and to see how I've really changed but I also really want to because I want to see myself as others see me."

In response to my question, "Did you ever postpone using the videotape after you had made the offer to your patient to use it?" she said that except on one occasion she did not postpone videotaping. That patient built up tremendous advance anxiety and had a very difficult week wondering why the therapist had now postponed using the video self-image confrontation. Goodyear always attempts to elicit in advance the patient's anticipatory reactions. She finds that "For the most part, 90% of the time, people assume that they will look worse than they really do. They are actually amazed that they looked as well as they do and act as intelligent as they do. It has always been extremely helpful in terms of helping a patient obtain a more realistic sense of his or her current body image and emotional bearing, no matter how deteriorated that status might be."

In regards to the frequency of use and duration she states,

> With patients like mine I would recommend video be used on an average of one time each month or if possible for a few minutes every session or every other session as it is such a very good medium to help people get in touch with their anger.

She, like myself, has found that the gestalt technique of having the patient look at and talk to an imagized someone—a relative, a doctor, or even God—by looking straight at the camera lens is very helpful. When the patient sees the replay the fact of whether the inner anger is being adequately expressed or not becomes very clear and in the atmosphere of the therapy session and relationship the anger of the dying person can be more completely and satisfyingly expressed.

> If I only tape the patient for five or 10 minutes I play back the whole five or 10 minutes. If I tape a whole session then I play back about 30 minutes at the beginning of the next therapy session. I focus on the content of what they were saying for working through of certain defense mechanisms such as denial, repression and projection in order to enable them to see and experience more objectively their anger, projection, denial and emotional withholding and withdrawal. I don't press any defense mechanisms that I don't believe the patients are ready to give up. The expression of deeper feelings is

150   *Videotape in Psychiatric Training, Treatment*

helpful for self-esteem, self-acceptance and insight during this difficult time. Patients are pleased to give up their projections onto doctors, relatives, friends and people in general. They are interested in getting a clearer picture of how self-destructive they actually are and what they are doing with their feelings so they can more easily express and work through their basic anger. They can also give up residual angers based on general mistrust and poor self-esteem established long before the onset of the terminal illness and enhanced by their illness and general loss of control.

It is important to note that she never had any major negative reactions with her use of video playbacks with 20 terminal patients over a five-year period, although a great deal of sadness was evoked. She believes that most terminal patients do have the ego strength to integrate what they are experiencing even if for only brief periods of time. She sees videotape as a valuable and perhaps necessary tool in working with those terminal patients who are interested in gaining insight into their physical and emotional state of being.

In Chapter 21 Carl Whitaker shares his use of videotape in family therapy in its special relationship to the therapeutic impasse. A pioneer in therapeutic approaches with families, Whitaker has also been a proponent of co-therapy since he and Malone first published their conceptualization of the roots of psychotherapy.* When a co-therapist is not available to him, videotape has served for him as an effective feedback system in working with whole families, particularly if the video is begun in the earlier sessions. While advocating the taping of the first family interview if possible, Whitaker is more guarded and tentative about its use during that same session. However, sooner or later he and the family elect to review part or all of that first session which is so very important in presenting the family system. However, he respects the family's veto rights in order to avoid escalating excess anxiety. He states clearly, "I am most concerned with its function as consultant with the family as the patient. I, of course, like to use it as consultant to me, the therapist, who is participating, and thus it becomes part of that larger family we call the therapeutic family. But I also use it as an extension of me—the manipulator. The machine has the capacity to increase the feedback to me so I become objective about my own subjectivity."

The chapter by Stoller on videotape feedback in the marathon* and

* Whitaker, C. A., and Malone, T. P.: *The Roots of Psychotherapy.* New York: McGraw-Hill, 1953.

* Stoller assisted Bach in developing the concept and structure of the marathon group. See Bach, G. R., The Marathon Group: Intensive Practice of Intimate Interaction. *Psychol. Rep.,* 18:995-1002, 1966.

encounter groups was prepared for this section to bring to the reader some awareness in depth of what transpires in these types of groups which may have growth and therapeutic benefits for participants. Stoller has made significant innovations with videotape (see Chapter 15, this section) and has clarified in this chapter some of the similarities and differences between the basic encounter group, the marathon group and regular psychotherapy groups.* Stoller has had a major influence in recent years in moving forward the growing edge of group approaches by combining his knowledge of psychotherapy with ways of accelerating interaction in time-limited intensive groups where he can use videotape for focused feedback.

Constance Nelson reports in her brief chapter on a long-term experience with an open-ended group of chronic schizophrenic outpatients taped once weekly. These patients also experience a replay once weekly just before each session. I believe her work to be especially significant in that she touches on the impact of "belonging" to a viable, interested, caring and connected group of significant others in undermining the separateness, alienation and loneliness of most chronic schizophrenic patients. Her long-term work reveals that in working with such chronically ill patients it takes a long time of consistent caring with at least one trained authority-figure continuously present to allow for trust, mutuality and eventually for change in such a patient population. But it is important to note that that change can occur. This report refutes the work of many young researchers who spend short periods offering one or two video replays to schizophrenic groups and then publish reports of how they see little evidence of change or hope for change through the use of video playbacks with chronic schizophrenics. It takes dedication, time, consistency, patience and the development of trust— but it can be accomplished.

In Chapter 23, "Multi-Image Immediate Impact Video Self-Confrontation as an Adjunct in the Growth of Self," I am reporting on my discovery and use of a method to more rapidly reach repressed introjects from the earliest years and to elicit free associations to experiences associated with early introjections, incorporations and identifications which do not ordinarily come through in psychotherapy for a long, long time, if at all. Examples of its use with patients and seminar participants are

---

* See Similarities and Differences Between Group Psychotherapy and Intensive Short Term Group Process Experiences—Clinical Impressions, by Berger, M. M., *J. Group Psychoanal. and Process*, 1:11-30, 1968, in which attention is paid to comparative definitions, goals, criteria for selection, motivation, resistance, commitment, size, drop-outs, compatibility, sub-groups, termination and benefits.

included as the data to validate the existence, impact and influence of multiple inner selves as brought forth through an innovative use of the capability of the video equipment. The report covers the basic equipment required, the actual technique and verbatim statements of what it stimulates.

The last chapter in this section by Metzner concludes this overview of well-tried and innovative new approaches to treatment. The approach presented by Metzner which he calls the videoscan technique (videotape self-confrontation after narcotherapy) involves the videotaping of a patient being interviewed under the influence of an hypnotic drug and then reviewing this taped material, which usually contains ideas and behaviors the patient doesn't remember, during later psychotherapeutic sessions for insight, integration and working-through. The reader should also review the work done over a period of years in the use of recordings and playbacks with alcoholics by Carrere, Paredes, Cornelison and others.

Clinicians with much experience as psychotherapists as well as with the integrated uses of videotape in treatment have found it important to emphasize the prognostic value of video usage. Patients who seem to be grossly unreactive to their initial exposure to playback of self-image and reveal little impact are generally more difficult to engage in therapy and are more detached from an awareness of their feelings.

14
TELEVISION AS A THERAPEUTIC TOOL

Floy Jack Moore, M.D.
Eugene Chernell, M.D.
and
Maxwell J. West, M.B., B.S.

INTRODUCTION

O wad some Power the giftie gie us
To see oursels as ithers see us!

—ROBERT BURNS

These lines are from a poem written almost 200 years ago by Robert Burns. We feel that giving patients a chance to see themselves as others see them will have a marked and beneficial effect on their degree of improvement. To this end, every patient admitted to the private psychiatric inpatient service at the University of Mississippi Medical Center beginning in August of 1963 became a part of a survey project. At selected times during the hospital stay each patient had an interview with a psychiatrist which was video taped in progress. These tapes were then viewed by alternate patients, giving them a chance to see and hear themselves interacting in a way that they had never experienced before.

A study by Cornelison and Arsenian (1) in 1960 reported the response of psychotic patients to self-image experience, employing photographic self-images. They were impressed with the responses and changes in the psychotic state accompanying self-confrontation. To our knowledge, there have been no controlled experiments attempting to evaluate the benefit of visual confrontation as a therapeutic experience for the psychiatrically-

Reprinted from *Archives of General Psychiatry*, 12:217-220 (Feb. 1965). Read before the American Psychiatric Association Meeting, Los Angeles, May 5, 1964. This investigation has been aided by a grant from the Foundations' Fund for Research in Psychiatry.

ill patient. This paper represents such an attempt and it is our feeling that audiovisual confrontation was a meaningful and corrective experience for the patient and, as a consequence, produced some therapeutic benefit.

MATERIALS AND METHODS

Within 24 hours of admission every patient, regardless of diagnosis, had his first interview with one of two psychiatrists working on this project. This interview was carried out in a special room with television cameras concealed behind one-way mirrors, thereby giving the impression of privacy. All patients were aware that they were being televised. The cameras themselves were in a control room which surrounded the interviewing area and were manned by experienced technicians. Each session was video taped. The first session lasted approximately 12 minutes and was designed to cover certain broad areas. Each interview was structured, but allowed for individual variation.

Immediately following this session alternate patients were taken to the viewing room where they saw a replay of what had just happened. This is possible because there is no delay in the process between recording and playing back the video tapes. This eliminates one of the major difficulties experienced when working with motion picture film. This viewing took place in a small room with complete privacy, only the patient and the interviewing psychiatrist being present. At that point, and on all subsequent occasions, the patients' comments were recorded by the psychiatrist who sat with them, but offered no comments of his own. Follow-up interviews were done four days after admission, and then at weekly intervals until discharge. These follow-up sessions lasted approximately five minutes and concentrated on how the patient was progressing and on his comparison of the present with his condition on admission as he remembered it. Half of the group (having the experience of seeing the video taped sessions) always saw the current segment plus all previous segments in sequence, giving them a chance to compare the reality of their earlier status with their stated memory of it. The alternate patients in the nonview group had exactly the same experiences but, of course, had no comments to be recorded.

The initial sample consisted of 80 consecutive patients admitted to our neuropsychiatric (NP) unit: 40 saw themselves on video tape and 40 had the same television interviews but did not see themselves on video tape. Records were kept by one of the two psychiatrists working on the project after his consultation with the resident assigned to the particular patient. Any clinical evaluation made by the resident was always done by him after consultation with his supervisor. Insofar as was possible, neither the resident nor the supervisor knew to which group the patient had been assigned. However, it was realized that on certain occasions this information had inadvertently become known to the resident, often because of the reaction of the patient to the experience.

After the patient's discharge, his discharge diagnosis and degree of improvement while in the hospital were then recorded by the psychiatrist after consulting with the resident who, in turn, had discussed these evaluations with his supervisor. Also, the resident was asked whether he knew to which group his patient belonged. The degrees of improvement were set up for the project in the following way: clinical judgments ranged from unchanged to minimally improved, moderately improved, or greatly improved to cured, thus providing three categories which were amenable to statistical analysis. Without exception, all patients in this study participated in the ward activities and received any necessary treatment(s) according to their individual problems and as prescribed by the ward physician. Thus, the only difference in the first 80 patients was that alternate patients (in half the group) saw their video tape interviews in a manner previously described. This video therapy required an average total time during their hospitalization of only 60 minutes.

RESULTS

In this sample of 80 patients, 75% were women. Most of the usual diagnostic categories were represented with a predominance of depressive reactions (30%) and schizophrenic patients (25%). The balance included a representative sample of patients usually seen on such a unit as ours.

The data concerning therapeutic results of the 80 patients are summarized in Table 1.

These results are significant beyond the 0.01 level by using the χ^2 analysis of two independent samples.

Fifty percent of those patients in the view group were judged to be maximally improved clinically. In the nonview group approximately 50% of the patients were clinically judged to be only minimally improved. Comparing the view group versus the nonview group, the view group showed very striking improvement. This suggests that the viewing experience does alter the clinical course of the patient and has an effect on the degree of patient improvement.

Referring to Table 2 we see that, in the group of depressive reactions, 11 out of 12 patients in both groups improved clinically as a result of

TABLE 1

Data Concerning Therapeutic Results of 80 Patients

	View Group	Nonview Group
1. Cured or maximally improved	19	5
2. Moderately improved	13	17
3. Minimally improved or unchanged	8	18
Total	40	40

their hospital experience. However, the 11 patients in the view group improved to a far greater degree than those patients in the nonview group. In the schizophrenic patients a significantly larger percentage showed clinical improvement in the view group as opposed to the nonview group.

The average length of stay for a patient in the view group was 24 days as opposed to an average of only 18 days for those patients in the nonview group. In addition, in the view group there were six patients who left the hospital in less than ten days, while in the nonview group there were 11 patients who left the hospital under ten days. One possible inference is that the viewing experience for the patient helped to involve him in therapy and was influential in his remaining in the hospital long enough to become involved in the total treatment situation. On the other hand, several patients in the view group had marked reactions to this experience after the first interview and were able to leave the hospital markedly improved in a very short time.

It was considered essential that the residents be independent observers in their evalutaion of the patients' clinical course and not be involved in the project per se. Of the 80 patients, on only 24 occasions did the resident actually know to which group the patient had been assigned. Analysis of this data showed that this knowledge concerning patients did not seem to influence the clinical judgments made. One other interesting result that was a tangential outcome of this study was that the two interviewing psychiatrists involved in the project both noted changes in their own interviewing techniques as the study went on. Both psychiatrists felt that they became more relaxed after using the television medium for several interviews. They also felt that they were able to recognize their interviewing faults and deficiencies as they viewed the playback and were able to correct them.

TABLE 2

Reaction Groups

Depressive reactions	View Group	Nonview Group
1. Cured or maximally improved	7	1
2. Moderately improved	4	10
3. Minimally improved or unchanged	1	1
Total	12	12

Schizophrenic Reactions		
1. Cured or maximally improved	2	0
2. Moderately improved	3	2
3. Minimally improved or unchanged	1	5
Total	6	7

COMMENT

The main finding of this study is that those patients in the view group, as opposed to the nonview group, showed significantly more clinical improvement as a result of the one added factor in their therapeutic regimen, namely the video-therapy experience.

In our research we were not directly concerned with the questions of if, how, or why psychotherapy works. In fact, it may be erroneous to try to explain or think about what happened to our patients in the context of any of the various kinds of psychotherapies, or even of using theoretical concepts, models, or ways of describing what occurs in psychotherapy. Certainly the video-therapy experience is a unique experience compared to any that a significant number of patients have experienced in the past. It could be so different that it requires a new approach to its understanding. For example, there seems to be a universal reaction by all who hear themselves on audio tape for the first time to be surprised, often displeased, and usually somewhat disbelieving. "Is what I'm hearing *me*? Is that how I really sound?" While we have not investigated just this aspect of a patient *seeing* oneself for the first time, it is truly a new and often unsettling experience for all the various people who watched themselves on video tape. However, our study itself was *not* a study of the self-image experiences of patients, but rather an investigation of the impact of a series of relatively structured interpersonal reactions (television interview and playback) during an emotional upset severe enough to require hospitalization.

Video therapy, as we call it, is *not* psychotherapy that is video taped and played back to the patient. Rather, it has several components—first, there is the structured interview done with no therapeutic attempt, per se, and recorded on video tape. This is followed immediately by the interviewer and patient seeing and hearing their interactions, and with subsequent interviews the interactions sequentially over a period of time.

The responses the patient made on a verbal level to the viewing experience seemed to fit in a fairly general pattern. It was noted by both psychiatrists that on the first viewing experience the patients uniformly referred to it as unpleasant and wondered why we were making them endure such a harrowing experience. However, on subsequent viewing occasions, usually after the patients had begun to note improvement, they reversed themselves and verbalized their feelings that this was no longer an unpleasant experience but had become a very meaningful and beneficial one. They also stated that they could see reasons for the viewing session and were no longer angry at the "unpleasantness" of the first exposure. Individual differences in responses were noted. For example, schizophrenic patients tended to pick out isolated parts of their behavior which they realized were sick behavior. Also, they called attention to their own loose associations and autistic thinking and made definite efforts to change this. On the other hand, the most dependent patients responded in a more dramatic way as far as their appearance and total behavior were concerned, usually with a marked emotional reaction often followed shortly by considerable clinical improvement.

A criticism raised was that the residents might have been biased, either consciously or unconsciously, and thus might have influenced the results. To control for this possibility we tried not to have the residents know to which group the patient belonged. We were successful in this except for approximately one-quarter of the cases, and the interesting thing noted was that in this quarter, as compared to the other three quarters, the scatter was comparable. Therefore, whether the resident knew or did not know did not seem to change the results obtained.

It must be emphasized that this was not a study of video therapy per se. That is, the patients were on an active, semiprivate teaching unit of a university hospital and received all of the usual therapies and attentions they might otherwise expect. The viewing was an added experience. The residents on our unit are the primary therapists, though they are very closely supervised. Individual therapeutic contact with the patients on the unit on the part of the staff members is discouraged. The two project psychiatrists doing the interviewing had no other scheduled individual contacts with the patients. Also, to our knowledge none of the patients knew that they were participating in any kind of a research project, or that they were being studied in any special way. With our extensive experience (since 1960) with patients of all types being televised, we cannot emphasize strongly enough how little difference this television interview seems to make to the patient. Only one patient admitted to the unit during this study refused the television interview.

One of the reasons why more elaborate rating systems were not used was that a large and extensive research project might have had an adverse effect on the patients and staff. Practically the only additional data we collected that is not routinely obtained on our patients was a record of the residents' knowledge of their patients' classification into the view or nonview group.

The degree of improvement was gauged at the time of discharge and the project did not take into account any adequate follow-up studies. How long the patients in the view group maintain this improvement is an important question that can only be answered with time and further studies. However, within the time of our study there was no increase in the readmission rate in the viewing group.

The final phase of this study will include an additional 80 patients. Forty consecutive patients will be studied at a time when patients are not routinely interviewed on television and none are undergoing the viewing experience. The last group of 40 patients all will have videotape interviews and all will see themselves on videotape.

SUMMARY

A total of 80 patients of varying diagnostic categories were randomly selected to be studied as a part of a survey project. These patients were interviewed by one of the two project psychiatrists in front of concealed television cameras, and videotape recordings were made of these interviews. The interviews were carefully structured with definite goals in mind. Of the 80, 40 saw themselves on the television screen immediately following the first interview, and after each subsequent interview they saw all prior segments in sequential order. The view group showed significantly $(0.01 \ \chi^2)$ more improvement than the nonview group. Improvement was gauged by independent observers who were unaware of the group to which the patient belonged. In addition, the experimenters involved in this project were not engaged in any therapeutic way with the patients on the unit.

It is acknowledged that there may be variables in this study which have not been adequately controlled, but it is suggested that a trend has been established. By design we did not change our protocol from patient to patient in any way for any reason. Thus, our video therapy technique suffers from a certain rigidity or lack of flexibility that can be eliminated when we have better criteria for its use. This might produce even more significant results. With present day technical advances in television and videotape equipment, this technique might greatly aid in the treatment of patients at a very small cost in terms of money or the time of scarce professional mental health personnel.

Further studies are in progress utilizing the television image as a specific part of therapy.

Technically, or even literally, video tape interviews can be the "giftie" in Robert Burns' poem. Can patients (people) given an exact replica of a sample of their behavior perceive this without significant distortion and utilize it? If so, then Robert Burns' stanza could summarize some possibilities.

> *O wad some Power the giftie gie us*
> *To see oursels as ithers see us!*
> *It wad frae monie a blunder free us,*
>   *An foolish notion.*
> *What airs in dress and gaid wad lea'e us,*
>   *An' ev'n devotion!*
> (From "To a Louse" by Robert Burns)

REFERENCE

1. Cornelison, F. S., and Arsenian, J.: Study of Responses of Psychotic Patients to Photographic Self-Image Experiences. *Psych. Quart.*, 34:1-8 (Jan.), 1960).

15
GROUP PSYCHOTHERAPY ON TELEVISION:
An Innovation with Hospitalized Patients

Frederick H. Stoller, Ph.D.

A recent innovation in the conduct of group therapy in a mental hospital setting took advantage of the presence of a closed-circuit television system. Regularly scheduled group therapy was conducted within the television studio and the proceedings broadcast to the television sets on the various wards. Participants in the groups were chronic hospitalized patients who, in the opinion of the staff, were not making any progress toward leaving the hospital. These patients were fairly representative of the largely chronic group of patients who have not responded to most efforts at rehabilitation. This paper will deal with the initial experience of conducting psychotherapy under such circumstances and will explore some of the implications of psychotherapy in an open, public setting.

A few words about the closed-circuit television station are in order and will provide an appropriate background for this innovation. Within the last few years, Camarillo State Hospital set up a television studio, operated under the auspices of the Rehabilitation Service for the purpose of creating and broadcasting programs of its own. The entire operation is handled by patients supervised and trained by two staff members. During the morning and afternoon hours of weekdays, this station has a regular schedule of programs imparting information, participant enter-

Reprinted from *American Psychologist*, Vol. 22, No. 2, February, 1967. The author wishes to express his gratitude to Tom Emmitt, supervisor of CSH-TV, whose active cooperation and encouragement made this innovation as successful as it was. The patient staff of CSH-TV also deserves particular commendation for the enthusiasm and resourcefulness they displayed in what was a novel and extremely difficult technical task. Special thanks is also due Larry Fielder who, in his former capacity of helping supervise the hospital television station in its formative years, also played a special role in helping set up this innovation.

tainment, and similar programs. Its purpose has been to serve the special needs of the hospital population rather than to supplant the programming of commercial television. It has a double role: a highly successful industrial therapy detail for a number of patients who work at the studio, and as an increasing part of the educational-recreational-therapeutic program of the hospital.

The idea of utilizing television for psychotherapy emerged from the author's experience in conducting a series of discussion groups on television. These groups followed the filming of movies on mental illness and consisted of rather abstract discussions of some of the problems outlined in the movies. Patients who participated in these discussions were relatively articulate and more likely to be in various stages of remission than in a chronic phase. In the experience of both the author and the participating patients. it was noted that the anticipatory anxiety so common with public performance was soon overcome once the actual performance commenced. The participants tended to conduct themselves in a highly creditable manner, somewhat to their own surprise. It would seem that performances of this sort tend to bring out the potential of individuals; that people tend to rise to the occasion when they are on public display. Within the context of providing continuity between behavior and self-expectancy, a successful series of performances could contribute to a dramatic alteration of the self-image held by individuals with histories of repeated failures.

With the idea that exposure plus the excitement involved in the conduct of television would provide an enhancement for the persons involved, a group of patients was sought who it was felt would particularly benefit from such an arrangement. The chronically hospitalized individual, particularly the chronic schizophrenic, constitutes a group whose characteristic self-debasement and retreat from social engagement represent elements which might be particularly well modified in such a setting. Initially, a group of 10 female patients was assembled, all of whom were chronically hospitalized, and many of whom were quite severely regressed. The public nature of the setting was exploited and interaction between the members of the group and the television staff was invited. Wards were invited to watch the proceedings, particularly the home wards of the patients. Initially, hand microphones were used and these had to be held up close to the mouth. It was felt that the close proximity of the microphone and television camera had a compelling effect and so would make withdrawal and silence less likely. At the beginning of the session, each of the participants was asked to introduce himself to the audience. This helped break the ice immediately.

Because of their unique quality, physical arrangements require a special note. The patients and the therapist sat in a tight circle and two television cameras constantly circled around the periphery of the circle, shifting to the various members of the group. In addition to the two cameramen, cable handlers accompanied each camera and another man handled the overhead microphone. Directors and other television staff occupied a control booth and, at any particular session, many visitors might be present. More often than not, 10 or more people were in the immediate environment of the group.

For the most part, the therapist focused the direction of therapy toward enhancing the interaction between individuals in the group and toward others in their environment, toward their static situation in the hospital, and toward steps they could take to remedy this as well as the self-image they had of themselves. Individuals were urged to take specific steps such as pursuing off-ward work details or approaching appropriate personnel concerning the initiating of leave planning. It was repeatedly emphasized that their present predicament was a function of their own passivity.

It should be emphasized that these patients were among the more regressed on their wards. Some had been hospitalized for as many as 14 years, others had rarely spoken for almost as many years. Some were actively delusional and all had exhausted the therapeutic efforts of the staff. As an example of the level of maturity at which they tended to function, one patient suggested, as an appropriate activity for the first session, that they pretend they were part of a big department store and that the therapist play he was the store owner and tell everyone what to do. For a number of patients, saying anything at all was an achievement. One young woman of about 24 years of age, who had been hospitalized since the age of 11, rarely uttered a word at any time.

Anyone who has attempted therapy with patients of this genre will know how difficult it is to obtain response of any kind from them. It was, therefore, quite gratifying to note the nature of the response induced through the modality of television. There was no question that a marked enhancement in the response of these patients over and above the usual format had occurred. Everyone responded to some degree and, as time went on, the increasing involvement of some individuals was quite marked. The response that they received from their home ward was one of excitement and recognition, a feature which was hardly part of their usual routine. Both ward personnel and fellow patients remarked on how well they had done and looked. The staff's perception of many of the patients changed remarkably because their actual behavior contradicted expectations most vividly.

As the number of sessions increased, and although novelty of the television medium wore off, its effectiveness as a therapeutic adjunct continued on a high level. The therapy session became the highlight of the week for the patients in a way in which routine group therapy rarely achieves. Concrete evidence of movement was apparent, not only in the manner in which the group functioned, but also in individual acts outside the therapeutic sessions. Some moved into off-ward work details and began to explore activities in the hospital about which they had not previously evidenced any awareness. Others began to seek out some ward activities in contrast to their previous inactivity. Some have left the hospital or are working on plans for leaving the hospital.

As some of the patients dropped out, a number of male patients were added so as to make a mixed group. As a group, the males received less feedback from their home wards than the initial female patients had and showed less dramatic evidence of movement. But even here, they responded in ways which were more gratifying than would have likely been the case had they been engaged in a group within a different context. One of these men froze the first few sessions, and appeared unable to say a word. Gentle pressure was exerted upon him every session, both by the therapist and by other patients who began to become adept at stimulating their fellow members into responding. After about three or four sessions in this manner, he suddenly began to talk in a free and open manner, to everyone's surprise.

Uncomfortable incidents were quite infrequent. At one time one of the patients began to cry openly and the therapist encouraged the group to handle her feelings in a very supportive manner. On many occasions patients have openly spoken in delusional fashion. However, it was the therapist's observation that psychotic verbalizing tended to decrease in frequency as the sessions became an established part of their routine. Most striking of all was the increased spontaneity of the group. During the initial session, the therapist did most of the talking and would direct himself toward individual patients a good deal of the time. The cameramen would maneuver their cameras wherever they saw the therapist direct his attention and so were able to focus the cameras on the appropriate speaker with relatively little difficulty. However, by the fourth and fifth sessions, the amount of spontaneity had increased to such a degree that the cameramen and director had difficulty anticipating who was going to speak next and often missed the initial parts of an interchange. While this was partly in response to the therapist's insistence that the members of the group address themselves to each other and the emphasis he placed on mutual help, it was also a function of the increasing ease with which these patients saw themselves in the framework of the television studio, broadcasting, and their growing involvement in the activity.

Subsequently, another group has been initiated with some slight changes in format. This group, while almost as chronic in terms of the number of years of hospitalization, tended to be somewhat younger in age and not quite as regressed. However, they were equally hopeless in the eyes of the staff and their status had become pretty well stabilized. Four males and five females constituted the second group and their spontaneity has moved with even greater speed than the first. Because of an improved sound system, the hand microphones used with the first group were dispensed with at no noticeable loss to the group's responsiveness.

A further innovation was attempted with this second group which shows very important promise. The first four sessions of this were videotaped and following the third session the group was invited to remain and view themselves. They accepted the invitation with great enthusiasm and watched a playback of the whole session. No attempt was made to deal with their feelings or impressions as they viewed themselves, but the matter was taken up with them during the next week's session. One patient remarked that he thought that he was speaking too much (he was) and he made a marked attempt to moderate his defensive verbosity. Another patient felt she had not spoken enough and made a visible attempt to increase her spontaneity. The use of videotape presents a possibility for immediate self-viewing and self-evaluation of one's impact on others which is unequalled by any other modality. The urge to look at oneself is apparently an irresistible one and even patients who seemed to have abandoned a considerable amount of their self-esteem cannot turn away from this. Its use in this fashion, although rather crude, would seem to hold a great deal of promise if accompanied by meaningful group discussion.

Subsequent work with videotape feedback has utilized what can be termed "focused feedback." It had been noted that when self-viewing is done in a passive fashion, patients tend to concentrate on aspects of their physical appearance rather than on meaningful elements of their interpersonal impact. By having the therapist focus on what he considers to be significant aspects of their manner of interacting, it was found that patients had the opportunity to see themselves within a meaningful framework. Under these circumstances, the opportunity for self-perception is unsurpassed. Videotape has the distinct advantage of immediate playback; the more this is delayed, the more chance of diluting the immediacy of this type of self-viewing.

One of the more surprising features of group therapy in a television studio is the degree of concentration which the members of the group tend to give to the group itself despite the multitudinous distractions which are an inherent part of the scene. Considering that we are dealing with chronic schizophrenics, whose general tangentiality, limited attention span, and tendency toward avoidance of interpersonal situations are such prominent characteristics, their degree of involvement suggests that some relatively unique phenomenon is operating.

In analyzing social functioning, Goffman (1) has used the analogue of the theatrical performance, pointing out that social roles can be likened to performances before an audience. He refers to groups of individuals banded together to maintain a common impression before a larger social group as teams. In this sense, the chronic hospital patient can be viewed as a one-man team rather than as belonging to a multi-individual team. It may be that the television group compels the patient to participate in a team which is literally performing before an audience. Such a multi-individual team is concerned about maintaining its performance and collective impression so that individuals within the team who damage the team image tend to be corrected by the other members. This phenomenon greatly resembles Bach's (2) observation that groups tend to push their members away from pathology. While this phenomenon is not absent in psychotic groups, the context of television seems to enhance it.

In this kind of an analysis, the therapist is very much a part of the team. He differs from the others only in that he may be more explicit about maintaining the performance and also provides a model for doing this. It should be emphasized that, in Goffman's terms, team performance is a ubiquitous and natural social phenomenon and the schizophrenic differs only in the degree to which he tends to avoid such participation. Viewed in this context, the presentation of group therapy in open sessions, before seen and unseen audiences, may not be as far removed from actual life situations as a first impression might imply.

Open therapy, that is, therapy conducted in a public forum, as opposed to the conventional closed-door private setting, has many implications for the manner in which the therapy is conducted. Moreno (3) has utilized audiences in psychodrama and very often the observers were used as part of the interaction. However, in television therapy, the only immediate interaction is with the studio staff and some observers within the studio. In Goffman's terms, the therapy group and the studio staff form a team for presenting a particular kind of social performance and, therefore, participate in mutual efforts to support a particular impression before the larger audience. The unseen viewers represent an audience with which no immediate interaction is possible but does, in many ways, represent the larger social scene we all face. Participating in the televised group gives the patient the opportunity to cooperate with others in performing before the world at large.

Mowrer (4) is one of the few who has seriously questioned the implication of privacy in the therapeutic endeavor. He has noted that privacy implies withdrawal and denial, a practice most patients have been engaging in for many years. He portrays conventional therapy in terms of a patient revealing long-hidden sins to another individual who will be equally as secretive about them as he was, perpetuating the attitude towards these sins. In actuality, a good portion of the psychotherapeutic movement has veered away from what Berne (5) has referred to as the game of "Archaeology," namely "digging up significant material." As Rotter (6) has stated in looking at recent trends:

The general overall trend is toward less emphasis on investigation of the past and interpretation of symbolic manifestations of the unconscious and more emphasis on dealing with the present, using the patient's relationship to the therapist in therapy as a source of learning. More recently, there has been increased interest in conceiving of the patient's difficulties in terms of inadequate solution of problems (p. 821).

This is particularly true for the field of group therapy, about which Rotter states:

The tendency is no longer to regard group therapy as a kind of mass situation with the same goals as individual psychotherapy. Rather it is regarded as a special situation where the patient has the opportunity to learn group norms, where he can be reinforced for social interest, and where he is able to learn about others' reactions to his own social behavior (p. 819).

Under the circumstances thus enumerated, the necessity for privacy and confidentiality can be challenged. In much of contemporary psychotherapy there is little attempt to unearth embarrassing facts about the patient nor to have him reveal aspects of himself which are ordinarily secretive or taboo. Rather, the kind of image he presents to the world is made explicit to the patient together with its consequences in terms of the kind of treatment he generally receives from the world (this is one specific reason why the use of videotape has such attraction as a possible technical enhancement to group therapy). With this approach to therapy the need for privacy and confidentiality is greatly reduced.

An undesirable concomitant of the usual secretive circumstances under which psychotherapy is generally conducted is the often negative misconceptions of the process that many individuals develop. It would be an impossible task to determine the proportion of persons who could profit from certain features of group therapy but who veer away from it under the mistaken impression that their personalities will be taken away from them or that their inherent weaknesses and inadequacies would be revealed in a destructive manner. The open exposure of psychotherapy, as it is actually conducted, would demonstrate to many that the process is far different from the general conception and that it is hardly the devastating and mysterious experience they anticipate. Unwittingly, many psychotherapists have perpetuated the conception of therapy as an arcane art so as to perpetuate their own omnipotent and magical image.

The impact of televised therapy on the audience is now being investigated. Informal inquiries have suggested there is an appreciable impact upon the audience that regularly observes group therapy. In many ways, television, with its intense close-ups that view the individual from a far closer vantage point than is customary in ordinary interaction, can foster intense identification. One should not underestimate the possible effect of this identification by chronic hospitalized patients when observing a group like themselves who struggle with their own inarticulateness and passivity and move toward more effectiveness. It has been observed that the patient TV staff has a tendency to respond to increased tension in the group with more erratic functioning in their various jobs, suggesting considerable impact.

There is much likelihood that, by having patients regularly observe televised group therapy, a more efficient utilization of trained therapists could be achieved. However, the probability is that it would be most effectively utilized if integrated with some more inclusive program. Television can only be a medium which educates and influences. It cannot be a substitute for personal interaction.

Group therapy on television is an innovation which has already shown evidence that it enhances the effectiveness of psychotherapy with the chronic schizophrenic. Exploration with a wider range of groups and the development of techniques exploiting the unique features of videotape are being undertaken. Training in psychotherapy as well as general education about therapy is also being explored. Perhaps most important of all is the light it casts on group processes by wrenching this common technique from its customary seclusiveness into an open, public setting.

REFERENCES

1. Goffman, E.: *The Presentation of Self in Everyday Life.* New York: Doubleday Anchor, 1959.
2. Bach, G. R.: *Intensive Group Psychotherapy.* New York: Ronald Press, 1954.
3. Moreno, J. L.: Psychodrama and Group Psychotherapy. *Sociometry,* 9:249-253, 1946.
4. Mowrer, O. H.: Payment or Repayment? The Problem of Private Practice. *American Psychologist,* 18:577-580, 1963.
5. Berne, E.: *Transactional Analysis in Psychotherapy.* New York: Grove Press, 1961.
6. Rotter, J. B.: A Historical and Theoretical Analysis of Some Broad Trends in Clinical Psychology. In S. Koch (Ed.), *Psychology: A Study of a Science.* Vol. 5. *The Process Areas, the Person, and Some Applied Fields: Their Place in Psychology and in Science.* New York: McGraw-Hill, 1963. Pp. 780-830.

AFTERTHOUGHTS*

"Group Psychotherapy on Television: An Innovation with Hospitalized Patients"

Frederick H. Stoller, Ph.D.

Reviewing a paper written some years ago gives one a strange feeling, particularly in terms of how much more candid one can be about past work. I find myself taken aback by the degree to which I had incorporated the values and goals of the mental hospital system and how I attempted to weave a web of justification through theoretical sanctions. Viewed from the vantage point of some years of subsequent experience I would now place much greater emphasis upon how one can affect the particular setting involved and the implications of open therapy for practitioners. The potential of videotape requires no further amplification here.

I no longer can view the mental hospital in as sanguine a fashion as I had. It is clearly a setting in which the very condition which we have

---

* The editor asked the author F. Stoller to write these "afterthoughts" because of the provocative nature of material in the article.

been trying to deal with (that is, chronic institutionalization rather than chronic mental illness) is fostered. Withdrawal, apathy and passivity are enhanced through the years by a massive dose of blandness: the surroundings, the routinization, the suppression of anything resembling excitement, passion, significant movement between people. The mental hospital is a deadening environment; as a space in which to exist it is somewhere between an emotional desert and an experiential slum. From time to time a new therapeutic movement enters the scene and things happen: an air of excitement has crept into the environment.

It should be clear that, in some way, this was being attempted through televised group therapy but became tempered by caution. The initial selection of patients for whom the staff held out little hope can now be seen as an escape clause on my part. An all too typical staff attitude had been adopted: there is nothing much you can do to harm these people and therefore it is alright to experiment with them. Besides, if you fail, who can blame you? The initial sessions did have an excitement about them—after all the endeavor was new and no one knew whether it would work or end up in disaster. But this impact abated as the sessions became matter of fact and it is now clear to me that I tended to play it safe and risk relatively little in what went on during these sessions. What might have been an attempt to alter the environment, to provide a richer emotional input and to color the atmosphere in a particular way became much too attenuated.

We all tend to find equilibrium for ourselves and much of what we watch on commercial television allows us to remain minimally touched. Yet when we become witness to such events as both Kennedy assassinations, television has the capacity to move us visibly. It is this capacity which I would utilize to the fullest in the hospital situation were I to repeat the experiment today. Instead of being so careful of what was revealed upon the screen I would exert myself to the utmost, both through the selection of patients and through what I introduced into the group sessions, to make them as impactful and stunning as I possibly could. I would not hesitate to have the group members touch one another, hold one another, cry, lash out in anger, even physically, express their loving feelings in a physical as well as in a verbal way, and in general create the most forceful experience I could manage. Since all therapeutic groups require time for development when impact on viewers is likely to be minimal, I would not hesitate to take advantage of the editing capabilities of videotape.

Watching television is much too passive an activity for such patients and it is only when we make it a stirring event that we change the context of such an experience. In addition, the very environment of the hospital setting does things to people, and in this I include the staff. Consequently, I would bring in therapists from outside the hospital and would seek out impactful individuals whose personal style was distinctive. I would encourage the formation of therapeutic groups which would use these sessions as points of departure. But above all I would try to alter the flavor of what took place in the hospital.

Whether or not anyone actually watched the therapy sessions, they *could* be watching so that I, personally, always felt my behavior under surveillance. This experience turned out to be one of the most frightening and growth-inducing of my career. Since I have moved away from the hospital setting and the open therapy made possible by the television station, I have found myself more willing to reveal myself to my patients. Thus, I do not hesitate to acknowledge difficulties in which I currently find myself if they should be kicked off by group members.

My own movement toward greater openness was not caused by my television experience but it was certainly enhanced by it. It is my conviction that it is the therapist who has the most immediate gain to be made by engaging in open therapy. It is therapists who are really much more anxious about revealing themselves and letting themselves be seen by their colleagues than the general public. In actuality, it was easier to get patients to volunteer for this activity than it was to get other therapists to do so. It should be obvious that therapists learn their art under supervision where a high degree of critical evaluation is fostered. Once outside the training situation, practitioners attain and maintain their reputation by how well they "talk therapy." They describe their own work to each other in a highly colored fashion that is clearly competitive and designed to impress. It is well known that there is considerable discrepancy between what therapists say they do and what they actually do. There is, finally, the relative invulnerability of remaining unknown. The more one presents a version of one's self rather than an actual sample, the more easy it is to defend one's self.

Given my subsequent experience, I would stress that every therapist who has access to a television system which would enable him to function in an open therapy situation owes it to himself to take advantage of it. Just as I am convinced that the most serious effects of our total institutions are not on the inmates as we like to think but upon the staff who choose to remain in such environments, so I think that the most serious effect of secretive therapy is upon the practitioner. Given experiences in open therapeutic settings, they are much more likely to be flexible and free in their subsequent work. The ultimate beneficiary would, of course, be the patient. But a closed, tight person pays a considerable price for his caution and, if his work enhances this tendency, the price is even greater. It is as true for therapists as it is for patients.

Ultimately it is necessary to make the distinction between the therapeutic model in which one does something for people as well as to them and the experiential model in which people explore ways in which they choose to live. Given the latter model it no longer becomes a question of obligatory secrecy or openness. Rather, it is opportunities to explore and try new ways of living which should be provided. To the degree that therapists do not explore, for themselves, new possibilities for conducting themselves, they tend to remain fearful for the patients with whom they work. If we can conceive of a world in which people have greater options to pick and choose how they want to conduct their lives and are provided with the opportunities for such exploration, we can see the open-therapy situation as a potentially freeing one in which people do not *have* to hold on to secrecy if they do not want to. However, it is inconceivable how therapists can lead people to move further than they themselves have moved. While therapeutic caution may reflect concern for people's welfare, it also reflects an extremely restricted view of life and living.

16

THE USE OF VIDEOTAPE IN THE INTEGRATED TREATMENT OF INDIVIDUALS, COUPLES, FAMILIES AND GROUPS IN PRIVATE PRACTICE

Milton M. Berger, M.D.

As more and more private practitioners realize the almost boundless potential for the constructive use and flexible integration of video into psychotherapeutic practice with individuals, families and groups, I predict its use will expand rapidly within the next decade. Personal communications and correspondence with colleagues throughout the country have indicated that there is a heartening interest in, but still somewhat limited use of, video in the private practice of psychiatry.

Video enhances the clarity of one's psychic, emotional, behavioral and body identity. In addition, the practitioner's interest in using this new modality constitutes a communication to the patient that the therapist is actively involved in risk-taking and experimentation towards greater therapeutic effectiveness. The impact of the therapist as a model for his patients, a newer and healthier model than they have heretofore been closely involved with in relationships, has often been documented. As patients can identify with the therapist's capacity for acting with responsible freedom and flexibility, they become potentially enriched as they develop and incorporate the concept of new options for themselves.

Videotape playbacks can be used in psychiatric treatment by a therapist with any theoretical view of personality dynamics which acknowledges: subconscious or hidden motivation for one's behavior or attitudes; the significance of signs and symbols which regulate and arrange relationships; resistance; transference and the impact of the concomitant communication of emotion, behavior and thoughts through multiple levels and multiple channels in human relationships. Therapists interested primarily

173

in modifying behavioral states by suggestion, direction, education or desensitization methods can also utilize video constructively to some degree.

More and more manufacturers have entered upon the production of low-cost videotape recorders and it is possible to install a useful, mobile system in one's office for a minimum price of two to three thousand dollars. When one considers that general practitioners as well as other medical specialists and dentists spend many thousands of dollars for technical equipment in their professional offices, whereas psychiatrists have to spend little or nothing for the purpose of professional equipment, it becomes then a matter of simple education and alteration of habit pattern for psychiatrists to realize that it is in their interest to add special equipment not only for the welfare of their patients but also for their own heightened satisfaction and fulfillment in the practice of psychiatry. It is also important to remember that the cost of special equipment is tax deductible. For an inexpensive installation to be used primarily in private practice the one-half inch Sony system is probably the best at this time. However, video cassette systems are most prevalent in the United States at present, particularly in institutional settings.*

It is not only through self-confrontation with a single immediate or past experience in psychotherapy that patients are constructively affected via videotape. Therapeutic impact is also made in a deeper and more effective manner through repeated opportunities to observe, perceive and integrate the image or picture of self alone or in interaction with others over a period of time. Despite my 36 years in psychiatry, it is my opinion that the component processes in working through towards emotional as well as intellectual insight and change in psychotherapy are not completely known. They go beyond recall, free association, abreaction, catharsis, connecting past and present, transference, reality testing, corrective emotional experiences, identification, universalization, education and maturation. The aforementioned processes and systems which are mediated through various communicational media and channels as well as those processes and systems which are operant but still unknown to us function more effectively in the service of working through when the psychotherapeutic process has incorporated in it the intermittent benefit of closed circuit or television playback.

It is worth repeating the axiom that the "hardware" must function in the service of the patient rather than the patient's interests becoming

---

* See Chapter 28, this volume, for a more detailed statement by a video specialist on the nature and use of equipment involved in audio and visual recording.

subservient to the equipment. The "hardware" must not dictate therapeutic strategy nor interfere with the basic relationship of trust between patient and therapist. It is important, too, to remind the private practitioner of psychiatry that the professional, ethical, moral, personal and legal concerns for his patients' welfare include attention to the issues of privacy and privileged communication. Though written permission is not usually required in a private office for use of a videotape which the patient is assured by his therapist will be destroyed afterwards or not shown to anyone else, it is considered crucial to obtain a signed statement of permission if the tape is to be used for teaching, research or demonstration purposes. Although a narcissistic, hysteric, masochistic or exhibitionistic patient may give signed permission in advance for use of a videotape whose reproduction or replay to others is clearly not in the patient's interest, it may rest on the therapist's judgment and integrity to decide not to share such a tape with others. (In Chapter 26 of this volume, you will find a detailed statement concerning the issues of privacy and privileged communication by Rosenbaum who expresses specific concern that the rights and welfare of the patient not be violated.) Such determinations go far beyond simple legal considerations, involving as they do deep humanistic concerns. (See Chapter 25 by Fields on legal implications and complications.)

INTRODUCING VIDEOTAPE TO PATIENTS

There are various methods of introducing the use of videotape to patients:

1. *"Res ipse loquitor"*—means "the thing speaks for itself." With videotape cameras, recorder and microphones fully exposed in my office, it is most unusual for a person coming into the room not to notice them and not to question their purpose within the first few sessions. When I notice the patient looking at the equipment, I may ask, "What reactions are you having to the presence of this equipment?", thus flushing out what may otherwise remain unspoken and preparing the patient for the time, perhaps even in our first encounter, for using this adjunct to psychotherapy.

2. *The "fait accompli"*—the lights, cameras, videotape recorder and monitors are placed in operation just prior to asking the patient or family or group into my office. As they walk in and notice the equipment is working, I may say (a) "I thought you might enjoy getting a more complete look at yourself today, okay?" or (b) "Do you think you're ready to risk a more open look at yourself? I think you are and it will speed up our work together, okay?"

3. *The "advance notice"*—as a psychotherapeutic session is coming to an end, I may say, "I'm hoping you'll agree to our using the videotape equipment in our next session. How do you feel about it?" Nearly 100% of the time the response is "Okay, if you think it will be of any value," or "Okay, but I want you to know I'm anxious about it." I usually respond with questions such as, "What are you anxious about? What do you fantasy?" The response to these questions may reveal much that has not been so clearly stated and made available before concerning the patient's self-image, degree of narcissism, and fear of "really" being known or seen by someone else, even the therapist.

4. *The "seduction"*—is brought about over a period of time by the therapist intermittently making suggestive, intriguing remarks in different sessions such as, "It's too bad we don't have the video system in operation today. It would be of real value if I could replay the last few minutes of what's gone on between us." Or, "I sure wish I could play back your facial and hand movements as you said that!" Or, "I've just been using the video with my last patient, would you like for us to use it today?" Or, with a couple or group, the therapist may suggest using the video while remarking, "It'll help us to really see what goes on between you to trigger off the difficulties you're having with each other."

It is of marked therapeutic value to elicit the patient's reactions or fantasies in anticipating his first audiovisual self-confrontation. Significantly laden, though mostly unpredicted, free associations are often expressed by patients just prior to self-confrontation via closed circuit television of videotape playback in response to the question, "What is going on in you now as you are about to experience yourself in this new way?"

The usual advance reaction of adults has been to use the imminent self-confrontation as a social situation calling for self-criticism. The examples which follow support the conclusions of Bahnson, which differ with the notion formulated by many theoreticians that the self-image is "a kind of homunculus existing within the person, ready for inspection on command—very much like a photograph, which at will can be pulled out of a hip pocket, looked at and then put back." Bahnson emphasizes that, "such concepts of self-image as a circumscribed cognitive phenomenon may be comfortable to work with, but they are a far cry from the complex and intricate experiences people have of themselves" (1).

For example, Clarissa, a 20-year-old, shy, immature, single, bright, attractive art student who is inhibited to the point of being at times frightened when with people, responds to my question about her reaction to the possible use of the videotape equipment by saying: "When

I walked in I assumed you must be interested in photography—maybe motion pictures. Then I thought maybe it's of use in your professional work. Then I thought it might be to take pictures of me. Then that that was stupid. (long silence) The idea absolutely terrifies me. (What idea?) The idea of being watched. (What about it?) It has to do with hiding. I tend to build up little fronts which aren't really me—and if someone is *really* watching, they're bound to see the *real* me. (silence) I know logically I don't have anything to hide. (So what do you hide?) I hide feelings—negative feelings—hate feelings—tense feelings—anxieties. When my feelings are hurt, a lot of times I don't show that—I can't take criticism—I react like inside I don't want to react and I try to hide that. I act very blasé—when I was younger people used to think I was self-assured but inside I was a nervous wreck and I show it more now. I also don't show love or liking. I'm embarrassed to show I like a boy a lot. Then there is the other thing about hiding my body. I never wear very tight clothes—that's hiding—but there is a little part of me that wants to be found out and hopes I'll still be liked. (Liked is the same as being accepted?) Yes . . . (she said as she continued on about being understood). (I commented, I have a feeling that you're confused about being liked—understood and accepted.) Yes, and I explode once in a while because I'm so angry and confused at being this way. Then I feel guilty and feel terrible but I can't help it. I realize I am that way."

She sits silently, looking dejected, with her eyes getting red and moist, but unable to cry. I point out to her how almost all feelings seem to be forbidden—are negative for her and that she has little inner permission to cry even in rationally appropriate moments like this. She then cries a little and I ask for her associations—her feeling reactions—to what has emerged. She continues: "As a kid my parents would be pleased if we were well-behaved, which meant being non-reactive—sitting like little statues. My mother has told me she realizes now how foolish this was and that what she thought was healthy wasn't really so and that she's realized how ridiculous it was to expect us to conform to the world. My father doesn't come into the picture (stated disappointedly). He allowed my mother to raise us—my brother and I. (He just wasn't there for you. You had a father and yet you didn't. What are your feelings now?) I love my father and don't feel it right to be angry with him. I wish my father were more manly. He lets my mother take over. He'll just sit by and watch and say nothing as my brother, mother and I have a big argument. I realize too that my father is the real puritan in the family. (silence) My father thinks sex is more like the icing on the cake—whereas my mother thinks it's more natural. I think my father is terribly inhibited and my mother is less so." Her train of associations reveals an interconnected mixture of superficial and deep thoughts and feelings involved with her I and her not-I, her self and her family, their attitudes and values and hers in past and present.

Some verbatim responses to the question, "What do you anticipate the effect of video playback will be?" have been as follows:

Michael, a handsome, well-built, 25-year-old, intensely driven, single, American-born male whose Dale Carnegie compulsively helpful approach to psychotherapy stirs up an image of the last of the Wild West cowboys galloping after the last of the Western steers, says: "It's gonna be exciting to see ourselves as others see us. It'll be quite an adventure! My immediate thought just now was that I'd try to impose a more attractive audiovisual personality on myself. It's funny, but I'm more excited about it for other members of the group—like Randy, who's been told of her sullen, pouty, removed posture. This might shock her out of it! I'm excited for myself too. So much of the time I assume a little crouched off contracted posture and it'll be interesting seeing when I feel it if I do assume it and how much. I think there's so few times when I just feel big—feel all there—like a man. There are times when I'm able to relax into that after I ask myself why am I crouching over. What bothers me most is my passivity, which I feel is feminine. . . ."

Aron, a self-effacing 34-year-old, intellectual, repressed, detached, bachelor accountant raised by a typically dominating, overprotective and guilt-provoking mother and an ineffectual, submissive, undemonstrative father, said: "I feel it'll be experimental and am afraid it'll add something artificial which would interfere especially at the beginning. Positively, I think it'll bring home to the people how they react to people and situations—to see how they sit like turds. I'd like to see how I react to thoughts and communications and to listen to my voice and change in timbre. And if I do change in group I think I'll bring these changes into my outside life. At the beginning I think the changes will be artificial; that is, if I see I'm sitting in a slovenly position I'll pull myself up and together. It won't be coming from within but it'll be good for me to change my position. It'll help me in my business, and seeing how I hold and carry myself and how others see me—and I want to change and give me more confidence in myself. Also the fact that I can look at a screen will bring the other group members into a perspective I can't get now. It'll be easier to see everybody else in the group that way."

A 28-year-old attractive, detached, markedly alienated, compartmentalized and extremely intellectual mother of a sickly child, who is separated from her actor-puppeteer husband and who has sought solutions for her underlying depression and loneliness through LSD and hypnosis, spontaneously remarked on first seeing the newly installed videotape equipment in my office as she came into her group session: "I'm angry about it. I'm afraid it means more mechanization and more depersonalization and distraction. I immediately think of Orwell's *1984*." She then pulled into herself with a disparaging belittling frown and almost hid her presence in the pillows of the couch as she looked down and away from others in her group, taking occasional peeks at them and me from the corners of her eyes.

Andy, a 33-year-old, alienated, untrusting, suspicious, bachelor psychologist raised by a hostile, paranoid father and an inconsistent, frequently absent mother, reacted to the possibility of our using videotape playback by saying: "To be observed means failure. It means to look stupid, inept and that I'll be the laughingstock as I was a child—and I truly feel stupid. (Do you though?) Sometimes I don't, but 95% of the time I feel I'll be laughed at—held in contempt—ridiculous—idiotic—untrained—a phony—a fool. . . ." Andy functions in therapy like a classical help-rejecting complainer (2).

Joshua, a 27-year-old psychiatric resident, saw the new audiovisual equipment in my office as he walked in for his group session and said: "I don't see it as being of much potential value. I believe I know and see what I do and how I am with others. I feel I need to know more of what's going on inside me which keeps me as I am. I see it as a spectacular gimmick which doesn't get to what really bothers us." He said all this without actually going through an experience with the equipment and in fact was attempting to discourage me from using it with him.

However, a few days later, Joshua was much taken with the videotape playback during his individual psychotherapy session. Initially he stated he felt overwhelmed with the impact of the awareness of how much of an adolescent child he still is. He noted and commented upon the fact that whether he is angry, smiling or happy that he is consistently speaking like, looking like, pleading like, cajoling like and feeling like a child. He could now begin to question with much deeper and healthier motivation his need to send nonverbal cues with his boyish "Please don't hit me, I'm lovable" head tilt and smile, so that he would arrange for others to treat him as a boy and not as a man. He said: "I see myself coming through so subdued and watered down I could vomit! I cover up feelings and dress them up with words. It's sickening how I look so winsome and helpless." In a session months later he remarked, "The videotape has certainly helped me to expand my observing ego!"

IMPACT TO SELF-IMAGE

It is quite common for a patient being self-confronted on the monitor of a closed circuit television system for the first time to make an immediate attempt to reconstitute his idealized image of himself by sitting up straighter, or pulling in his waist or straightening out his hair or tie. He then turns his head in different directions to self-experience how he comes through to others from those vantage points. I use a two-camera system with four monitors and often move the cameras and monitors into positions to give the patient the most opportunities to simultaneously experience his body and self-image that he has ever had. Following the initial self-critical reaction and the acts of self-image restoration, a patient who is not too overwhelmed with self-hate may begin to note and comment on some favorable aspects of himself. This is a favorable prognostic sign.

Immediate impact image reactions occur when the patient is able to watch himself on one or more television monitors during a psychotherapeutic session. In my office, with its one mobile camera and its fixed-to-the-wall remote control camera as well as four monitors, I can easily arrange the patient's chair position so that he can look at me or himself on the monitor while a camera is recording a full view of him. He can thus observe his face, hand and body movements and expressions while he is talking. I ask patients to observe whether or not their facial and body expressions are in harmony with their verbal content and inside feelings and to share with me reactions concerning their disharmony as the session goes on.

A variety of responses to such immediate closed circuit self-confrontation can occur and I tend to use this approach cautiously in suicidal patients or those whose self-hate is narcissistically or realistically based on their body image. The use of this equipment is different at times in private practice than in institutional settings.

There are different types of reactions to immediate image confrontation the first time it is experienced and when it is experienced on later occasions. An example of a profound reaction was registered by Mildred, a 35-year-old single teacher whose self-effacement and high standards for herself have caused her much pain and little real self-esteem despite her physical endowments of a good figure and good looks, her high intellectual potential and her artistic, esthetic talents in sculpturing and interior decorating. She came to therapy because of her inability to create a sustained relationship with a responsible loving man which might lead to marriage.

During our second individual session, she agreed to the use of the videotape system as I suggested it would be of marked value for her. She sat silently looking at herself in the monitor, twisted her head from side to side while looking herself over critically and commented: "I don't look as stiff as I usually look. The muscular tensions don't show as much as I feel them. People have often said I looked very calm when I wasn't, when I felt scratchy and tense. So it seems I think I show more about myself than I really do. (How do you feel about this?) It's all right. (Just all right?) It's fine. I feel like I still have a hiding place. (What do you have to hide?) My private room, my privacy, my thoughts I don't want to share and my feelings I don't want to show. It seems I then have more charge of me. More of me is at the disposal of my will. (You feel not as vulnerable, not as frail . . . to what?) To public exposure. (She smiles now.) (You smile like you've got a big secret.) The words sounded so loaded, like I was carrying around a big secret. (What's the secret?) At that moment I was thinking about a man in my office I've got a crush on and that if the office gets hold of this they'll have a lot of fun. (You mean ridicule you?) Yes, it'll get on the wire. Many times in life I felt very self-conscious and thought here I am making a perfect ass of myself and yet maybe others never think of me that way at all.

"When your feelings are known to others you can, that is, I can, be hurt and I often expect to be hurt and I anticipate it. It's not a very vigorous kind of attitude. Other people avert so they're just not hurt. Or if they're hurt, so what? It doesn't destroy them, but I for some reason feel destructible. (Are you?) (she smiles) No, I'm not, literally. I tend to survive. I don't think I'm the kind who'd have a complete nervous collapse unless things were really terrible. (Like what?) Like if everybody I loved died right away and I woke up the next morning without a family, without friends. I don't know why this feeling of being exposed—I always relate it to being humiliated, that's not like nervous collapse—like being destroyed—just humiliated. (What do you recall about being humiliated?) I don't recall. Oh, I'm sure this has to do with my father. The only time I can think of is probably not the crucial time. In adolescence when I started to wear makeup all wrong, at thirteen, he'd suddenly attack me and call me 'liver lips' and accuse me of rolling in the flour barrel because I wore too much make up. He obviously didn't like it and he was saying in his way 'What an unattractive girl you are' and here in my own way I was groping to be attractive and be pretty. I'd just get up and leave the table in tears. (What are you feeling now?) Sort of sad. Feeling sorry for the girl who fled from her family's dinner table because her father scoffed at her. Mother was there. She agreed with Daddy. I always wondered what on earth they thought they were doing. I put on so much powder because I had so many pimples. I always wondered why they didn't try to help me do it right. Mother's attitude was that one shouldn't call attention to oneself. I got confused about contradictory messages they gave. I saw Mother and Daddy nude until I went away to high school at age 16 or 17. I'd see them nude swimming in Maryland at our island in summer and at home nude in their bedroom and in the bathroom. They were quite casual about it. (Were there sexual feelings between you and your father?) I don't remember having any. (pause) One time when I was 16 he patted my breasts and I was slightly shocked. Now I'm thinking 'Well, that nasty, sly old man, poking his daughter to see how she was developing, sort of investigating.' (Did it occur to you that perhaps he was doing more than objectively investigating; that he was perhaps doing something for himself?) Oh, no. It surprised me because it was without any precedent. He is an old exhibitionist even now at 70. One time he came to New York City to visit me—I had a roommate. My father was sitting around in his shorts with his penis hanging out—serving drinks. I was shocked and after a while said: 'Is that all you are going to put on?' and he said he'd put more on if I wanted him to."

The basis for Mildred's coming through to me as perplexed and not trusting was amply defined. The background for her confusion and denial about her sexual and other feelings became increasingly clear to me as being grounded in parental double-binding, oedipal ambivalence and conflict as well as guilt and anger which had to be denied or repressed. It has been difficult to help Mildred to gain insight leading toward a healthier self-image as well as to move toward greater self-assertiveness and self-esteem because of the tenacity of her defensive systems.

WORKING THROUGH

Videotape playback of a portion of an individual psychotherapy session can be profoundly helpful in working through. In the following example, the playback helped to expose underlying dynamics which had impeded constructive growth in the patient for a long time. Her seeming passivity and guardedness with me in psychotherapy sessions were the transferential expression of a security stratagem which literally and figuratively was life-preservative for her.

Dorothea, 33-year-old single, American-born, self-effacing, quiet, unobtrusively dressed, passively sitting social worker, whose voice was usually flat, controlled, drab and colorless, was transfixed as she watched herself during the first playback in an individual session. For 15 minutes we watched the monitor revealing the stillness of her body as she sat rigid, fixed, almost as if paralyzed except for some movements of her hands, face and neck. This brought her to quiet tears and almost expressed anger, and she remembered and talked about having been raised in 12 different homes of relatives from age two to seven. Her father had died when she was two. She recalled hearing her mother say to her over and over again, thousands of times: "Be good! Be obedient! Mind! Don't give anyone any trouble. I worry if I were to die, and it could happen maybe tomorrow or the next day or next year, then who would take care of you? If they had trouble raising you, you'd go to an orphans' home."

Up to this point, I, as therapist, had been encouraging her to move towards greater mobility in her personal and interpersonal living, not knowing that, unconsciously, greater mobility for Dorothea meant the threat of abandonment. We had both been stimulated to react to the degree of her physical immobility when I presented the playback without sound at both regular and fast-forward speeds.

Herb, a 32-year-old aggressive, alienated, argumentative university instructor had come for psychotherapy one year previously during a hypomanic agitated state. His cynicism and distrust had diminished enough to allow him to participate in a playback of his individual session without insisting it would be "just a waste of time." He stated in a subdued and poignant manner, "I didn't realize I'm in such agony. I'm really suffering! I didn't know I could be so serious. I'm not as bad looking as I thought I was. I see I'm alert and as fast as I thought I was. I respond to you. And, (laughingly) I don't have as bad a Brooklyn accent as I thought I had. I see the way I'm closed-minded, opinionated and manipulate things 'cause I'm in such pain. I see how I have no tolerance for you; I'm so queasy and restless. I'm also heavy, I didn't realize I was that heavy. Have to do something about that.

"This has given me a lot of confidence in myself. I didn't realize I express myself as well as I did. Though I'd like to have alertness and sparkle in my eyes—not so much pain. I didn't realize I grimaced so much, though people have told me. I thought I'd show more disdain and found I didn't.

"And did you notice? (gleefully) I don't chew my glasses as much. In fact, I didn't chew them once today and I used to chew them all the time."

Another patient, John, observed himself intensely and then stated quietly with marked control:

"I don't recognize that guy as myself. I pity the poor soul. I saw him as cold—like a Mediterranean punk, with sort of a conceit and complacency—even a blandness to him." (John, the third child in a wealthy, alienated family, raised mostly by governesses, gave up early, ruled out love and emotion in his life.) "I felt I'd climb on top of the world, so they'd have to respect me. I lumped together my mother, father, sisters and others—'friends' who had rejected me. I went for intellect. I feel this terrible hatred for my parents (said real coolly). I really feel guilty about this. I have the school kids' admiration for the Bogarts—the cool—the strong—the unfeeling—the tough—and it's how I used to fancy myself too. A few years ago I'd have admired that punk. Now I saw the agony in his soul. Now I'm in a state of changing values about feeling. Before it was intellect—intellect—intellect! Now it's being a mensch and feeling."

Henry, a 25-year-old furniture designer struggling with homosexual conflicts, responds to his first videotape playback by remarking, "My voice is deeper and perhaps more masculine than I thought. It's interesting—I do not get any pleasure from it—it's interesting. (How do you feel about how you look?) I don't like the way I look—my forehead—my eyes—I never realized how slanty and slit they are—they're ugly. I don't like them—I feel nothing more than describing—like I am editorializing. I do smile a lot. (How do you feel about that?) I think it's strange—I don't know why I'm doing it—it's strange."

"I don't like some of the motions I make with my eyes—movements—motions (What are they?) the closings, the openings—just that they seem so effeminate. I don't like the motions—there is just too much fluttering. The whole face is too—it—uh—is it overreacts—too much—so many inflections to every sentence—to every word—it's overreacting in my face—the eyebrows keep moving—there's so much expression—it's an overexpression. I talk phony too—I drag with a drawl. I think it's amusing to sit here and see myself.

"I move around a lot like a player piano according to one of my friends. My life is like that—I'm at the wrong speed—like I go so fast. I saw this on the television—I saw all these fast movements—the hands, the mouth, the eyes. (I cringe as I listen to you contrive to disown yourself.) I never realized how fast and jerky these movements are—the way I live must be like that too. I'm just so anxious to get on to the next thing—the next event—I never spend a quiet moment. . . ."

Another patient, Harold, a bright, "eager-beaver," 31-year-old single "up and coming" executive in an advertising agency had come into therapy primarily because of homosexuality. His often absentee, self-effacing and ineffectual father had not served as an adequate male model while his guilt-provoking, aggressive mother had raised him as her bedmate until he was fourteen and her confidante until he went off to college. Following his first videotape playback he sat stunned, astonished and silent while tears welled in his big sad eyes. Suddenly he shouted exultantly: "I look like a man! I sound like a man! I'm not really a fag at all." A common immediate reaction to the playback is to be pleased or displeased with the evidence of one's masculinity or femininity.

An example of video's long-term impact in working through is seen with Sandy, a 24-year-old, intellectual, alienated, single college graduate who saw herself on videotape replay in her group after not having seen herself on video for three months. She commented: "I saw how much I operate as a therapist, trying to analyze what goes on in others rather than feeling or reacting to or in myself in a personal way. Although I still saw more facial glumness than I'd like to see and my hair looked raggedy, I had a stronger feeling of liking myself than ever before. I remember initially how I had cringed as I watched the playback, not believing it was me. Though I still felt disconnected with the me on the screen I was fascinated with what I saw. Instead of being overwhelmed as before with the discrepancy between the me I saw and the me I envisioned myself as, I now saw and felt the me in the playback was a real, alive person with whom I could identify. I saw myself as intelligent, sometimes attractive, gesturing a lot when I talked, sometimes whining yet sometimes with a sense of humor, holding back quite a bit of frustration and anger which I saw coming out in movement—a physical boundness I remembered feeling at times during the part of the session played back which was the way I felt a lot in my childhood. But mainly I was glad to be meeting again with myself, a person I now was feeling I liked a great deal."

Insight which is more than intellectual may be promoted and integrated through repeated playbacks. For example, a real "Ah Ha!" experience can occur when a patient can see and hear how his repeated help-rejecting complaining leads his peer group members to wind up irritated and frustrated with him, finally refusing to focus on him any longer during a specific group meeting as he dismisses, puts down or otherwise wipes out their suggestions, advice, reactions or interpretations. Alger and Hogan emphasize the "second-chance" phenomenon through the use of videotape playback which allows patients to become aware that the feelings experienced at the time of the original interactional situation were actually not clearly conveyed to others. As an individual becomes aware of this during replay and realizes the discrepancy between what seems to be shown by his behavior on the screen and what he actually remembers feeling, he can clarify through a second communication the feelings he had inadequately expressed before with a resultant improvement of the relationship between those involved. Alger and Hogan, who are also markedly impressed with the value of videotape in the private practice of psychiatry (see Chapter 20), have noted that the emotional insights enhanced through videotape playback, when added to the more common intellectual insights achieved in psychotherapy, are more likely to bring about significant behavioral changes in patients (3).

Geertsma (4) has pointed out that those of us involved in work with videotape, whether it be referred to as "self-image experience," "focused feedback," "self-confrontation," or "self-observation," are operating "on the assumption that externally mediated self-cognition is potentially a powerful technique in psychotherapy and behavior modification." To the degree that video provides for greater depths of observation, perception and cognition which are interrelated processes basic to psychotherapeutic progress, it is indeed a powerful technique.

The process of bringing about awareness in the service of working through and furthering motivation towards change, following emotional as well as intellectual insight, is enhanced when a patient is given the opportunity for intermittent self-confrontation via videotape playback.

An example of the impact of *focused feedback confrontation* with videotape is revealed in reviewing the progress of Aron, the previously mentioned 34-year-old successful accountant suffering with emotional illiteracy, who has severe relationship problems with men as well as women because of his distrust and fear of intimacy. He came to therapy in a panic at the prospect of consummating marriage with Rhonda, whom he felt had guilt-provoked him into giving her an engagement ring after they had been dating and having an affair for six months.

Three months after beginning combined individual and group psychotherapy we agreed to look at closeup films of his face taken by me during his group psychotherapy session the evening before. His interest in the playback was intense because of his desperation to learn what keeps him running compulsively to and from unsatisfactory, clutching relationships with women. During the playback he made the following remarks and observations:

"I see my father's face, my father's eyes, and I get sad and get the same feeling he had—that life is bad—don't trust people—don't have any friends unless they can do something for you. I'm still holding on now to what I had in childhood—the same impassivity in my face—and the ways of controlling my mother and father to get what I wanted by getting sick.

"There I look like my father sitting by the window—looking out at the world—apart from it—isolated. He had the same pursed look of his eyebrows and his eyes were sometimes expressionless and sometimes yearning. He didn't know how to smile. One of his eyes seemed to face outward and one inward, and yet they seemed to merge.

"I learned to use words to get what I wanted—like my mother. She was very voluble, very quick witted, very adaptable to any circumstance.

"As I keep looking at the picture of myself, I'm reminded of a time when I was 20 and went to the wedding of a friend as best man. I remember talking to his mother a few days before and that I asked his mother, 'Why does he want to get married instead of going to college?' She went to his closet and pointed to a wooden tie rack and said to me, 'That's you—a schtick holz' (in Yiddish). When she pointed to the wood, I knew what she meant and I was very, very silent. As time has elapsed since then I've realized that that was my father too—a piece of wood. Once at home we were drinking—toasting to the New Year and I toasted to 'love' and my father responded, "I don't know what that is—what love is—or even if it exists.' Everybody laughed including myself and I said inwardly to myself 'Fool! That's how you are—you have no understanding of life—and that's the reason no one understands you and you understand no one.' Feeling the tremendous gulf between us I was thinking 'You'd be better off dead.' The gulf between us was always felt but never expressed.

"Years later, after his second heart attack, he said to me, 'Take a vacation—enjoy life' and I had the feeling that he realized then the type of life he'd led and was telling me in his way not to live the way he did.

"I was thinking now of the positive things I did get from my mother and suddenly began to see her in a different perspective. Yes, she was smothering, domineering and directing, but my father had no capacity to enjoy life and my mother did. She had a capacity to enjoy life, to live . . . and she blamed my father for denying her that. Last week I realized my sister married a man just like my father and my sister is doing to him and to her kids and herself what my mother did to her and to me. She is absolutely controlling him and still trying to control me . . . and I resent it."

One month after his first playback experience with videotape, Aron remarked during an individual session, "I got angry inside when I saw during the playback my stillness and passivity and non-feeling when I was in group the other night. I see now how come people tell me I'm such a nice guy, but don't react very much to me. Jesus—look at the lack of expression in me. And yet, with all the inside thoughts and feelings that were going on in me, I sat there with a masked face and still body and finally I moved my lips into a pout!"

One week later he talked of how upset he was to have such a wooden or stone face and added, "My eyes lack luster. They're just not active. I close off and rarely come alive."

Three months later Aron asked me to turn on the videotape equipment so that he could observe himself concomitantly through the closed circuit television monitors. He free associated aloud as he watched himself during this individual session: "I still remember the first time I saw myself on the playback. I was flattened, masklike. I think I used the word 'stone-faced' as if there was no movement. Now I notice a little more mobility and a more relaxed and a more expressive face. My face before was formless and now there is form. My face before was closed and now it's beginning to be a little more open." There was a minute of silence as he observed himself. . . . "My eyes are a little more open, more expression-filled. I'd still like more mobility, more expressiveness in *the* eyes, and a more relaxed look on my face. I still have the overall impression as I look at *the* face . . . tense . . . (As if what?) . . . as if I am expecting an attack, wary. . . . (Anything else?) . . . non-committal, very non-committal." (Note the pattern of shifting from "my face" to "the face" as an expression of Aron's pattern of alienation as well as a statement of increasing anxiety as he confronts that which he sees in his eyes and face with antipathy.) (Anything else going on in you?) "No, I have been busy watching the camera. (The camera?) The picture. (The picture?) Myself. I have always felt the ocular vision was a truer vision than the camera vision. I'm not interested in photography or in seeing pictures of myself unless someone says, 'Gee, he's handsome.' But if they say nothing like that, I'm not interested in looking at a picture of myself. I feel more uncomfortable in the group when we have the camera on than when we don't, particularly as we're talking and watching the screen at the same time. I feel I'm missing the full impact of the vocal and visual imagery. I feel I miss some of the vocal while I'm catching the image on the monitor. I feel the best aspect of the videotape is the playback, when we can watch how we look and sound without interruption.

"I see a change, especially around *the* eyes. (*The* eyes?) My eyes are beginning to open up. I hope they stay that way. My lips are more relaxed and not drawn and tight. My forehead is more relaxed. I think I'm noticing my strides in therapy in recognizing some of my old and present traits and hangups in others . . . more forcefully . . . noticing feelings in others or their relations to others which I never noticed before."

Aron's repeated self-confrontations with the aid of videotape playback have helped him to accept and partially work through many facets of his alienation from self and his distancing or self-isolating maneuvers which are expressions of the distrust of others which his parents, through nonverbal as well as verbal channels, had so thoroughly inculcated in him.

With Aron we found that utilizing video closed circuit and playback over time increased his motivation to work cooperatively in therapy towards change. In addition to increasing perception of his reaction patterns and his impact on others, it also facilitated his verbal communication to his therapist—all this more rapidly than might otherwise have been likely.

CLARIFICATION OF FAMILY ARRANGEMENTS

The use of videotape playback in private practice to demonstrate the patterns and systems of unconscious arrangements, as well as the responses of family members to each other, can expedite insight, understanding and motivation to change better than any previously used modality. Typical repetitive, regulating patterns which may be revealed and played in a focused feedback are:

1. *Placate*—"You're right" or "Yes, I'm wrong about that."

2. *Blame or provoke guilt*—"But you made me do it that way" or "It's your fault because. . . ."

3. *Preach*—"When I was a child . . ." or "I can't understand how a child who's been given everything like you have can sit there and say that. . . ."

4. *Change the subject to something irrelevant*—"I'll get back to that but I want to point out that the other day. . . ."

5. *Withdrawal of one or more family member(s) into silence, resignation and a* "What's the use? It won't make any difference anyway" attitude.

6. *Denial*—"It may have looked that way, but you just don't understand."

7. *Psychosomatic response*—"Since I've been sitting here my heart is pounding like it's going to break" or "I'm getting a splitting headache now—you get me upset when you say those things."

8. *Discounting*—a family member used a dismissing type of head nod to the side and down or hand movement with palm down to indicate that what was being expressed by another family member is being "put down" or "discounted."

9. *Being realistic*—the family is open, truthful and conscientiously attempts to recognize, accept and resolve realistic conflicts of interest or problems while being congruent in communicating or relating.

Some additional values of video usage with families follow. More families who come for help believing their problems are unique can be helped when together they watch a playback of another family with similar difficulties. The experiential process in the here-and-now encounter of a family interview allows the family's reality problems and its distortions and neurotic interactions to be more truthfully perceived in a much shorter time. The family sickness can be approached therapeutically with more directness and effectiveness and with less chance of the therapist's remarks and intent being distorted by one individual family member. The capacity of the therapist to identify with and empathize with each family member as well as with the family as a whole can educate, stimulate and help the individual family members to identify and empathize with one another. The members of a family may be taught to look at their problem from one another's point of view. They may more readily face up to the paradoxes and contradictions and incongruities of life in general and family life in particular, and learn that these paradoxes and contradictions and incongruities exist for all of us.

Video can aid in the clarification of the ways in which family members use communications to conceal as well as to reveal truth to one another. For example, some may speak with so many words or so rapidly that the listener cannot really understand what is really going on in the speaker. Or, the nonverbal smile that accompanies the words may reveal the opposite of the actual words spoken. Frequently the tone of voice is so much more important in family communications than the content. Mary, furious at the way her husband, Jack, had spoken to her, said, "His tone was sheer martyrdom and accusation and indicated a very deep dislike for me, and when he asks questions I feel he's asking not for information but to accuse me." Repeated playbacks were required before Jack could acknowledge the validity of his wife's observations and the impact of his tone on their relationship. A wife may complain of her husband retreating into silence, and say, "I get so annoyed when he just won't say anything to me for a long time." She is denying that his silence is in fact saying a great deal. His silence may communicate that if he opens up he will have to become explosive, violent and abusive, and would rather not. On replay, video revealed the tremendous angry pressure in the husband's use of his finger to tamp down the tobacco in his pipe while his face and clenched fingers around his pipe revealed his squelched inner fury. His silences may indicate his feelings of futility—that he feels at such a time there is just no sense in talking, as he is aware that she does not want to have a conversation but to convince him of her point of view or to justify her position or her actions.

CLARIFICATION OF NEUROTIC CLAIMS

Clarification of the neurotic claims that people make on one another can be accomplished. A neurotic claim exists when we expect what we only have a right to hope for* (5). The lack of knowledge of this seemingly simple but oh-so-profound fact has caused untold human misery and despair. When our excessive expectations, which we had no right to have in the first place because we only had a right to hope, are not fulfilled, we tend to feel abused and angry, sometimes even furious. Certainly we feel much more than the kind of disappointment that ensues when a hope is not fulfilled. Many of our abused reactions can be quickly mollified and dissipated if we will ask ourselves, "Am I expecting what I only had a right to hope for?" Neurotic claims, silent as well as verbalized, particularly when they are subtle as they so often are, can be acknowledged in the more objective silent participation of self with others during a playback than in the more hectic, anxiety-laden interaction of a family, couple or group session.

The use of video may help to clarify the tendency to project or externalize onto one's spouse or children or others that which is really in oneself. Such projection may have to do with responsibility or a thought or a feeling or anything else. Blind spots can be exposed. I have found in my work with groups of married couples that there are many deep similarities in the character of the partners. The partners, however, being blind to this, may be quite hostile to their spouses for possessing traits that exist in themselves. It is easier to see distasteful aspects of ourselves in others than it is to see them in ourselves, but video playback forces us to remove our blinders.

DIAGNOSIS AS PROCESS

Diagnosis is too often conceived of in static frames of reference—whether this diagnosis be made in a social service or psychiatric setting. To conceive of "the diagnosis" as a static fixed entity is analogous to thinking and conceiving of "the unconscious" as a fixed entity or geo-

---

* See T. S. Eliot's "The Cocktail Party" for a statement of the human condition which requires giving up excessive expectations. I frequently refer patients to this work.

graphical location. Each is to be equally and vigorously attacked and denounced. *Diagnosis,* just as the contents of one's unconscious, whether one be a patient or a psychotherapist, *is a process.* It is in movement. It changes as inexorably as the days of our lives, as the tides and atmospheres. The changing battleground of inner and outer conflict is a person, a human being with soul included, in relationship to his whole self and to the selves of others. At any one moment healthy constructive forces may be in ascendance, and at another moment these forces may be eclipsed by the forces of destructive neurosis or psychosis.

The changing diagnoses of the family members and of the family as a unit when it is together present a challenging kaleidoscope of myriad interaction patterns which reflect intrapsychic and interpersonal health and sickness in varying degrees. These patterns will present themselves differently and in different order, intensity and variation with different therapists. These diagnostic patterns will frequently be more evidenced by nonverbalized communications than by what is said. These nonverbalized communications will often contradict the verbalized content of the family. When such contradictions occur with consistent inconsistency in the majority of the communications in a family which is unable to truly be with one another, where the child exists primarily to extend the parents' infantile and unfulfilled self-images, then we have a fertile family background for the development of schizophrenia or other serious personality disorders.

When videotape playbacks reveal such contradictions between verbal and nonverbal communications to be only occasional in a family, they may serve to reflect or express the multiple paradoxes of life itself or of the double-standards which exist in many of our ways of life. They reflect the general pathology of our culture. To function within the framework of this general pathology is in fact to appear healthy. We must be careful to distinguish between the kind of strategic duplicity necessary for living within the general psychopathology of our culture and the kind of compulsive duplicity or pathology which is an indication of deep inner character neurosis.

In experiencing the family unit in a therapeutic session, collusion between parents, or between children, or between the mother and daughter against the father can be sensed and interpreted or otherwise used by the therapist as it is expressed. He may decide to not focus on it until it has been revealed in playback. The use of this collusion to undermine family unity and maintain isolation and conflict can be explored and worked through. Which mother has not silently given a look to her daughter or son as a little head nod or partial benevolently patient smile as she quietly waits out her husband's tirade against the child's behavior? Does this collusion serve to castrate the father in the child's eyes so that Mama is experienced as the real power behind the family throne?

ROLES

Through the playback of an individual, family or group session patients with massive blind spots or other denial techniques can be confronted repeatedly with the self-defeating, self-isolating or otherwise self-negating arrangements or "games" they establish and maintain with others. They can be helped more rapidly to recognize and to come to grips with the values of their unconscious compulsive need to enact such roles as:

Jester	Frail Tyrant
Referee-Umpire	Teacher's Pet
Catalyst	Prosecutor
Don Juan	Seducer
Cockteaser	Guardhouse Lawyer
The Idiot	The Scapegoat
Injustice Collector	Rejection Collector
The Abused Type	Saint
Missionary	Fashion Plate
Crisis Creator	Innocent
Story Teller	Advice Seeker
Clock-Watcher	Virtuously Honest Sadist
Whiner	Overprotective Mama
Leader of Opposition	The Judge
Nitpicker	Kill Joy
Planner	Egghead
Self-righteous Critic	The Baiter
Expert	The Doctor's Assistant
Provocateur	Martyr
Fragile Baby	Ombudsman-Guardian
General	Negativistic Clique Creator
Intellectual	Help-Rejecting Complainer
Flirt	Runt of the Litter
Sophisticate	Strong Silent Type
Cockroach	Compulsive Helper
Troublemaker	Can't Say No
Magician	Manipulator
Monopolizer	Competitor
Charmer	Ostrich
Iconoclast	Fair One
Victim	Pollyanna
Vindicator	Castrator
Prima Donna	Guilt Provoker

CLARIFYING TRANSFERENCE IN MARRIAGE

Following the first 10 minutes of a session with a young couple whose marriage was threatened by dissolution, a videotape confrontation was provided. Prior to this session the wife, Stella, had been seen twice in individual sessions and the husband, Melvin, had been seen once. Stella, now 28, has been working as a researcher for a market research corporation since their marriage two years ago. Melvin is a 27-year-old graduate student working for his degree in business administration. I chose to replay on videotape moments of this couple's interaction in which he seemed to wear a particularly significant, serious, and anxiety-provoking facial demeanor. We learned that behind this demeanor is a judgmental person, somewhat detached in the service of intellectual objectivity and non-involvement, who presents a facade which can be at least anxiety provoking to his wife if not downright frightening. The net result is to produce a feeling of being ill at ease in people who are with him. Asked if she is familiar with this "face" and how it complicates her life with him and is a source of difficulty, Stella immediately responded in a knowing manner with, "Yes! That is what gives us so much trouble! When he looks that way I don't know where I am with him then. When he looks that way I feel very insecure, very anxious."

Talking to her husband directly during the session, Stella said, "Melvin, I don't know where I stand with you at such times and it drives me to ask you for approval, attention or reassurance, particularly reassurance which I seem to then want and need—reassurance that everything is okay between us. Somehow I try to involve you at such times with food questions, stories or sex even though I know it seems to annoy you. It's like I've got to get something from you to know where I am with you and where I am with myself."

Melvin, when asked what goes on in him at times when he is expressing this demeanor, said: "I am weighing what whoever I am with is saying. I am kind of asking, 'Does it make any sense?' 'Does it have any basis?' If it does not make any sense to me, I then have a feeling that the person talking is stupid." Melvin was then informed by me that this particular demeanor has a distancing quality which serves to separate as well as to provoke anxiety. It expresses aloofness and bears a judgmental quality.

As Melvin was able to gradually acknowledge, understand, and free associate to this "look," he stated that he had learned this look from his father. At the dinner table in his childhood home there were often many silences as it was not "de rigueur" to talk unless you had something very worthwhile to say—something intelligent. He recalled that he had to learn to watch what he was saying at the table because he was constantly being put down—"taking grief." He continued with, "I constantly felt I was on trial with everything I said or did when I grew up." Melvin was able to understand that he had incorporated this very look of his father's which had in fact given him so much trouble. Asked by me whether or not he was aware he "wore" that particular face, his wife interrupted and answered for him, saying, "He wears it more with women than with men because he thinks women are more irrational—like his mother. He has told me so many times. He also finds it much easier to be animated and to have fun and let go with men than with women."

During the remainder of the session, Melvin, Stella, and I reviewed the additional dimensions of his "look." We concluded that his "look" is a statement of being in abeyance and yet not of being in neutral abeyance as much as being in malignant abeyance. It is a look of being noncommital at the moment because he had not learned it is all right to have multiple feelings about or between himself and others at any one moment. So he keeps the mixture of feelings, attitudes and judgments going on in his inner world private, while he edits and sifts out one feeling or one judgment which he may then feel safe enough finally to state or act upon. When Melvin realized increasingly that this "look" of his was and can be a powerful tool to turn other people off or to make them squirm, he smiled with great pleasure. For despite his veneer of aloof self-sufficiency, he felt inadequate and insecure underneath and was delighted to learn the strength and impact of this weapon which he had been using for years without awareness.

This illustration clearly validates the reports of Mendell and Fisher on the passage of neurotic values and behaviors through multiple generations in the same family (6).

VIDEO DURING GROUP THERAPY

Some examples of the use of videotape playback during group therapy sessions are:

Fritzi, a 32-year-old, smilingly ingratiating mother of two children, who separated recently from her husband, a biochemist provoked by her to great rages, remarked quietly, after experiencing a playback of herself during a group session: "I could see how I come through phony, as if I'm reciting, which is what I do when I'm talking to Jack. I also picked up that I come through as not telling the whole story. I'm so used to hiding my true feelings I'm afraid to be open. But I didn't think it showed."

Sam, one of her peer group members, who is angered by her manipulating tactics with himself and others, says, "You come through as if you are trapped and afraid to express your anger or any other feeling straight."

Another member of the same group, Mike, said sadly with surprised recognition, "What I see is that what I hate so much in my brother and nephews is in me too. And I finally can acknowledge the bitterness you've told me I come through with."

Jimmy, a hard-core passive-aggressive character neurotic, still plagued with deep anger towards himself and others, commented, "I see I need to go to another therapist . . . to take elocution lessons. I could hear my Brooklyn accent. But at least I did sound sincere, direct and warm and felt I came through more with the group. I'm feeling more part of the group these days and I'm feeling more involved with my family at home too. . . . I had a fantasy, Milt, that you're gonna get electrocuted 'cause I feel you're inept with electronics." This last statement was a clear-cut projection of his own self-hate for feeling he was an inept bungler at physical tasks including his sexual impotency with his wife whom he hated but did not have the courage to leave.

Another group member, Mark, insisted that his outer physical appearance is not important. He insisted that the fact that he is unshaved, unkempt, wearing sloppy, dirty, unpressed clothes should not effect his relationships and that only what he is underneath should count. He was helped to understand the tremendous neurotic claim he was making on others, "Love me, love my smell!"

The first playback experience in group therapy is one in which individuals focus interest primarily on themselves. Though narcissism and neurotic egocentricity are a common basis for this initial focus on self-image, there may also be aspects of healthy curiosity and real self-interest in operation. In later playbacks there is less self-image preoccupation and a greater interest in pathological interactions as well as in characteristic styles of being and relating to one another. In these playbacks there is often a different quality of nonverbal communication amongst the members than in the usual interaction. In the intimacy of the playback there may be seemingly insignificant but very important expressions of caring amongst members. Sometimes patients who have difficulty in letting go their tears during regular group interaction can cry during the playback in a manner similar to those people who can only cry while in a theater watching a movie or play. The lessening of pressure to relate to and with others through words allows for a different kind of involvement to develop which is more in the direction of communion and communing.

INSTANT REPLAY

During a psychotherapeutic session in which a videotape recording is being made it is *sine qua non* to inform all participants that each has the right to request an *instant replay* at any time during the session. This availability of videotape replay is one of its most unique assets and distinguishes it thoroughly from the use of sound movies of a psychotherapy session. It is easier to arrange to use instant replay in private practice than in an institution where sessions being taped are often used for teaching and research purposes. The reactions of each participant to a second chance to reexperience and examine what has just transpired may bring out evidence of multilevel contradictions, compartmentalizations and blind spots and offer individuals an opportunity to study, explore and more clearly understand what one person does which triggers off a reaction in another person. Instant replay can also be employed to make especially difficult or sensitive confrontations without the therapist verbalizing the implication of the full interpretation. There is a reliance here on the concept of "res ipsa loquitor." This helps to assess the patient's capacity for awareness of the implications of his functioning and fosters self-reliance.

Resistance to the use of video or audio equipment should be listened to and respected while an attempt is made to understand and undermine the basis for the resistance. As pointed out earlier, the elicitation of fantasies as to what its use may reveal is of significance as is the flushing out of subtle paranoid trends or needs to maintain secrecy around one major area of concern or another. If a patient is too upset to watch an instant replay it may be best to postpone the replay while working through the basis for the upset or fear of replay. There is such a state as a patient being just too raw and vulnerable inside to risk a further confrontation at certain moments and in the spirit of helping him the therapist should not force him to face what he is not ready to face. This is an individual, delicate matter which depends so much on the skill and art of the therapist to bring to successful fruition. Such self-encapsulating behaviors by patients need to be responded to with empathy and deep understanding of the dynamics in operation in order to work through such blockages.

In psychotherapy groups, cohesiveness, intimacy and esprit are heightened during a playback which all members are interested in experiencing. However, when the timing of the playback is not in tune with where the group as a whole is and where the individual members are at a particular moment, the playback is reacted to with disinterest, boredom, impatience and irritation at the therapist.

During a playback individuals or members of a group may be more open to experiencing compassion for themselves or others than during the regular session. The playback allows for a reflective, feeling experience untarnished by the usual defensive interactional patterns of patients with their therapist or group.

Patients with a paranoid coloring, who through their suspiciousness and projection of malevolent intent to others manage to repeatedly ruin the potential for successful relationship while maintaining their isolation and detachment, are easier to reach with reality through repeated playbacks of a taped segment of interaction revealing their compulsive distortions and projections. In the context of the therapist's consistent, sincere interest and willingness to replay a segment of tape over and over again in order to work through his patient's pathology, the patient may receive enough transferential and/or realistic gratification to motivate him toward giving up his neurotic trend (s).

The development of trust in the therapist is a cornerstone for the evolution of intimacy and mutuality in a successful psychotherapeutic relationship. Videotape playbacks allow individual or group patients to perceive through many sensory inputs who and how the therapist is for them. They are quietly able during playback to more clearly perceive and integrate the therapist's capacity for empathy, rapport, support and whether and to what degree he really understands and is with them. They are able to perceive his literal, figurative or metaphoric communication of "I support you, I hold you in my arms, I cherish you, I nourish you. I care about you. What happens to you is important to me. I have an investment, a personal investment in what becomes of you; I am myself emotionally involved in your fate. . . . I keep you within bounds; I do not allow you free indulgence of impulse, of love or hate. You must respect my position of authority on these grounds. I am strong enough to stand out against your pressures and importunities, your temptations and briberies" (7).

The video recorder captures for repeated replay and understanding that characteristic, nonverbal, behavioral or physical stance of a person which tells others his mode of being in this world. In my experience, I have found that in watching the replay, I have at times been able to spot and comprehend an individual's life stance as expressed in this fashion either for the first time or more clearly than ever before. For example, some patients have a way of sitting forward with head crunching into neck and shoulders in a modified turtle fashion, their head partially drooping forward in a helpless fashion while they are pleading to be loved. This plea is in harmony with a repeated nonverbalized statement being made with hands held forward with open-fingered palm held upwards in a "love me, give me—because I have suffered so" fashion. This stance paraphrases at times the underneath attitude of "the world owes me a living and a loving because I've suffered so!" (See Chapter 2, p. 00, this volume re attitudes.)

The use of video both compels the therapist to see more of what goes on nonverbally than he had previously realized and demands of him an increasing alertness to the nonverbal signs and communications which are ever present so that he can more adequately use focused feedback as a therapeutic intervention. To just play back a long segment of videotape is sometimes experienced with boredom by an individual or group who considers it a therapeutic interference to here-and-now interaction, experiencing, associations or awareness. The frequent use of the video heightens the therapist's sensitivity to cues having major or minor implications which other therapists are not able to discern as well.

The increasing interest in perceiving, understanding and utilizing nonverbal behavioral activities in both the understanding of what psychotherapy is as well as in expediting therapy has received a profound impetus since the introduction of videotape into psychiatric training and treatment. There are many references to it in this volume, as it applies to the impact of self-image confrontation, to perception of the self by therapists in training as well as in ongoing practice, and to the awareness that what individuals have thought to be private or secret information about themselves is really very obvious to others, even when they are relatively nonastute observers.

THE PATIENT AS CAMERAMAN

In my experience, the person who moves the camera to zoom in on or focus on a person or interpersonal interaction sees more of what is going on nonverbally than the other observers and participants present. In watching the monitors, vision becomes focused on the central person or bodily action in the observer's field of vision without the usual degree of distraction by what is seen through peripheral vision. In private practice I have noted that patients who are encouraged to use the camera to take pictures of others developed a heightened awareness of what is communicated by hand and other bodily movements.

Sandy reacted with feelings of childlike delight and excitement to the opportunity to be able to "play with a complex adult technological toy." The following day she informed me, "As the other group members came into the office my predominant feelings were of playful fun and a sense of being special as cameraman. I was also feeling an immediate sense of incompetency, saying to myself, 'I can't handle these controls,' although I really wanted to do so. When Sharon mentioned that she too had wanted to use the camera in response to your invitation but had been afraid to speak up, I was so glad that I didn't hesitate despite my conflict.

"Then an increasing sense of responsibility took over and I started to focus less for fun and more on what seemed important, what was really happening. My attention, and therefore the camera lens too, was focused primarily on hand, leg and body movements. I noticed how often hand, leg and foot movements were not parallel with verbal expressions. I have a sense that although I was not consciously concentrating on what was verbalized I still was somehow receiving and responding to what was said. Although later in the session I was able to better hear what was said as well as see what was going on, I feel a more total emotional remembrance and impact from the early portion of the group meeting.

"Although it's now a day later, I retain a clear visual image of what people looked like—what I was picking up on the camera. . . . Mary's pained, holding-back face showing strong emotions inside which she was not expressing and how long she sat this way so very controlled but looking as if she might explode like dynamite at times and not knowing or able to control the continual slight movement of her foot. I recall, too, feeling how Sharon needed support as she kept looking at you or the floor, was so self-conscious and could never seem to get comfortable. I remember how she'd make small facial movements like turning down the corners of her mouth like she wanted to cry and giving off such an air of self-deprecation.

"I had the same feeling of somehow not participating fully with the group that I usually have with any group of people . . . of being quiet . . . of not saying anything yet very aware of everything going on.

"Then I remember feeling a sense of isolation at the camera and a feeling that I must be trying your patience because I was probably focusing on things you wouldn't and not focusing on what you'd want me to as you'd want them on the tape. It was when these self-critical feelings became strong that I stopped using the camera.

"The strongest impression I'm left with is how much significance I've placed up to now on what people were verbalizing and yet how small a component of their total expression that is."

This illustration reveals Sandy's difficulty in remaining joyously involved in a creative new experience. From freedom to participate in a childlike fashion she gradually moved not only to a mature sense of responsibility but a few minutes later to an exaggerated super ego-driven sense of responsibility. In this condition she externalized her own self-critical operations until her anxiety and discomfort became so great she stopped what she was doing. In addition she was able to become aware of how unaware she had previously been of the importance of nonverbalized nuances in relationships as she had overemphasized the importance of the spoken and written word.

IMPACT OF NONVERBAL COMMUNICATIONS OF PATIENTS AND THERAPIST

Darwin, in *The Expression of the Emotions in Man and Animals* (8), noted that movements or behaviors which are serviceable in gratifying some desire or in relieving some sensation, if often repeated, become so habitual that they are performed, whether or not still of any service, whenever the same desire or sensation is felt, even to a very weak degree. In understanding nonverbal attitudes and gestures it is necessary to keep in mind that such behaviors usually occur involuntarily and unconsciously and may therefore communicate to an observer what in the expressor may still be subliminal or in another level of unawareness.

It is important that therapists keep in mind not only that movements and gestures are subservient to long-range values in each culture but that values and attitudes may be expressed differently in varying cultures nonverbally* (9).

Most patients are more or less unclear about their own facial and bodily appearance and expressions as well as about the impact these have on others. There are some patients whose facial expression arranges for a profound interpersonal barrier, somewhat like a thick plexiglass shield, to be set up between themselves and others. They are usually unaware of this and unaware of how this barrier serves to perpetuate their isolation and inability to satisfy their social hunger. They know only too well that poignant, internally voiced, frequent self-question: "What's the matter with me? How am I different from others? How come people shun me despite my conformity to the usual customs?"

---

* Reusch, J. and Kees, W. amplified this in 1956 in their book, *Nonverbal Communication*. They point out how amongst Americans gesture is largely oriented towards activities such as keeping occupied, being enterprising, striving for achievement and being entertained. Amongst Italians, gestures tend to be emphatic, redundant and flamboyant, serving the purposes of illustration and display for people living in a climate of passionate emotional expression where there is a desire to express bodily and emotional needs in elaborate and somewhat outspoken terms while simultaneously maintaining warm interpersonal contact; amongst Jews, gesture serves as a device for purposes of emphasis and for inter-punctuation, being predominantly discursive and with a jerky tempo. Contactual movements such as grasping, poking, pulling and shaking are frequently employed.

There are multiple ways in which such patients ward off other people: by wearing their face as if it were a wax mask as in Madame Tussaud's museum; by wearing a menacing facial expression and body manner which says, "On guard! Be careful what you say to me. If you sound like you're stupid I'm gonna really cut you into ribbons"; by wearing such a judgmental, haughty and omnipotent face that only someone with a fairly healthy ego would risk offering an opinion in their towering presence (see example of Melvin and Stella, page 000); by wearing a facial smile which keeps pleading "gimme more—gimme more—gimme" while it is obvious to others that the demand for "supplies" is insatiable; or by wearing a facial expression or facsimile of a smile which is more "an arrangement of the face rather than an expression of the heart," as Jean Stafford, the short-story writer, has stated.*

I might add here parenthetically that many attempts by individuals to obtain psychotherapy have failed due to the nonverbal impact of the therapist's nonempathetic masked "professional face" offered to frightened, anxiety-ridden, self-hating and self-rejecting patients at a time when they most needed human warmth, contact communication or a supportive interpretation.

In a playback session patients not only have an opportunity to observe with an expanded ego their distorted transference reactions toward the therapist but also to quietly observe and assess who he really is as a person. They can assess the degree of his capacity for continuity, constancy and caring or the lack of it. They can observe and assess the degree of his interest, sincerity, involvement and integrity or the lack of it. One therapist who watched himself on playback for the first time was shocked as he realized how his patients had been experiencing him. He stated, "I didn't realize how aloof, detached and intellectual my manner was. I seem to have a superior attitude. I had no idea of the way I had been acting until after seeing it on the screen and hearing the tape" (10). Just as it is with acknowledged patients, therapists often have difficulty in believing or accepting what is said about them by patients, colleagues or supervisors. It is not easy to maintain such denial tendencies when confronted with oneself audiovisually. In the therapist's ongoing search for his own identity and his own struggle for authenticity, the impact of videotape self-image in interaction is a meaningful and enriching experience which enhances his personal and professional growth.

Who and how the therapist is for his patients is reflected in his seeming lack of haste as he empathetically enters into, remains in and departs

---
* Personal communication.

from the patient's presence, in his sensitive countenance and outstretched hand as he greets his patient. The therapist's capacity to apply "tincture of tact" with all of his verbal and nonverbal communications enables the patient to retain his personal dignity while he undergoes the process of disillusionment which is inherent in psychotherapy.

There are many nonverbal communications registering with each patient which serve to inform him whether he is being experienced as an object or thing or case rather than as an individual patient-person or person-patient. I have found that he will react to treatment accordingly. Rosenbaum has repeatedly expressed concern that the practice of individual psychotherapy often makes the procedure barren and reinforces the therapist in his feelings of omniscience, resulting in an I-It rather than an I-Thou relationship.*

Just as doctors with different personality makeups will bring forth different results in the same patient, so too will different personality makeups of patients stir up reactions in a therapist which may interfere with the curative process. The patient's nonverbalized attitudes, emotions and transference distortions may stir up countertransferential and other reactions in a therapist which he is unaware of until he experiences a video playback. Nonverbalized aspects of character structure which may affect the therapist are: 1) the patient who is demanding, pushing, controlling and irritable, 2) the patient who is scared, shy, bunny-like or withdrawn, 3) the patient who is clinging, helpless, complaining, dependent and childlike, 4) the patient who is independent, standoffish and pain-denying, 5) the patient who is a coy, seductive, narcissistic charmer flinging sexuality about openly and provocatively, 6) the patient whose abused attitude of being an injustice collector is used to make claims for special attention from the therapist via an unstated implication that life and the therapist owe him or her a living and a loving because he or she has suffered so much, 7) the patient who is obsessive-compulsive and perfectionistic, or 8) the patient who is aristocratic, arrogant and just above-it-all. Video repeatedly demonstrates for us that nonverbal communication, alone and in conjunction with lexical languages, serves not only as a medium for expression, communication, and imparting information, but also to establish, maintain or regulate relationships (12).

REPLAY TECHNIQUES

When a replay of part of a psychotherapy session is used during the actual encounter it represents, it is worth repeating here that most thera-

---

* Personal communication.

pists experienced with videotape find it advisable to play no more than ten to twenty minutes of the tape. Because of the tremendous amount of data communicated in the playback, to go beyond this time usually results in a self-protective loss of interest or in a decreasing emotional involvement or in confusion. If it is possible to tape the patient's spontaneous reactions to the playback, at least on audiotape if not with videotape, both therapist and patient will find the free associations at this time an important aid to the therapeutic process. While it is more common to have a second video recorder in institutional settings than in private practice, the cost for this purpose is very much worth it as the results are so valuable. Another method I have found practicable is to ask the patient to withhold his remarks until the playback is concluded and then to subsequently record him audiovisually on the same tape, as the machine is now available again for recording. Such a record for five to ten minutes after self-confrontation may be reviewed more than once and used for working through.

Another method of utilizing either instant or later replay is to play back the picture without the sound so the patient can more objectively experience the impact on others of his nonverbal behaviors and posturings as he sees himself for the first time from others' point of view. He can perceive and began to understand how his nonverbals influence and help bring about the reaction of others to him.

Stopping the playback at times when a characteristic facial, hand or body movement or position of a patient is presented may allow the patient and therapist to focus in on this behavior which has had impact on you the therapist or on others and which the patient has been either unaware of or aware of only to some marginal degree.

At other times it is important for therapeutic progress to stop the replay to examine or replay a second or third time a portion of the tape which reveals something about the patient's functioning which is a surprise to both the patient and therapist. Such moments are found to be common with videotape. It encourages humility in the therapist to realize how much really is transpiring that he is not conscious of, yet which is significant. Such experiences serve to prove that how we react to one another is profoundly influenced by subliminally perceived expressions and communications. It is, of course, significant from a psychodynamic viewpoint that a particular statement or behavior was not remembered by either therapist or patient. Exploration of such a transaction may reveal significant transferential and countertransferential implications or may represent denial or a blind spot because what is being expressed represents a source of anxiety and/or conflict being avoided by patient and therapist.

While watching a playback one frequently observes the presentation of a patient's typical neurotic values, attitudes, mannerisms or hang-ups. The appearance on playback of such hang-ups which the therapist has heretofore been unable to successfully motivate the patient to acknowledge offers an excellent opportunity for the therapist to achieve his therapeutic aim. The representative segment of tape can be played over and over in focused feedback style until the patient finally grasps the impact of its meaning. Such a working through requires the utmost artistic as well as scientific skill on the part of the therapist so that emotional as well as intellectual insight can occur. One of the great values of videotape is that the playing back of such a segment of tape can be accomplished in a matter of seconds and the repetition does not affect the life, stability or reproductive qualities of the tape itself.

At times during playback it is of value to turn off the video picture in order to accentuate for the patient in the context of what comes before, and what comes after, the impact on others of such vocal variables as tone, inflection, pitch, speed, juncture points, enunciation, accent, volume, rhythm and degree of articulateness. This is of value in helping a patient comprehend how it is that others react to him the rejecting way they actually do when he believes he is speaking and functioning in a warm, benevolent, kind or friendly fashion. This technique is of particular value in working with patients who are arrogant, accusatory, pompous, dogmatic, tyrannical and who demand from, demean and belittle or discount others. Many patients have blind spots and other resistances to acknowledging these aspects of their personality despite the evidence of it in their disturbed relationships with spouses, children and others. Video confrontation sometimes forces patients to accept the truth or to insist that the therapist, the group and the videotape are distorting and do not really understand or see them as they really are and so they terminate therapy with this therapist.

An interesting technique to flush out latent or borderline paranoid processes in a patient who is a member of a therapy group is to ask a patient who comes late to a group meeting which is being videotaped to share his fantasy of what he believes the group said about him prior to his arrival. If a person airs his belief that his peer group members either ignored his absence or talked against him for one reason or another, it may have a salutary effect for him to hear in the playback of the early portion of the group the expressions of concern and caring that were in truth expressed. Such an experience may lead him to give up some of his distrust of others. If there were in fact negativistic, rejecting remarks made it might be more an expression of psychotherapeutic skill and judgment to neither ask the patient for his fantasy nor to play back the first portion of the meeting as these would only serve to whet his paranoid systems. At other times such a playback offers an opportunity for the latecomer to catch up on what was going on earlier in the group meeting as well as to offer more objective reactions or interpretations of individual or group process than the other, more subjectively, involved participants.

A valuable use of playback is to review a patient's participation in a former group or family meeting during his individual psychotherapy session. This allows for maximum use and benefit from the technique of focused feedback (see Chapter 18 by Stoller in this volume). Analysis and working through of resistance patterns can be accomplished more expeditiously this way than through regular individual sessions and the patient can be encouraged to risk being different in his next group or family encounter.

A successful 28-year-old television scriptwriter who was singularly ineffectual with interpersonal relationships reviewed the tape of her last group experience during her next individual session. She said through quiet tears, "What bothered me was this smug attitude I have on my face —like I know it all—and I really don't... also this very affected speech I seem to have. I noticed a few sibilant s's that were creeping through and it bothered me. I associate it with being theatrical. If a man did it, it would be the mark of a homosexual. The not moving around is more natural for me. The other attitudes are more studied and affected—the smugness, the speech.

"I wasn't participating that much. (Where were you? Did you see what you do with people?) I was just watching what was going on. (Yes, you have been doing that for months.) This isn't new. I sit and watch a situation and figure out my part in it and then I may go into it. I may take six minutes, six months, six years—maybe never. (How do you feel about that?) Frankly I don't feel this is as important as other things that have happened since I was last here. I keep going back to the psychological evaluation and the statement that I am still tied to home. I thought, 'I'll show them'—I just won't go home for months.

"I feel nothing I have to say is important so I have to soup it up by saying it with my mouth and mind but not with anything else. (Certainly not with real feelings.) It seems to be the way I've learned to get attention with this unusual tone—inflection and changes in my voice—I use them to make what I say important and what it does is to make it unimportant as if it were not to be believed. (That's what your group members have told you, isn't it?)"

The replay of a psychotherapy session of a patient meeting with her mother who had come to visit her for a short time was seen by the patient one week later. A week after this playback she came into her session remarking, "I've been grumpy all week realizing how much I hate my mother. Last week and the week before I just didn't feel it. I wasn't really aware of how much I kowtowed to her presence... that that's what I've been doing my whole life. I've become progressively more annoyed that she wasn't truthful and that I was confused. At first I was fascinated by what I saw in the playback—having a schizophrenic-like reaction in which I was confused and detached and didn't feel it. But all the past week I realized how I hated her for the way she is whereas in recent years I had felt guilty for not being able to communicate and relate to her. They had convinced me it was my fault—that I was the catalyst for any antagonism between us. (Just what did you come to now that's different?)

"I was in a blue funk because I wasn't expressing my hatred or anger and was depressed 'cause I hadn't expressed it—not to her alone—hadn't even expressed it to you. It's still hard to see how I could express it to her or even if it's desirable to do so. I was tearful because I knew I couldn't say anything to her without crying and afraid that if I did start to cry I wouldn't be able to stop. And that's exactly what I went through in childhood. And then I felt terrible 'cause I couldn't stop crying...."

Just as we've experienced definite value in bringing a tape of a group, couple or family encounter into a patient's individual session, it is of value at times, *with the permission of those on the tape,* to bring the tape of a couple or family session into a patient's group meeting. It can bring more reality concerning key relationships to the group than a patient ordinarily brings with his verbal statement of what transpires in his life outside group.

The following verbatim statement was made by a 33-year-old, self-effacing, married college graduate who had been raised in a puritanical righteous-minded family in which she was constantly led to believe she was to feel guilty, wrong or insignificant. In her marriage she had tried constantly to appease her husband through compliance and self-abnegation in the expectation of being loved and appreciated. To her husband, Herb, however, her compliancy and inability to risk differing or being disagreeable stamped her as a passive nonentity which served as an irritant to his grandiose image of himself and his wife who should be his social and intellectual partner. Although she was in fact still the intellectually bright person he had been attracted to initially, in marriage he now reacted to her self effacing qualities as a mark of "weakness." This compulsive paradoxical reaction occurred despite the fact that Nellie offered him the kind of unquestioning warmbreasted giving which he had not had earlier from his mother and which he was so desperate to receive. The prospect of a divorce brought her for psychotherapeutic assistance. She was seen in individual sessions twice weekly, one double session with her husband once weekly, and in one group session weekly. After three months' participation in a group, during which time she had functioned mostly as a silent, passive-dependent, other-directed person, she agreed it could be beneficial to allow her peer group members to watch a videotape playback of herself and her husband made during their first couple session three months earlier so that they could gain some more-or-less first-hand understanding of her marital "arrangements" and relationship. Her husband had previously given his permission for this film to be shown to her group. The following comments were made by Nellie in the individual session which immediately followed the group session in which the playback was shown.

"I realized that a lot has happened in these months. In the beginning of that tape we were sitting silently hating each other in that awful atmosphere of picking on each other. Since then we have learned a lot about what makes for our hostility—anger—tension. As the tape progressed I had feelings—as if the group was—as if I was being revealed to the group. I felt scary. They were seeing me in a different light than they had seen me in the group. It may make it easier for me to be more myself in the group—less guarded. The fear had no form at first as to what they would think. It was the very basic fear of being revealed to somebody and the expectation they would not approve. They'd disapprove of some of the things I said. When I realized what was coming next on the tape, that I'd lose my temper and was really involved with what was going on with Herb, I was sure that they'd disapprove of me.

"There were parts of the replay that were very touching in watching this struggle going on between us. It was sad in a way. Yet encouraging that we are growing more aware, learning things. At the time of that session I was so angry and tense, but watching it now it was different. I could see now how he really didn't know then, and also now lots of the time, what he's feeling and I thought he did! I had seen him as absolute with his pronouncements. Now I could see his confusion and his not knowing was like mine—my not knowing!

"At first when I came here I felt Herb was fairly sure of what he was doing and that he was hurting me. I didn't see we were hurting each other. He was just as mixed up. When you asked what he feels when he sits aloof and detached, if he felt pleasure and power—he didn't know! When we first came I thought he did. I hadn't seen the amount of conflict and unsureness in him or his pain which was so clear on the tape and it wasn't clear to him that he had pain which his face showed—and he didn't know it—how his face looked and showed it.

"I guess that I felt the group's response would be that I'd be wrong when I said something—that I had to always be right. But they didn't respond that way and that was relieving. (That's one of the things that's been holding you back in group, isn't it?) Yes. I hear Herb say things—tossing things into the room and I feel it's just so risky for me if I were to come out with something that was obviously hostile and someone would jack me up on it. That's scary to me and yet that's how I'd learn something."

A properly-timed videotape playback can serve many purposes. In this illustration we see that a relatively silent, dependent group member who was extremely fearful of the possibility of criticism because of her active transference to the group of her fears of criticism from her primary family was able to share a replication of her marital dialogue. In the supporting atmosphere of the group she was finally able to risk exposure of her private life. During the playback she could more objectively assess and accept some of her projections to her husband and the consequences of these distortions. She could also realize through reality-testing that the group and others do not automatically react to her with disapproval and criticism as she expects or anticipates all too often to her own detriment.

In order to assess movement or non-movement of a patient in psychotherapy it is of profound value to review a tape taken weeks, months or years earlier. With some patients I have taped five minutes of one of their individual sessions every month for one year in order to have a record of as well as to review change during psychotherapy. The replay of the tape of a group session taken six months or more earlier evokes much nostalgic warmth and interest as each group member spots the persistent neurotic foibles of other members more readily than his own.

Another method of using video equipment involves the presence of one or more monitors which present immediate, simultaneously-produced camera-eye pictures of what is going on through the closed circuit system. While some patients initially complain that this is distracting to them, it is noted that gradually patients gain a good deal from this additional approach to self-awareness and self-appraisal at the moment of involvement in interaction with others. It was an experience referred to as serendipity when I learned that by focusing one or both cameras on a silent member of a group so that he could see himself on two or three monitors simultaneously, I could stimulate or catalyze him into verbalizing 95 percent of the time.

On two occasions it was possible to prevent patients from consummating their plan to undergo plastic facial surgery by the use of repeated television close-ups of their nose, chin, eyes and face. They were helped to accept that they had displaced their general self-hate onto some physiological feature of themselves to externalize and simplify their more complex conflicts about their self-image and their difficult relationships with others. It was helpful for them to experience closed circuit self-image confrontations while with peer group members who could validate or invalidate their impression of the grotesqueness of their hated facial feature.

While some therapists using video believe in hiding or disguising cameras, monitors, microphones, videotape recorders and similar special equipment, it has been my practice to keep everything out in the open. I concur with Wilmer's use of the camera as a participant-observer (13) and believe that an open use of such equipment further undermines the focus on secrecy mixed with privacy which is commonly part of the underlying attitudinal system in psychotherapy. The emphasis on openness and the statement of truth undermines not only paranoid potential but self-defeating notions of unhealthy personal uniqueness (see introduction to section IV, this volume).

The study of the dynamic implications as well as the regulatory functions of nonverbal behaviors is made more easily and immediately available to psychotherapists and patients with videotape than with conventional sounds films so often utilized by researchers such as Scheflen. For example, in psychotherapy, as a result of the development of skills over time, a therapist can correctly interpret for a patient that the manner in which he reaches for a package of cigarettes, takes one out, tamps it, lights it, blows out his light and inhales or exhales his first lungful of smoke has become a duplicitous pseudo substitute or fascimile for the poise the patient does not feel. He can help his patient see through repeated videotape playback of such a sequence how his cigarette ritual is used as a time and space filler while the patient fumbles for a reply which will appear to be replete with wisdom or knowledge or at least will sound correct. The patient can learn how he uses automatic or compulsive smoking not only to relieve anxiety but also to serve as a small procrastination in the face of a difficult or distasteful task. Scheflen attempts in his research to discover and identify and interpret units of regulatory behavior in relationships by grouping elements in the communication systems of a culture along a time and space dimension. This is done while relating such units to the multiple behind-the-scenes contexts within which such events take place. An example is reported of repeated context analysis of a sound film in which "the therapist turned out to be taking out a cigarette ... bringing it and a pack of matches to her lap ... waiting until the patient finished a story ... putting the cigarette in her mouth ... watching until the patient looked away ... lighting up ... discarding the match." A simple test used by Scheflen to prove that each element belonged in a structural unit was accomplished by sweeping back and forth through the film and noting: if each element in a proposed unit appears each time every other element appears and does not appear when the others are absent, then all elements are interdependent and represent an entity. In the aforementioned illustration Scheflen interpreted the unit referred to as one "structuring therapist-patient reciprocals." In this situation this patient and this therapist shift the dyadic context from free-ranging conversation to the typical relationship entailing free association and interpretation. The shift into this context may begin during a conversational lull when the therapist lights up and begins smoking and then proceeds to other unitary behaviors (14).

Through videotape the private practitioner can also research and refine and more clearly define for himself and his patients the nature and kinds of verbal and nonverbal mutual or reciprocal regulating patterns which occur between them and the influence these patterns or systems have in the life of the patient. Therapists are able to also learn more about their own regulating patterns while making such process observations.

To alleviate anxiety amongst private practitioners concerning the possible harmful effects of repetitive self-observation by videotape playback, I cite the reports of: (a) Cornelison and Arsenian (15) who noted that psychotic patients who were confronted with an instantly-developed polaroid photograph of themselves a short time after they were admitted to a mental hospital seemed considerably more amenable to subsequent therapeutic intervention and acceptance of reality than patients who did not have this opportunity. Their study has stimulated many of us towards the use of videotape in psychiatric treatment.

(b) Geertsma and Reivich (16, 17) who researched 64 psychiatric inpatients to elicit its impact on them. Although 77% experienced initial anxiety, 68% responded favorably to the experience. While a smaller number of patients, who were more upset by the experience, tended to dislike it, there was in no patient evidence of sustained negative effect.*

In my experience with outpatients in private practice as well as with inpatients on a community mental health service (10) the impact of playback confrontation has generally been positive even with severely ill patients. For example, Sally, a 27-year-old schizophrenic female who has avoided close relationships with males remarked immediately afterwards, "I didn't know how scared and quiet I looked. I just sat there. I looked much sicker. It was a surprise. I knew I was tense but not that bad. And yet I looked like I could be a woman and not just a little girl." Her last remark was a hopeful sign prognostically reflecting as it did a recouping and regrouping of her constructive inner forces to go beyond her level and way of functioning to date.

Another patient, Susan, a 29-year-old woman who is divorced and works as an editorial assistant, suffers with frigidity and multiple psychosomatic symptoms. After experiencing a playback with her psychotherapy group she said, "I didn't really talk. I just talked about things. Not that they weren't really true, but I avoided the really big questions and feelings going on inside me." With the directive support, encouragement and interest of her therapist and group, Susan could now be helped to open up and explore those intimate matters she had previously resisted sharing and looking into because of difficulties in trusting others.

Marion, an extremely attractive and well-structured 38-year-old college graduate with an M.A. in art history who had been thrice engaged but never married, was a bit startled and commented after a playback, "When I saw myself on videotape playback with our Tuesday group, I was fascinated by the fact that I could feel such clear-cut feelings inside myself and yet would project a watered-down bland version of myself which had no piercing quality! When I see myself on your television I see the blandest kind of cream of wheat type person—just a terribly nice person—as if my personality had no cutting at all. It sickens me. As if I wasn't in focus—was not a clear-cut personality—as if I had no well-defined edges—like Sara who had been in our group had and could project without saying a word—just with a look!"

It required many months of repeated self-viewing for Marion to give up some of her fear of unexpected hostility from her peer group members and to risk direct expression of her own irritation and hostility with them and me. Working through her transferential fear of her irrationally double-binding, seductively incestuous and unexpectedly angry father was necessary to help her emerge as a more clear-cut personality with her own

---

* For fuller account of this research see Chapter 2, this volume.

identity. Over time, clarity emerged concerning Marion's deep sinister fear of marriage and the way and degree to which she was unconsciously driven to sabotage or avoid the possibility of a really loving, non-exploitive relationship with an eligible man which could actually lead to marriage. This working through occurred during her concurrent participation in one individual psychotherapy session per week plus once-a-week participation in two different psychotherapy groups in my private practice. One group was composed of patients who were more on a sibling level with her. The second group had in its composition a 65-year-old male who could remind her of her father and a woman who reminded her of her detached, onlooking mother.

This other woman, Fay, also had major problems in being closely involved and her detachment was also in the service of avoiding anger. Through her childhood Fay had repeatedly heard the family myths concerning the legendary angers of her maternal grandfather. What she remembered was how viciously he had teased her older brother while she managed to fade into the woodwork. Fay remembered that her mother's angers were completely inconsistent and irrational and would be expressed with high-pitched screaming. Such outbursts would go on and on and on and on until they would suddenly stop as her mother settled into a period of punitive silence towards her which could last from two hours to a week. In reacting to the playback images of how quietly removed and bland both Marion and she sat in group, Fay remarked, "By the time I was nine I no longer heard her anger. I would dismiss it knowing it was irrational. From my mother I learned how futile anger was as I saw how little it accomplished with me. I never had a model of realistic anger which was expressed realistically to accomplish something successfully. And you know what happened with my father. He'd sit quiet or depressed when he was angry. And finally he got so angry he committed suicide when I was a teenager. In the past I've panicked at the idea that I might get so angry I might do what my father did and then I'd be abandoning everyone—especially my kids. So I've just not felt my anger even at times when I knew with my head it was appropriate."

The use of videotape playbacks with this group enhanced the processes of identification, sibling support and peer encouragement to risk change as well as the working through of transferential hangups. Patients whose observing ego is enhanced and who become more cooperatively and enthusiastically involved in the psychotherapeutic process experience in a deeper fashion and function more holistically.

Patients treated in my private practice volunteered to participate in a psychotherapy group which was to be regularly videotaped by me with the aid of a professional cameraman for the purpose of making a training film on group psychotherapy. When the meetings of the group were to be terminated as planned, the group members were insistent on working out arrangements with me to continue the life of the group as they had benefited so much from the experience. The group held its termination meeting eighteen months after we had begun the project. There were no harmful results from participation in this project. Other patients have asked from time to time if they could be considered for participation in such a group and we have looked into their motivation. To date we have produced the 16mm sound-motion picture film "The Scream Inside— Emergence Through Group Therapy"* which was shown at the 1969 annual meetings of the American Psychiatric Association and the American Group Psychotherapy Association, as well as a thirty-minute edited videotape on nonverbal communication and one on video replay.

The use of video renews our sense of humility and decreases our omniscience as we learn how much more has been going on in the therapeutic relationship than we heretofore realized. To learn more of the subtleties of what is involved in establishing, maintaining and regulating relationships is an aid to the ongoing growth of the therapist as well as to his patients.

In this chapter I have presented some of the richness and variety of manners in which the revolutionary new tool of video can be utilized in the private practice of psychiatry. A practitioner who flexibly integrates its use in working with individuals, couples, families and groups according to appropriate timing and context can enhance and expedite a more holistic and successful psychotherapy for all who come to him for help. I am sure that creative therapists will add many valuable new ways to its use.

REFERENCES

1. Bahnson, C. B.: Body and Self-Images Associated with Audio-visual Self-Confrontation. *J. Nerv. Ment. Dis.*, 148:262-280, 1969.
2. Berger, M. M., and Rosenbaum, M.: Notes on Help-Rejecting Complainers. *Int. J. Group Psychotherapy*, 17:357-370, 1967.
3. Hogan, P., and Alger, I.: Impact of Videotape Recording on Insight in Group Therapy. *Int. J. Group Psychotherapy*, 19:158-165, 1969.

*This 45-minute black and white film made with assistance from the filmmaker Edd Dundas and Dr. Robert DelVecchio, Medical Education Director of Sandoz Pharmaceuticals is available without charge, for showing to professional audiences only, by application to Dr. DelVecchio at Sandoz Pharmaceuticals (Route 10), Hanover, New Jersey 07936.

The Use of Videotape in Private Practice 215

4. Geertsma, R. H.: Studies in Self-Cognition. *J. Nerv. Ment. Dis.*, 148:193-197, 1969.
5. Horney, K.: *Neurosis and Human Growth*. New York: W. W. Norton & Co., 1950. Chapter 2, 40-63.
6. Mendell, D., and Fisher, S.: An Approach to Neurotic Behaviour in Terms of a Three Generation Family Model. *J. Nerv. Ment. Dis.*, 123:171-180, 1956.
7. Coleman, J. V.: Aims and Conduct of Psychotherapy. *Archives of Gen. Psychiatry*, 18:1-6, 1968.
8. Darwin, C.: *The Expression of the Emotions in Man and Animals*. New York: Appleton Press, 1872.
9. Reusch, J., and Kees, W.: *Nonverbal Communications: Notes on the Visual Perception of Human Relations*. Berkeley, Calif.: University of California Press, 1956.
10. Berger, M. M., Sherman, B., Spalding, J., and Westlake, R.: The Use of Videotape with Psychotherapy Groups in a Community Mental Health Service Program. *Int. J. Group Psychotherapy*, 18:504-15, 1968.
11. Cole, J.: Evaluation of Drug Treatment in Psychiatry. Paper presented at the annual meeting of the American Psychopathological Association, New York City, Feb. 23-24, 1962.
12. Scheflen, A.: Communication and Regulation in Psychotherapy. *Psychiatry*, 26:126-136, 1963.
13. Wilmer, H. A.: Television as Participant Recorder. *Amer. J. of Psychiatry*, 124:1157-1163, 1968.
14. Scheflen, A.: The Sound Camera Breakthrough in Research, Training, Therapy. *Roche Report: Frontiers of Hospital Psychiatry*, 6, No. 11, June 1, 1969.
15. Cornelison, F. S., and Arsenian, J.: A Study of the Response of Psychotic Patients to Photographing Self-Image Experience. *Psychiat. Quart.*, 34:1-8, 1960.
16. Geertsma, R. H., and Reivich, R. S.: Repetitive Self Observation by Videotape Playback. *J. Ment. Nerv. Dis.*, 141:29-41, 1965.
17. Reivich, R. S., and Geertsma, R. H.: Experiences with Videotape Self-Observation by Psychiatric In-Patients. *J. of Kansas Medical Soc.*, LXIX:39-44, 1968.

17
THE USE OF VIDEOTAPE IN GROUP PSYCHOTHERAPY

Nazneen S. Mayadas, D.S.W.
and
Donald E. O'Brien, A.C.S.W.

INTRODUCTION

In recent years the group process as an agent of change has attracted considerable attention in the behavioral sciences. This has been demonstrated by the proliferation of group movements, of which group psychotherapy is only one part. Broadly defined, group psychotherapy is that process of behavior change which is initiated in persons through the structured medium of group interaction, and with the planned intervention of a professional therapist(s). Also gaining popularity in the behavioral sciences has been the use of videotape equipment in conjunction with both individual and group psychotherapy. Our discussion here will address itself to attempting to link, both theoretically and practically, the group psychotherapy process with videotape usage. Our focus shall concern itself only with the traditional model of group psychotherapy, i.e., verbal communication and mutual interaction of members in groups of single individuals, couples, and families (1). Models of encounter groups, T-groups, sensitivity groups, etc., are viewed as outside the concern of this paper.

Psychotherapy, which earlier followed the Freudian dictate of esoteric communication between therapist and patient as a necessary prerequisite to analysis (2), has now opened its doors to the rigorous study of phenomena such as therapist behaviors and interactional processes in groups, as viable channels to understanding the therapeutic process and its effects

Reprinted with permission from *Group Psychotherapy and Psychodrama*, Vol. 26, No. 1-2, 1973. This paper was presented at the 31st Annual Meeting and Psychodrama Training Institute of the American Society of Group Psychotherapy and Psychodrama, April, 1973, New York, N.Y.

on patient outcome variables (3, 4, 5, 6). This movement toward inquiry and scientific research into both individual and group psychotherapy methods has led to the comparison and investigation of the respective gains achieved in patient outcomes through the use of these two methods of behavior change. Since the emphasis of this paper is specifically on group psychotherapy as a change modality in dealing with the individual and his subsequent social interactional patterns, the focus will be on those processes which occur in group settings and exert influence on members' behaviors.

Perhaps the major contribution of the group method is its approximation of the social context of interaction, i.e., the patient has the opportunity to try out new behaviors with a range of different persons, just as he does in real life. In addition, the group provides the individual with the opportunity of forming multiple interactional patterns and receiving feedback from a number of persons regarding his actions. If there is agreement between group members with regard to his (the patient's) behaviors, group consensus would magnify this convergence of opinion and bring the stated behaviors more clearly into focus, thus stressing some of the advantages that group psychotherapy tends to suggest over those of individual psychotherapy. This concept of consensual validation (or group consensus) stands out as perhaps the single most potent variable in mirroring members' behaviors. An individual will find it difficult to continually deny behavioral modes if there is consensus within the group regarding particular behaviors emitted by him (7). Hence, the group can act as a powerful agent of change to the extent that the members create for each other an awareness of emitted behaviors and reactions to these behaviors. On the basis of this new insight the members can use the planned facility of the protected group situation to try out new behaviors in a simulated social environment. This is a rare opportunity which is available to the individual, only within the structured context of a psychotherapeutic group.

The process of group interaction does not take the responsibility of the therapeutic relationship away from the therapist (8). The therapist is there, but the intensity of the dyadic interaction is diffused, and the pressure to establish and maintain a relationship is shifted from just one patient-therapist dyad to the total group. The group milieu also provides the therapist with the opportunity to observe the individual patient in direct interaction, instead of just "hearing about" his interpersonal behaviors. Also, there is greater reliability in diagnostic assessment, since both the therapist and the patient receive feedback regarding the patient's behaviors.

This facility of feedback is enhanced when the processes of group psychotherapy are further accelerated by use of videotapes. The instant replay capability of this technical device adds a self-corrective dimension to the already stated advantage of consensual validation. With the feedback received from the taped self-image in interaction, the group member is in a much better position to verify his behavior against three given criteria: 1) his self-perception, 2) others' perception of him, and 3) the actual image on the television screen. In the authors' experience, when the method of change initiated by the group process is further defined by the introduction of direct undistorted videotaped feedback, the probability of denial is reduced to a minimum and resistance to change is considerably lessened (9).

This paper will concentrate on the use of videotapes in group psychotherapy, and will discuss the 1) general parameters of group therapy, and 2) specific theory, techniques, and usages of videotapes in implementing behavior change within a group setting.

GROUP PSYCHOTHERAPY AS A CHANGE PROCESS

The rationale for group psychotherapy gaining prominence within the last two decades may be attributed to many causes, such as time-cost benefits for both patient and therapist, greater flexibility by the therapist to practice new methods and techniques of operation, a safer, more secure environment for the patient to try out new behaviors, and the empirical evidence supporting small group dynamics as a change facilitator (10, 11). In the context of our present day society where rapid changes in norms and values lead to alienation of self and identity diffusion, the group serves both as a context for, and a means of, change (12). In the group setting, the patient is able to see himself as part of an interacting system, in which members share, support, and help each other to meet existing needs and to improve adaptability to the demands of their respective interpersonal environment. As stated earlier, the influence of the therapist is present, but its intensity is diminished due to the many other relationships in the group. Neither the individual member nor the therapist carries the entire burden for the "success" or "failure" of the therapeutic encounter. The responsibility is jointly shared by the group, and members to a large extent determine the direction and goals for therapeutic outcomes. The transference phenomenon so essential to the traditional model of psychotherapy takes on a multidimensional perspective in group treatment. Thus, the transference of the object cathexis of the patient is not restricted to the therapist alone but is dispersed over a much wider range of feelings and attitudes transferred toward different group members (13). The therapist in the group situation intervenes according to his own frame of theoretical reference. He may view himself strictly as a facilitator or catalyst whose job is to move the group to the desired goal, or he may hold an opposite view and see himself as just another member of the group. Based on their orientation, therapists utilize groups on a continuum which ranges from working with the individual within the context of the unhampered group process to active intervention in the process and the ensuing interaction between members as a *means* of interpersonal behavior change. The present authors tend to set the parameters of group psychotherapy somewhere in the middle of the two extreme orientations mentioned. As such, the techniques of intervention discussed here are not limited to any one theoretical orientation but are based on a wider, more eclectic psychotherapeutic framework.

The skill of the therapist using this approach is evidenced by his recognition of spontaneously emerging interactions consistent or disjunctive with current needs of the group as a whole, or of some individual members (14). Since the criterion for the selection of the treatment method is effectiveness of outcome, the therapist has considerable facility to move from one stance to the next as the situation demands.

THEORETICAL CONSIDERATIONS IN THE USE OF VIDEOTAPES

One of the basic contributions of videotape recording is that it provides a virtually undistorted reproduction of the situation to be analyzed. A number of theoretical orientations have been advanced to account for behavior changes as a result of video feedback. These explanations draw upon concepts from learning theories, theories of symbolic interaction and self-identity, and theories of cybernetic feedback. However, no single satisfactory theoretical orientation has been put forward to explain the behavior changes arrived at through exposure to self-image viewing, either by itself or in interactional contexts (15). This paper attempts to synthesize these apparently discrete concepts into an internally consistent framework for explicating the rationale underlying the use of videotapes as a therapeutic tool.

Since eclecticism is the preferred mode of therapeutic intervention of the present authors, a varied number of videotape techniques are formulated with a view towards enhancing group processes such as feedback, confrontation, self-image exposure, and the testing out of new adaptive behaviors in interpersonal group relationships.

It is this flexibility of an eclectic approach in planning interventive activities which gives the therapist license to try new methods of facilitating and bringing to the awareness of members the processes of reciprocal interactional patterns, feedback of individual and group behaviors, formation of sub-groups and collusions, overt and covert methods of goal achievement, small group roles, and a myriad of other ongoing exchanges that take place between persons in any group situation. The recognition of these processes has been progressively sharpened over the last two decades with the use of videotape playback in group psychotherapy (16). This method of confrontation in groups acts as self-corrective feedback and as a minimally refutable device in the appraisal of social reality. In human interaction feedback is a response from "B" to stimuli sent by "A." This response is perceived by "A" as a function of his ("A" 's) behaviors, and as a consequence helps to shape "A" 's subsequent behaviors in relation to "B." In any interactional situation, then, the behaviors of person "A" elicit certain response from person "B," which again provides the stimulus for "A" 's behavior and vice versa. Thus "A" and "B" provide "feedback" for each other in interaction. As the number of persons interacting increases, as is the case in a group situation, this process becomes more complex. Feedback from interacting others also serves the important function of developing the individual's self-image, which is an internalized constellation of behaviors that a person develops as his unique style of performance based on how he perceives the "generalized other" in his life space expects him to act (17, 18, 19). These two dimensions can be further expanded into (a) the ideal self-image, or the image a person desires to project in social reality; (b) the perceived self-image or how he views himself; (c) the actual self-image or how he appears in social reality; (d) how others perceive him, and (e) how he views others' perceptions of him. The greater the congruence between these different levels of self-image perceptions, the less identity confusion in the person (20). In other words, to the extent that there is consensus in the feedback the person receives regarding his self-image from the above listed sources, to that degree it will support his self-validation and strengthen his self-identity.

The group situation provides the individual a unique opportunity to test out his hypotheses about himself in a structured, planned simulation of a social environment. This facility is further refined with the aid of videotape feedback. The feedback from the videotape reflects his socially projected image to the individual and confronts him with the discrepancy, if any, between his cognitively perceived self-image and the actual image on videotape. Each person has two dimensions upon which he bases his self-image: 1) how he perceives himself; 2) how he views others as perceiving him. The person with the benefit of instant taped replay cannot only conceptualize his self-image and wait for feedback from the group to validate it, but he can also get a full, minimally distorted image of his interactional patterns. With this device he can attempt to alter his physical and interpersonal postures so that they become more veridical with his ideal self-image. This visual impact of the self-in-interaction, along with the consensual validation of the group, can serve as an extremely potent device for confronting behavioral phenomena such as denial, discrepancy between affect and content, and incongruence between verbal and non-verbal behaviors (21). The instant replay capability of videotapes avoids a time lapse between emission of behavior and reviewing the taped segment of the interaction so that the memory recall probability is heightened and the person is able to relate with enhanced facility to the dynamics of his taped interactions.

Modes of videotape playback range from instant to delayed replay and various other usages of feedback by therapist and group members. (These methods are elaborated in the section on techniques.) Depending on the technique preferred by the therapist, the control of the replay capability of videotapes is potentially available to all group members and can be used by them and the therapist to enhance their sensitivity to environmental stimuli as they learn to differentiate between behavioral discrepancies and functional/non-functional interactional patterns in the therapeutic group milieu.

TECHNIQUES

While the theoretical issues discussed above are important considerations, there are also a number of specific techniques that have been developed which are of interest to the therapist who wishes to employ video tape as a treatment modality.

The first, and possibly the most important factor to consider in utilizing videotape is that it has an "instant replay" capability. Thus, any individual action, or group interaction, that the therapist wishes to comment on, emphasize, or recapture, is available for replay instantaneously when a group session is being videotaped. The therapist can make a much more powerful intervention when he possesses the capability to comment on the patient's action—and show it to him—as it actually occurred, by reproducing the event rather than being confined to just talking about a happening that is, of necessity, in the past.

The technique of using videotape in group therapy has been most widely advocated by Stoller (22) who developed the technique of "focused feedback." Briefly, Stoller's method emphasized instant replay, but specified that attention should be limited to a specific action, or behavior, that the therapist wishes to highlight. Further before viewing the replay the therapist explains to the patient just what it is that he wishes him to focus attention on, so that the patient is better prepared to profit from the replay. Focused feedback, as Stoller conceives it, can be utilized in at least two ways: 1) to emphasize maladaptive or undesirable behaviors that the patient exhibits but may not be aware of, and 2) to highlight and reinforce desirable patient behaviors which the therapist may wish to encourage. (See Chapter 18 this volume.)

A second technique is to tape a therapy session, and then at the start of the next session to play back about 10 minutes of the tape to the group. This method uses the tape as the stimulus for the new group session (23, 24). A third method similar to this is to tape a session and replay it for critique and comment during alternate sessions. However, this method can be very wasteful in time unless both the therapist and the patients are skilled in the use of videotape playback.

Closely related to this approach is a method whereby the therapist tapes the entire session but stops and replays as and when the patients request. In order to make effective use of videotape feedback in this method, the patients must be highly sensitized to picking up behavioral cues and must learn to interact with the tape rather than watch it passively as with a commercial television performance (25). The ability to spot behaviors, stop the tape and discuss the replayed interactions requires constant alertness and active involvement with the ongoing processes viewed on the tape. This is often a novel notion for the patient who has been conditioned to watch television as a passive mode of recreation. Hence, productive use of videotapes in therapy is a systematically acquired and learned process which requires a high degree of sophistication on the part of both the patients and the therapist.

A fifth method that is quite interesting and adaptable to group psychotherapy, is for the therapist to leave the room while the session is being videotaped. It has been reported (26) that this method can elicit certain material from patients that might not otherwise have been brought out. Since this technique assumes that the patients know that the session is being taped and that the therapist will view the tape, the dynamics involved in the production of the material seem to merit further investigation.

A sixth method is to videotape each group session and retain representative portions of each session on tape. After a number of sessions have been held, short (five-minute) segments of these earlier sessions can be played back to the group. This can serve as an indicator of group change over a period of time, and can also serve to make the group members more aware of changes that have occurred in their individual and collective behaviors. This process is called "serial viewing," and was originally described by Moore et al. (27) as a technique for use with individual patients.

If two or more cameras are available and the therapist has the use of a special effects generator, he can make use of a "split screen" replay technique, which shows a close-up view of the actions of one group member and, at the same time, the corresponding *reactions* of one or more of the other group members.

Another use which has been suggested (28) is to show naive (new) group members tapes of other group sessions. In effect, this method calls for using tapes as "models" by which new groups can pattern their future interactions.

Gonen (29) has reported using videotape in conjunction with psychodrama. He describes taping a psychodrama session and playing it back to the patients. He reports that this method can tap certain feelings and emotions that were not brought out at the time that the psychodrama was enacted.

Different feelings are expressed in the literature about what is regarded as the best time for playing back to patients their behaviors. Miller (15), in a review of the literature, found that almost all writers considered immediate playback to be the most effective, although Paredes et al. (30) in a study of individual patients had observed that if playback was delayed for a few days the patients seemed to be "more involved" at the time of playback. Miller, in his own study, however, found no significant differences between the effects of immediate or delayed playback to groups. (It has been our experience that when using "focused feedback" techniques immediate playback is most effective in terms of patient response.)

In the discussion above the implicit assumption has been made that the efficacy of the techniques described is highly related to the therapeutic skills of the user. The use of videotape is seen by the authors as ancillary to group therapy. Therefore, if the user is ineffective as a therapist, then it would not be expected that his employment of videotape would automatically make him an effective therapist (16, 23). For example, use of the focused feedback technique presupposes that the therapist knows which behavior to concentrate upon, with what specific group member, and that this be done at the proper time during the course of the therapy. The therapist intervenes in the situation on the basis of his knowledge and experience. If he does not have a good theoretical knowledge base and subsequent skills, then his use of videotape will be in vain.

This leads to another point that needs to be emphasized and which was touched upon when the use of videotapes by patients in therapy was discussed. This concern relates to the need to "educate" or "teach" group members the proper use of information available during a playback session. Moreno and Fischel (31) first emphasized this point in one of the earliest articles addressed to the many complexities of the interactions between television and knowledge gained through the behavioral sciences. He pointed out the value of "adjusting and educating the audience to the appreciation of spontaneous material," and the great loss of the potential value of the material when the audience is not properly primed. Even so it is not unusual today to read in the literature of patients seeing themselves on videotape for the first time and getting some tremendous insight into their behaviors (9, 21). However, it has been our experience that this acclaimed self discovery is not commonplace. Rather, the patient must be trained to "see" how he is really behaving, much in the same manner that a student must be trained to "see" the subtle nuances of patient behavior. In groups this training takes on two aspects: first, the patients' being taught to analyze their own behaviors and the effects these behaviors have on others, and second, they must be taught to analyze the behavior of others. If this orientation is successful, feedback becomes available to the group members on two levels: 1) the feedback available from the video image, and 2) the feedback available from other group members and the therapist, which can be confirmed by the videotape playback (16).

In the authors' use of videotapes in group therapy we have found that there are a number of factors that can influence the acceptance by group members of the session's being recorded. First and foremost is the degree of comfort that the therapist himself feels in recording the session. If the therapist is completely comfortable with recording his professional activities on tape, then his confidence will be communicated to the group members, and resistance will be minimal. Even with this confidence, it is extremely important for the therapist to communicate to the group when they are being televised, and what uses will be made of the tapes by the therapist. If there is any possibility that the tapes will be shown to others, this should be made clear to the members and their consent obtained. In cases where there is any question as to how the tapes will be used it is wise to have formal releases signed by all of the group members (32, 33).

It is felt by the present authors that this regard for the rights of the client will not only serve to begin the group sessions with a degree of openness that will reduce client resistance to the employment of the videotape equipment, but will also serve to increase the client's trust in the therapist which, in turn, should help to improve the client-therapist relationship—another factor which is felt to be important in making successful use of video playback in therapy (19).

PROCEDURAL CONCERNS

There are usually a number of procedural questions that arise when videotape is to be used with a group. For example, when should the videotape be introduced, should the camera be hidden, etc? An attempt to answer some of the more common questions will be made from the authors' own experience, and from the information obtained from the literature. First, it seems that there is more acceptance of videotape by the group when it is introduced at the onset of the group (16, 22). Although there are different opinions in the literature as to whether cameras should be hidden or in sight (9), the authors' own experience indicates that cameras can be used in plain sight of the group without in any way hindering the group process. There may be, of course, a short period during the first session when there is some self-consciousness about "being on television." But if openly recognized, this can be used as a point of intervention or as a beginning topic for group discussion by the therapist (34).

A question often asked is whether the cameraman's presence is a hindrance to the group process. Although a cameraman is not a necessity, his presence is a decided advantage when trying to tape groups, especially when lacking elaborate remote control facilities. Again, the authors' own experience in this area tends to support the contention that his presence will not be a hindrance, provided that it is presented in the form of a "legitimized role" to the group members, much in the same way that one would legitimize the role of a student observer at the sessions (35). In fact, the authors have often combined these two roles by placing students in the role of cameraman, with complete acceptance by the group members.

RELATED ADVANTAGES OF VIDEOTAPES

To this point we have discussed the usage of videotape as a therapeutic agent. However, it also has the capability of being viewed as an excellent training tool which was surprisingly enough predicted by Moreno and Fischel (31) long before the advent of videotapes or sophisticated production techniques. For example, for the therapist seeking to improve his techniques, viewing one of his group sessions provides an excellent method of conducting a self-critique regarding his own strengths and deficiencies. Along the same lines, viewing a group session can provide the therapist with new insights about the dynamics of the group, and provide him with new information that he might have neglected to notice during the session itself. If one plans to use videotape in this way it is wise to caution the reader that it is of most value when the tapes are viewed within a day or two of the actual session. This has the advantage of the session being recent enough for easy recall, and any new information obtained during viewing can be used at the next group session. If a number of weeks pass and a number of new group sessions are held during the period prior to viewing, much of the potential value of the tapes is lost, since studying raw footage of "past groups is a tedious and not very rewarding task.

Another valuable use is to employ tapes for consultation purposes. If one is having trouble with a group at a certain stage of development, or if one wishes an outside opinion of his own techniques, viewing a group session with a supervisor or a consultant is an excellent method of getting a valid opinion of another about the group in question.

On the opposite side of the coin, if one is responsible for supervising a group therapist there is no better way, short of being physically present during the sessions, of reviewing and critiquing his progress than to watch the tape of his therapy section (36). For, unlike verbal or written summaries by the therapist, videotapes provide accurate and complete information about the sessions, and allow for timely and appropriate commentary by the supervisor on points that might not otherwise have come to his attention by other supervisory methods (24).

Another advantage from the supervisor's point of view is that videotapes allow him freedom as to when and where he wishes to view the session. For example, Benschoter et al. (37) report supervising group work students from a distance of 100 miles by use of a closed circuit system. Hence both from the development of the therapist and from the point of view of the training consultant, videotapes are an invaluable device in enhancing theoretical knowledge of human behavior and acquiring practice skills.

SUMMARY

This paper has attempted to look at the various uses of videotape techniques that can be applied as a therapeutic tool in group psychotherapy. Videotapes in therapy came into widespread use in the sixties and gained considerable recognition in the past decade. The main advantage of using this device in therapy is the replay capability of tapes, which provides both the therapist and the group members with a virtually undistorted picture of the interactional processes that occur in the group situation. This videotape feedback provides the members with a recorded image of their behaviors, and acts as a confrontive, insightful, learning experience for those receiving the taped feedback about their behaviors. This feedback helps the person to recognize discrepancies between his ideal, perceived, and actual self-image. The therapist, within the context of his theoretical orientation, uses the replay process to intervene in the group situation and help members become aware of their desirable and undesirable behaviors and the interactional patterns that ensue as a function of exchanges within the group. The process of group psychotherapy and the feedback that members tend to provide each other in a group situation is further facilitated and enhanced by the added dimension of a reproduced situation on tape which is open to analysis by all, including the person whose behavior may at that moment be the target of change. Thus, videotape feedback tends to cut through defensiveness and denial with greater facility and acts as a powerful agent of change.

The use of tapes is not only of benefit to the patient but also a continuous learning tool for the therapist. By watching himself on tape, either alone or with a training consultant, he can sharpen his interventive skills and become progressively more sensitized to the complexities of verbal and nonverbal behavioral patterns of group members. The therapeutic knowledge of the therapist and his comfort in being televised are, however, prerequisites to productive use of tapes. A therapist who questions his own performance and lacks a sound theoretical grounding and repertoire of interventive skills would not benefit himself or his group by using videotapes. Hence, videotapes, though a viable tool for therapy and training, are only as good as the competence of the therapist employing this technical device in his practice. Tapes must always be used as adjuncts to facilitate the therapeutic process and never in lieu of the therapist's knowledge of human behavior and skills of intervention in group psychotherapy.

REFERENCES

1. Stein, A.: The Nature and Significance of Interaction in Group Psychotherapy. *Int'l. J. of Group Psychotherapy*, Vol. XX, No. 2, April, 1970, pp. 153-162.
2. Freud, S.: *An Outline of Psychoanalysis.* New York: W. W. Norton and Co., 1949.
3. Meltzoff, J., and Korneich, M.: *Research in Psychotherapy.* New York: Atherton Press, 1970.
4. Bergin, A. E.: The Evaluation of Therapeutic Outcomes. In A. E. Bergin, and S.

Garfield (Eds.), *Handbook of Psychotherapy and Behavior Change.* Wiley, New York: 1970.

5. Bednar, R. L.: Group Psychotherapy Research Variables. *Int'l. J. of Group Psychotherapy,* Vol. XX, No. 2, April 1970, pp. 146-152.

6. Strupp, H. H.: *Psychotherapy: Clinical Research and Theoretical Issues.* New York: Jason Aronson, Inc., 1973.

7. Asch, S. E.: Studies of Independence and Conformity: A Minority of One Against a Unanimous Majority. *Psycho. Mono.,* 70, 1956.

8. Gazda, G. M.: *Basic Approaches to Group Psychotherapy and Group Counseling.* Springfield, Ill.: Charles C Thomas, 1968.

9. Alger, I., and Hogan, P.: The Use of Videotape Recordings in Conjoint Marital Therapy. *American J. Psychiatry,* 123 (11):1425-1430, 1967.

10. Cartwright, D., and Zander, A.: *Group Dynamics: Research and Theory.* New York: Harper and Row, Publishers, 1968 (third edition).

11. Hare, P. A.: *Handbook of Small Group Research.* New York: The Free Press, 1962.

12. Vinter, R. (Ed.): *Readings in Group Work Practice.* Ann Arbor, Mich.: Campus Publishers, 1967.

13. Slavson, S. R.: Group Psychotherapy and Transference. *Int'l. J. of Group Psychotherapy,* Vol. XXII, No. 4, Oct. 1972, pp. 433-443.

14. Slavson, S. R.: Eclecticism Versus Sectarianism in Group Psychotherapy. *Int'l J. of Group Psychotherapy,* Vol. XX, No. 1, Jan. 1970, pp. 3-13.

15. Miller, D., The Effects of Immediate and Delayed Audio and Videotaped Feedback on Group Counseling. *Comparative Group Studies,* 1 (1):19-49, 1970.

16. Stoller, F. H.: Focused Feedback with Videotape: Extending the Group's Functions. In G. M. Gazda (Ed.), *Innovations to Group Therapy and Counseling.* Springfield, Ill.: Charles C Thomas, 1968.

17. Mead, G. H.: *Mind, Self and Society.* Chicago: University of Chicago, 1934.

18. Cornelison, F. S., and Arsenian, J. A.: A Study of the Response of Psychotic Patients to Photographing Self-Image Experience. *Psychiat. Quart.,* 34:1-8, 1960.

19. Geerstma, R. H., and Reivich, R. S.: Repetitive Self Observation by Videotape Playback. *J. Nervous and Mental Diseases,* 141:29-41, 1965.

20. Erikson, E. H.: *Childhood and Society.* New York: Norton, 1963 (second enlarged edition).

21. Berger, M., et al.: The Use of Videotape with Psychotherapy Groups in a Community Mental Health Service Program. *Int. J. Group Psychotherapy,* 18:504-515, 1968.

22. Stoller, F. H.: Therapeutic Concepts Reconsidered in Light of Videotape Experience. *Comparative Group Studies,* 1 (1):5-17, 1970.

23. Danet, B. N.: Impact of Audio-visual Feedback on Group Psychotherapy. *J. Consulting and Clinical Psychology,* 33 (5):632, 1969.

24. Onder, J. J.: *The Manual of Psychiatric Television: Theory, Practice, Imagination.* Ann Arbor, Mich.: Maynard House Publishers, 1970.

25. Shamberg, M., and Raindance Corporation: *Guerrilla Television.* New York: Holt, Rinehart and Winston, 1971.

26. Moore, F. J.: Unpublished lecture, University of Maryland, Fall, 1967.

27. Moore, F. J., et al.: Television as a Therapeutic Tool. *Archives of General Psychiatry,* 13:217-220, 1965.

28. Farson, R. E.: Self-Directed Groups and Community Mental Health. In L. N. Solomon and B. Bersom (Eds.), *New Perspectives on Encounter Groups.* San Francisco: Jossey-Bass, 1972, pp. 224-232.

29. Gonen, J. Y.: The Use of Psychodrama Combined with Videotape Playback on an Inpatient Floor. *Psychiatry, J. Study of Interpersonal Processes,* 34 (2):198-213, 1971.

The Use of Videotape in Group Psychotherapy   229

30. Paredes, A., et al.: Behavioral Changes as a Function of Repeated Self-Observation. *J. Nervous and Mental Diseases,* 148 (3):287-299, 1969.
31. Moreno, J. L., and John K. Fischel: Spontaneity Procedures in Television Broadcasting with Special Emphasis on Interpersonal Relations Systems. *Sociometry,* Vol. 5, No. 1, Feb. 1942, pp. 7-28.
32. Geertsma, R. H.: Studies in Self-Cognition: An Introduction. *J. Nervous and Mental Disease,* 148 (3):193-197, 1969.
33. Mason, E. A.: Filmed Case Material: Experience or Exposure. *American J. of Orthopsychiatry,* 39 (1):99-104, 1969.
34. Czajkoski, E. J.: The Use of Videotape Recordings to Facilitate the Group Therapy Process. *Int'l. J. of Group Psychotherapy,* 18:516-524, 1968.
35. Hadden, S. B.: Training. In S. R. Slavson (Ed.), *The Fields of Group Psychotherapy.* New York: International Universities Press, Inc., 1956.
36. Gruenberg, P. B., et al.: Intensive Supervision of Psychotherapy with Video Recording. *American J. Psychotherapy,* 98-105, 1969.
37. Benschoter, R. A., et al.: The Use of Closed Circuit TV and Videotape in the Training of Social Group Workers. *Social Work Education Reporter,* XV (1):18, 19, 30, 1967.

18

VIDEOTAPE FEEDBACK IN THE MARATHON AND ENCOUNTER GROUP

Frederick H. Stoller, Ph.D.

Introducing videotape feedback into the group highlights two important areas of concern that can easily be obscured: the data which the group members find relevant and the self-examining attitudes they will develop. In their own fashion the encounter and marathon groups, relatively new directions in the group sphere, shed fresh light on where and how groups can operate. Considering these novel approaches together is not only of interest because of their increasing use in a wide variety of settings but also because of the insight they bring to bear on more conventional group therapy.

THE DATA OF THE BASIC ENCOUNTER GROUP

The basic encounter group is a term fostered by Rogers (1) and is here used as a generic name encompassing sensitivity training, human relations laboratories, and a host of similar phrases. A unifying characteristic of all these groups is the assumption that the participants' basic motivation is to learn more about themselves and others, broaden reactivity and sensitivity, and get in touch with diverse segments of their potential. Such goals are considered as being appropriate in and of themselves without implication that the individual has psychological or characterological difficulties or that he finds himself with a major life problem.

Shifting the focus from problem to person makes an important distinction in the kind of material that becomes the essential data of the group. To a considerable degree group members are forced to rely on their own perceptions and reactions to one another as they meet within the group experience. By tying such reactions and perceptions to specific behaviors on the part of the group members they are encountering, considerable effort goes into the development of feedback. Participants learn about themselves both through the giving and receiving of feedback; extra-group data may be shared as ways of illuminating or countering the feedback but it is never the starting point for the encounter group experience. A number of important consequences can be specified:

1) By concentrating on their own internal reactions and perceptions for data rather than upon speculations based upon a particular theoretical approach to personality, group members benefit both in the giving and receiving of feedback. They can learn their own capacity for trustworthy perceptions as well as the distortions and blind spots they are likely to have.

2) Since the burden of tying personal reactions to the specifics of behavior is placed upon the person giving the feedback, concrete behavior is emphasized as one of the important targets of attention. Ultimately, it becomes understood that specific aspects of behavior are eliminated from consideration only through collusion: a determined conspiracy on the part of the group members to overlook the "obvious" in favor of the more "profound" as a way of avoiding what is most immediately painful in each other's conduct.

3) Relying upon in-group rather than out-group material allows group members to develop and explore a greater range of role relationships for themselves and each other. The usual therapeutic group immediately places a participant in the role of patient and/or therapist and by encouraging extensive case history development, tends to narrow the role explorations sanctioned by the group. Eschewing such a starting point, the encounter group is more likely to encourage a much broader range of roles to emerge. Also, by not establishing the individual's out-group situation as the important base of consideration the group is established as the essential reference group for the behaviors observed.

When feedback is seen as one of the important goals of a group, the introduction of videotape feedback will become a meaningful enhancement of such goals rather than a burden with which the group has to learn to deal. The shift from therapeutic orientation to encounter is an extremely important one for the implementation of videotape. Most psychotherapeutic groups, unless they have had videotape feedback available to them from the beginning, tend to react to its introduction as a disruption of their essential function: speculating about one another's life styles. But the television camera does not capture the more abstract, high level data which we label "problem." It will capture immediate behavior, particularly interaction between people, and it is only when the group is already attempting to deal with such data themselves that they see the videotape as enhancing their efforts. Because the encounter group deals with much more immediate data than most therapeutic groups, they are much more prepared to incorporate videotape feedback into their procedures.*

THE MARATHON GROUP AS AN ANALOGUE

While the marathon group represents a rearrangement of time and therefore could be conducted under a broad range of circumstances and settings, under its principle proponents, Bach (2) and the author (3, 4, 5) it has taken a position midway between the psychotherapeutic and encounter group. Marathon groups are often sought out as part of an individual's psychotherapeutic program and it can often provide an important shift of gears as a compensation for the accommodation which inevitably becomes a part of any continuing therapeutic relationship. Individuals will often enter the marathon with particular life problems in mind and there will be considerable effort to make bridges between the group experience and the life circumstances of the group member; there is an encouragement of parallels between movement through the group and movement through the world. However, many individuals enter the marathon group as part of their own search for growth and self-learning without necessarily being involved in a life problem. Should this be the case, there is little attempt to pressure the group member into talking about his life circumstances. For all participants behavior within the group is taken as significant data in its own right. Bridges between the group experience and the person's out-group life distinguish the marathon from the encounter group.**

Continuing as it does over a 24- to 48-hour period of time, the marathon group has a special psychological quality which makes it unique as

---

* It is of significance that the bulk of initial utilization of videotape in the sphere of psychotherapy has been in the realm of training. The field has been much more ready to expose therapists to self-encounter than patients. This is probably due to conventional psychiatry and clinical psychology's distrust of their patients' capacity for dealing with directness and honesty. Highly revealing fears and anticipations of patients' incapacity for handling self-confrontation have been expressed to the author from many psychotherapists; because such errors have been on the side of caution, the faulty image of people inherent in such expectations has not stood out as starkly as it should.

** The distinctions between psychotherapy and encounter groups are by no means exhausted by what has been outlined: it should be obvious that the therapeutic contract, with its emphasis upon obligations and responsibilities between client and therapist, is different. The marathon, consisting as it does mainly of a temporal arrangement, will depend to a considerable degree upon the orientation of the group leader. Therapeutic contracts concerning length of contract before and after the marathon experience also can differ considerably. Nevertheless, the heightened experiential aspect of the continuous session places it in a different dimension than routine psychotherapy.

a therapeutic experience. Group members come to such a special occasion with considerable expectations so that there is a psychological mobilization initiated prior to the experience itself. Within the session, as continuity and cohesiveness mount, the group becomes more and more of a world unto itself with its own flow and ebb and its own inevitability. Such concentration has a special value in that the world of the marathon group is miniaturized enough and compact enough for certain connections to be made by most participants. As the individual moves through the world of the marathon he engages in behaviors and emits signals which draw certain feelings toward him and which encourage others to construct a set of expectations about him. In short, each participant undergoes a *group career,* a set of acts and interactions within the group which constitute his particular history. At any given moment a participant's *group fate,* the cumulation of reactions, expectations, and behaviors which other group members have toward him, can be specified. Because the marathon has a unique combination of compactness and richness the group fate can easily be related to the group career of each individual.

It should be clear that there are important phases in a marathon group experience, that an intervention at a given point in the marathon's history has a very different significance and consequence than at another point. Such differential consequences have been found to be particularly relevant to the introduction of videotape feedback into the marathon group. The effect of such feedback, how it is received and used by the recipient is clearly a function of his concern about his group fate and is directly related to the development of his group career. Timing, therefore, is a prime consideration in how videotape feedback is used and while such timing will be dealt with in terms of the marathon experience, it is a necessary consideration for all groups. However, since the phases of the marathon are so clearly delineated, the intensive group will be dealt with as if it were an analogue for self-examining groups in general. However, before this is possible, a description of how the videotape equipment is used in the marathon is necessary.

THE RELATIONSHIP OF VIDEOTAPE EQUIPMENT TO THE GROUP

Self-confrontation through videotape within the group setting, as featured within this paper, has been described in considerable detail elsewhere (5, 6). However, in order to make the emergent strategy meaningful to the reader it is necessary to briefly describe the most important features of the system which has been given the name "focused feedback."

Videotape feedback is to be used by the group for its own purposes.

For this reason it has been found that the more readily the group members can have access to the equipment and the more control they can exercise over its replay, the more meaningful it becomes and the more integrated into the group interaction it becomes. Consequently the videotape equipment, along with camera and television monitor, is part of the group circle. For this purpose it has been found that relatively uncomplicated arrangements such as a single camera and half-inch video recorders lend themselves to unobtrusive inclusion within the group and to ready access by the group members. The price paid for such simplification is that only a portion of the group interaction can be recorded at any given moment and there is a loss of some detail. However, since the videotape feedback will be used in a highly selective manner this is not too limiting a factor.

Videotape is seen as containing an enormous amount of information so that it is quite easy to inundate a viewer with more input than he can deal with. Since the individual will exercise his usual frame of selective inattention, to use Sullivan's term (7), an essential decision must be made as to who is going to exercise the all important highlighting that must take place with the playback material. Focused feedback refers to just such selection on the part of the other group members and/or group leader: Small portions of the videotape are played back and only those portions which would appear to specify some particular point about an individual's behavior. Most of the videotape feedback is embedded within the group interaction as an integral part of the group feedback and, for the most part, involves immediate playback.

A strategy for feedback has been developed which borrows heavily upon the observations of Mead (8), particularly as developed by such writers as Shibutani (9). Within the process of role-taking, Mead speculated that before engaging in an act an individual rehearses it in his mind as well as the anticipated response of the audience. It is on the basis of the *anticipated* response that acts are completed. Therefore, wherever it is felt that a discrepancy may exist between a group member's anticipated response and his actual reception from others an opportunity for videotape feedback exists, concentrating upon specific aspects of his output which may contribute to the unexpected reception by others.

In order for the self-confrontation on videotape to be meaningful there must be a self-conscious appraisal of one's self which comes closest to what Turner (10) has discussed as reflexive role-taking. In this function, the other's perception of one's self is used as a mirror and the role-taker attempts to direct his attention as to how he appears to others. It should be obvious that this is a function which receives considerable attention in group. With the advent of videotape feedback, the role-taker for the first time has direct access to his image without it necessarily having to be completely mirrored through someone else. It turns out that reflexive role-taking is a difficult stance to internalize.

VIDEOTAPE FEEDBACK WITHIN THE MARATHON

Given the structure with which the videotape is utilized, it is now possible to specify the learnings which have occurred as a consequence of introducing such a tool within the marathon. Most importantly, it has been found that the development of the group and the position of the individual within the group, two closely related factors, are the most important considerations affecting the consequences of a particular feedback intervention. A particular person given the opportunity to confront himself on the television monitor will have very different reactions depending upon his own group career. The degree to which he will overtly make use of the feedback material is quite clearly a function of the degree to which he is thrown into disequilibrium by the group experience; it is only when an individual is off-balance in terms of knowing how to deal with input that overt movement will be seen.

In the initial phase of the marathon, generally lasting about the first third of the total session, group members react to confrontation on videotape with a lack of inner tension. It is immaterial whether or not they tend to be critical of themselves; they have little or no capacity to relate what they see with their group fate. What is lacking at this point is the capacity for self-examination; group members are generally markedly less perceptive about themselves than they are of others. It is much more important, at this phase of the marathon, to attend to how participants look at themselves than to look at the television monitor. It is almost inevitable that when they encounter themselves at this phase. people lack the physical signs of attention and struggle which invariably accompany self-examination and are much more interested in handling the material in a nondisturbing manner than taking it into themselves.

Despite the relatively little overt use group members can make of videotape feedback in the early phase, it is nevertheless a necessary part of the whole procedure. It is important that participants learn how to use the videotape, to come to accept it for themselves as a part of the armamentarium with which they are provided. It is also likely that the covert effect of videotape feedback at the early phase is more meaningful than might meet the eye, as the work of Robinson (11) suggests.

In the middle phase of the marathon, participants have moved from their initial self presentations ("let me tell you what I am like") to the development of specific group fates ("let us tell you what you are like"). In this phase there is a major struggle over how the individual will attend to the data being presented about himself. The group fate has achieved sufficient impact to make it of consequence to him. It is almost as if the individual cannot allow himself to feel how much the feedback he is getting really means to him and he must continue his defensive struggle. But it is an intensely more profound struggle than in the early phase because of the increased involvement with the group. Videotape feedback at this point can often change the way in which the group member conducts his transactions with the rest of the group; it can cause him to attend to the other group members when they are reacting to him in a very different fashion than had been formerly the case. That is to say, the group member is not so much ready to restructure his way of seeing himself *vis-à-vis* the world as he becomes ready to take in and consider what others are trying to tell him rather than put most of his energy into holding it off.

An illustration of a middle phase way of dealing with videotape feedback can be seen in the case of a man who was struggling with the group in their perception of him as being overly involved in his father's ubiquitous internalized presence in terms of his adolescent-like behavior. But most of his energy was invested into holding off the group's perception of himself. When he had an opportunity to react to himself on videotape he remarked that he could see himself as a weakling. His relationship to the group abruptly changed and one could see him attending much more carefully, not only to reactions to himself, but to what was taking place with others in the group. This marked a distinct turning point for him in the marathon.

In the final phase of the marathon, participants are often in a state of marked disequilibrium insofar as their group fate is concerned. This phase of the marathon is often marked by such rapid movement on the part of numerous participants that it is often difficult to anticipate.* Videotape feedback during this phase will much more likely result in dramatic reconstruction on the part of the individual. The self-confrontation comes at a point when they can make clear connections between their group career and their group fate and the individual is often ready for a very different kind of experience to take place. This is videotape feedback at its most dramatic—the fruition of the kinds of reactions

---

* One of the more remarkable features of a marathon is the way in which time seems to expand and contract. Certainly what can be accomplished within a given time during the later phases of a marathon cannot be anticipated through any other procedure.

that most who turn to this tool anticipate seeing: self-confrontation as a profound revelation to the individual.

Just such a self-confrontation took place with a young woman who entered the intensive group caught between her revulsion at her husband's infidelity and her inability to see herself in any independent role. After considerable struggle with the group, in the final phase of the marathon she was given videotape feedback. She was suddenly able to see herself as a person who clearly had many more options than she had ever considered and had an intense and immediate alteration of her self-image, to the extent that she commented on feeling lighter. Her changed self-concept persisted over time to contribute in a very significant manner to changes she subsequently initiated in her life-style.

Using videotape feedback within the context of a marathon experience allows one to see the range of reactions to this tool. The basic stance which the individual brings to self-confrontation is critical but it is also apparent that the group culture which has developed will aid and abet the self-examining stance to a considerable degree or permit a wide range of avoidance. It is also apparent that videotape cannot be used to bypass any of the phases of group development. It is, instead, a tool for enhancing what the group members are already attempting to do.

ADDITIONAL OPPORTUNITIES FOR VIDEOTAPE FEEDBACK
IN THE ENCOUNTER GROUP

Because the marathon experience is so powerful, it does not lend itself to post-examination. As a consequence, videotape has been used only within the marathon, rarely outside of it. However, in the ongoing encounter group there is ample opportunity for examination of the videotapes outside of the group session itself. This can be accomplished through a viewing period in which selected segments of the tape are viewed and reactions encouraged.

Inherent in the group is a heightened defensiveness. When the individual has an opportunity to react to himself without the necessity to deal with others at the same time, a different type of assimilation is possible. Whether more leisurely consideration of one's behavior is more effective than immediacy is a question still to be settled. In any case, since there is likely to have been so little experience in anyone's life in self-confrontation, there is some gain to be obtained through training group members in enriching their range of self-perceptions (12).

Still another dimension can be attained through the demonstration of change; movement is thus reinforced. Tapes showing behavior at one point in the group experience can be saved to be shown at a later time.

238 *Videotape in Psychiatric Training, Treatment*

When an individual is able to see the changes that he himself has accomplished, both his own potency and the value of the directions he has been taking can become very real to him.

In the final analysis it is behavior, particularly unaccustomed behavior, which, when captured on videotape, can provide the most important movement. Thus, it may be the giving and receiving of affection, not talking about it, which can add the most learning for an individual. In similar manner videotape provides an avenue for an individual shaping his own behavior, determining for himself how he would like to be and attempting to bring about his own changes. Thus, a young man was very ineffectual in expressing his anger toward his family. When he rehearsed this on videotape he acknowledged how unhappy he was with his own behavior and kept rehearsing and reviewing until he was able to express himself in a way that satisfied him.

It can be predicted that, to the degree that groups break out of their verbal traps, to the degree that they permit themselves behavior (as opposed to discussion), videotape will become a more meaningful and powerful tool. By pushing the boundaries in the direction of experience, marathon and encounter groups are contributing to a deeper understanding of this important new approach to self-confrontation.

REFERENCES

1. Rogers, C. R.: The Process of the Basic Encounter Group. In J. F. T. Bugental (Ed.), *Challenges of Humanistic Psychology*. New York: McGraw-Hill, 1967, pp. 261-276.
2. Bach, G. R.: The Marathon Group: Intensive Practice of Intimate Interaction. *Psychol. Rep.*, 18:995-1002, 1966.
3. Stoller, F. H.: Marathon Group Therapy. In G. M. Gazda (Ed.), *Innovations to Group Psychotherapy*. Springfield, Ill.: Charles C Thomas, 1968, pp. 45-95.
4. Stoller, F. H.: Accelerated Interaction: A Time-limited Approach Based on the Brief, Intensive Group. *Int. J. Grp. Psychother.*, 18:220-235, 1968.
5. Stoller, F. H.: Focused Feedback with Video Tape: Extending the Group's Functions. In G. M. Gazda (Ed.), *Innovations to Group Psychotherapy*. Springfield, Ill.: Charles C Thomas, 1968, pp. 207-255.
6. Stoller, F. H.: Use of Video Tape (Focused Feedback) in Group Counseling and Group Therapy. *J. Research and Devel. in Educ.*, 1 (2):30-44, 1968.
7. Sullivan, H. S.: *The Interpersonal Theory of Psychiatry*. New York: Norton, 1953.
8. Mead, G. H.: *Mind, Self, and Society*. Chicago: Univ. of Chicago, 1934.
9. Shibutani, T.: *Society and Personality*. Englewood Cliffs, N.J.: Prentice-Hall, 1961.
10. Turner, R. H.: Role-taking, Role Standpoint, and Reference-Group Behavior. In B. J. Biddle and E. J. Thomas (Eds.), *Role Theory: Concepts and Research*. New York: Wiley, 1966, pp. 151-159.
11. Robinson, Margot B.: Effects of Video Tape Feedback Versus Discussion Session Feedback on Group Interaction, Self Awareness and Behavioral Change Among Group Psychotherapy Participants. Unpublished doctoral dissertation. University of Southern California, 1968.
12. Stoller, F. H.: The Long Weekend. *Psychol. Today*, 1 (7):28-33, 1967.

19

A SIX-YEAR VIDEOTAPED PSYCHO-THERAPY PROJECT WITH AN OUTPATIENT GROUP OF SCHIZOPHRENICS

Constance B. Nelson, Ph.D.

My interest in the use of audio-videotapes dates back to my years at the St. Cloud, Minnesota Veterans Administration Hospital (1966-67) when I designed and carried out a study of videotape therapy with chronic schizophrenic patients (1, 2).*

It was startling and disappointing to find no significant differences between our AVT and control groups—especially so since the articles being published then by Cornelison and Arsenian (3), Moore et al. (4), and Stoller (5), were reporting such favorable results with this new technique. Dr. Morris Vestre, then at the University of Minnesota, who consulted with me on this project, advised me to reflect on and keep in mind our patient population.

In addition to the fact that all of the patients were on medications, which alters differential effects of new treatment modalities, there are some other insights I have had about our lack of proof for the superiority of AVT: 1) Our therapist for the AVT and control therapy group had no previous experience in group therapy with psychotic patients—nor had the co-therapist, the head nurse in the Unit.** I had many years' experience, both in state and in VA hospitals, with such groups and supervised his therapy during feedback sessions with him, but, in light of recent findings of Karon and VandenBos (6), when the therapist's own experience and motivation are not controlled, an important

---

Paper presented at the American Association for the Advancement of Science Meeting in Denver, Colo., February 1977.

* Nelson and Shardlow: Unpublished Report, 1970.

** A copy of Mr. Shardlow's evaluation (1967) of this experience can be secured by writing to the author of this chapter.

239

variable has been ignored. 2) Five months—the length of time for our inpatient study at St. Cloud—is not a long enough time span for patients such as these to have developed a therapy alliance with the therapists and with each other. (Time involved in forming such alliances with psychotic patients has been discussed by Sullivan (7), Fromm-Reichmann (8), and more recently by Kernberg (9), and Werner Mendel (10). 3) After completion of the study, I happened to hear from a staff person that the AVT room (where therapy groups met) was in the basement of the building where—years before—lobotomies had been done; it is quite possible that some or even all of the long-term patients (randomly found in each group) might have had a very negative and guarded reaction to the project. (Of course, none of the patients ever spoke of this!)

For the last nine years, my work has been with outpatients in the Denver Veterans Administration Hospital Mental Health Clinic. Since February, 1970, I have worked with a videotaped therapy group made up mostly of chronic schizophrenic outpatients—and have always worked with a co-therapist.* Each co-therapist is in training one year at our clinic and whether he or she is from psychology, social work, or clinical pastoral education, the phenomena are similar: 1) Initially there is suspiciousness of the new therapist, intense testing out, denial of hostility and attempts to split the therapists; 2) usually after six months the co-therapist is accepted as a therapist, and 3) when he or she leaves, there are genuine feelings of sadness and loss along with some vicarious feelings of "graduating" to new opportunities. Not only is this an excellent training experience for our students, but it is mandatory for me to have someone who can continue the group in my absence and I feel it is much more therapeutic for the patients to have two than to have one therapist. The inter-generational and sometimes sex and race differences between us are evident and that plus the fact that we respect and support one another seems to catalyze transferences rapidly. The group meets for one and a half hours each week and, whenever the AVT equipment has been in working order, each session has been videotaped. The group watches a replay of chosen excerpts from the preceding session for the first half hour each week, then goes into the adjoining room to have the day's session taped. Since June of 1974, we have been fortunate in having a technician to do the taping and replays for us. This has helped the co-therapists to get a "clearer picture"—actually and theoretically— as we have been freed up from trying to operate the hardware and can attend to the group process and the progress of each individual within

---

* Current co-therapists are Rev. David Latham and Mr. Douglas Kerr.

the group. Our present technician* has been extremely helpful in her astute observation of changes in patterns of relating within the group and this has helped us in choosing particular passages for replay.

The group is an open-ended group, heterogeneous as to age, sex, educational, occupational levels and physical problems; the average number of years' membership is four; one member has been there only six months; two are charter members, having begun in 1970. Each person has signed permission for the taping; those unwilling to sign have been screened out from such an opportunity. At this point, I am convinced that those who do choose to sign are not hurt by the process of being videotaped. Some of them appear to have been helped to the extent that they themselves and/or their peers have mentioned such changes as these (during and after the playbacks): "Your voice isn't as loud as it used to be." "Now we can see your eyes!" "You can interrupt other people when you want to say something; last year you couldn't!"

Definitive research is needed. Variables which might profitably be measured in pre- and post-testing and in follow-ups include: 1) ego development (Loevinger's (11) Ego Development test?); 2) authoritarianism (Levinson's (12, 13) "F" Scale?); 3) openness and awareness— together with more judgment about situations where each is appropriate and where they are not appropriate; 4) decision-making; 5) self-esteem; 6) self-object relations; 7) growth in communication between co-therapists who, like good parents, model how to differ yet maintain respect for each other; 8) the degree to which group and leaders share group history and culture which serves to counteract the "ahistoricity" of the individual schizophrenic.

If self-confrontation is a part of the therapeutic process, the visual and auditory playback of one's own participation week after week, year after year, ought to facilitate the process. When it does not, one can then look at resistance, negative transference, countertransferences, denial, and all the other defenses which clients, patients, trainees and staff use in dealing with very affect-laden material.

One might think that, especially with psychotic patients, the cumulative effect of seeing oneself interacting, attacking, or withdrawing within the group would challenge the psychotic's notion that forces outside himself control what happens to him. Wouldn't he grow less fearful of authority, seeing the therapist sometimes talk too much, sometimes misunderstand what the message really is? My experience over the years suggests that this will be true only if the patient is freed up to learn and

---

* Miss Laura Curtis who is studying for an M.A. in Communications.

242   Videotape in Psychiatric Training, Treatment

if the therapist's experience about timing and interventions can help facilitate growth at the teachable moment.

It may well be that some of our authority-oriented patients who early in therapy "think" only in stereotypes are quite threatened by the egalitarian nature of therapy where therapists and patients alike are seen during feedback sessions as being "simply more human than otherwise." If self-concept be based on defiance of an omnipotent authority and if the therapist ("omnipotent authority") be seen as not omnipotent, there may be in AVT therapy—as in any other therapy—a great deal of resistance and anger, rather than a giving up of the defiance. The patients who are able to become more comfortable with the therapist as a real person are freed up to be more active in decision-making and in trying new behaviors. Other patients dependently continue to demand that the therapist tell them what to do, insist that she read their minds and keep them from making mistakes. As with analysis of outcome in any therapy research, so with AVT therapy, we see different outcomes in terms of premorbid personality and defensive structures within different patients. Sinclair Lewis said in one of his novels: "The same fire that melts the butter hardens the egg." So playback, feedback, confrontation (terms used interchangeably in AVT literature), may promote emotional and interpersonal growth in some and harden resistance to such growth in others.

Research must be done to study the many variables which need investigation if AVT is to be used effectively in long-term therapy with chronic psychotic patients.

REFERENCES

1. Nelson, C. B., and Shardlow, G. W.: A Pilot Investigation of Videotape Technique in Group Psychotherapy of Hospitalized Chronic Schizophrenic Patients. V. A. Newsletter for Research in Psychology, XIII, (2), 122, 1970.
2. Shardlow, G. W. Evaluation of Audio-Video Tape Playbacks as An Adjunct to Group Therapy with Chronic Schizophrenic Patients. Unpublished manuscript, 1967.
3. Cornelison, F. S., and Arsenian, J.: A Study of the Responses of Psychotic Patients to Photographic Self-Image Experiences. Psychiatric Quarterly, 34:1-8, 1960.
4. Moore, F. J., Chernell, E., and West, M. J.: "O Wad Some Power the Giftie Gie Us": Television as a Therapeutic Tool. Archives of General Psychiatry, 12:217-220, 1965.
5. Stoller, F. H.: Group Psychotherapy on TV: An Innovation with Hospitalized Patients. American Psychologist, 22 (2):158-162, 1967.
6. Karon, B. P., and VandenBos, G. R.: Medication and/or Psychotherapy with Schizophrenics: Which Part of the Elephant Have You Touched? International Mental Health Research Newsletter, XVII (3), 1:8-13, 1975.
7. Sullivan, H. S.: Clinical Studies in Psychiatry (H. S. Perry et al., Eds.). New York: W. W. Norton, 1956.

8. Bullard, D. M. (Ed.): *Psychoanalysis and Psychotherapy. Selected Papers of Frieda Fromm-Reichmann.* Chicago: U. Chicago Press, 1959.
9. Kernberg, O.: *Borderline Conditions and Pathological Narcissism.* New York: Jason Aronson, 1975.
10. Mendel, W. M.: *Supportive Care: Theory and Technique.* Los Angeles: Mara Books, 1975.
11. Loevinger, J., and Wessler, R.: *Measuring Ego Development*, Vols. I and II. San Francisco: Jossey-Bass, 1970.
12. Levinson, D. J.: An Approach to the Theory and Measurement of Ethnocentrism. *American Psychologist,* 2:412, 1947.
13. Levinson, D. M., and Huffman, P. E.: The TFI and Its Relationship to Personality. *Journal of Personality,* 23:251-274, 1955.

20

FREEZE-FRAME VIDEO IN PSYCHOTHERAPY

Ian Alger, M.D.

Over the past decade technical improvements in videotape equipment have made its use so much more reliable and simple that thousands of small videotape production units are now operating in clinics and private offices throughout the country. The new thrust is towards the development of a broader, more inclusive, and more clearly defined therapeutic integration of video techniques. The application of "freeze-frame" intervention allows the therapist to work within his usual therapeutic framework and at the same time include new observations and material which the video camera has captured.

"Freeze-frame" is a term which describes the capacity of some videorecorders to stop the action at any particular moment. All of us see this demonstrated on commercial TV when the ice hockey puck is shown slowing in its path to the net and then is stopped, still-framed against the bulging webbing, past the goalie's glove, frozen on the screen. The "freeze-frame" technique is but one of many ways that video playback can be used in psychotherapy, but in this chapter a more detailed description of its use will be the focus.

It is somewhat paradoxical that the video method which so superbly allows for recording action should now be used to portray still pictures, a seeming return to the era of still photography. Clearly, video recording allows the viewer to distinguish sequences of movements, the flow of cued behavior, and the dissection of complex behavioral interaction. When it is used to identify single frames of behavior, however, it has the advantage over still photography of permitting a selection of the single frames from recordings of the entire sequence. Thus, one can discern exactly which member of a group initiates a sequence, and one can capture the exact nuance of expression which may have lasted only a fraction of a second. With the picture frozen on the screen, all participants in a therapy session, therapist included, can associate to the moment

244

and can examine and review, with no pressure, all of the feelings and ideas generated. The starkness of the frozen moment allows a stepping back from the situation, thereby providing a meta position for comprehending the interactions in a broader perspective. This phenomenon of the shift to a meta position is one of the particular advantages of the videotape method in therapy, because it encourages the development of a more equal and cooperative relationship between patients and therapist as all become involved in the more objective examination of the video data. In regard to this point, however, it must be kept in mind that the video images, whether in motion sequence or in still-frame, provide not only objective information, but also lend themselves to projection by the viewers. The still-frame perhaps more than the motion picture offers an enticing projective screen, and the participants and especially the therapist must continually explore the boundaries of subjective and objective experience.

The cliché of the picture and a thousand words finds particular support in the video experience. Visual images tend to have powerful retentive impact. But a further elaboration of this phenomenon is found in the freeze-frame technique. Once a particular therapeutic insight or awareness has been derived from the exploration of a freeze-frame image, that particular image retains the metaphoric quality for the total experience and derived conceptualizations. The calling up of such an image by any member of the therapeutic encounter thus possesses a powerful symbolic quality, which in shorthand way can communicate a wealth of emotional, ideational, and behavioral material. A father may say in a later session, "Remember the way you looked down while I was speaking to you?" and the son will recall that frozen frame and in this metaphor remember his own feelings of anger, the father's feelings of hurt, and the resolution which was made when each came to understand the other's fear of closeness. In this way, families and couples can develop a new and personal family shorthand containing freeze-frame metaphors which can have enduring usefulness in their human communication.

TECHNICAL CONSIDERATIONS

Details of basic video technology will not be reviewed here. Rather, those factors will be emphasized which relate to the relevance of the equipment for freeze-frame operation and to the ways in which the therapist can exercise control over the taping and the replay.

Most one-half inch reel-to-reel videorecorders have both stop-action and slow motion modalities. Even the porta pack has still-frame capacity.

Newer three-fourths inch cassette models also have still-frame features, but many lack slow motion action. The "search" feature on some cassette models is useful in that it allows the therapist to cue a particular spot as the recording is being made, thereby allowing a return to that particular spot later by merely depressing a button. However, the inexpensive reel-to-reel one-half inch model still provides a dependable and versatile working companion. It should be positioned near the therapist so he can operate it easily and at will. The monitor should also be placed within reach so the therapist can control the volume and eliminate feedback during the recording phases. Another monitor positioned across the room from the therapist allows him to focus the camera during the session. The camera can be set on a low tripod and operated with one hand by the therapist, utilizing the barrel of the zoom lens as a handle, and also permitting zooming and focusing at the same time. More elaborate units have a remote control camera(s), and the therapist can control pan and tilt, as well as focus and zoom.

If the therapist works with a co-therapist, the taping and decisions for the replay can be left primarily with the other therapist. However, the most total integration of therapeutic effect can be obtained when one person is able to decide on the camera shots, the moments of replay, with decisions on which images to freeze-frame, and the relationship of the video feedback to the other therapeutic interventions which are used. On first consideration the complexity of being camera operator, therapist, and video technician simultaneously may seem overwhelming, but surprisingly little practice will enable most people to become adequately proficient, and further use brings increasing ease. It should be repeated, however, that the same system can be used by co-therapists, and it should also be mentioned that some workers prefer joint leadership models.

Although in this method the therapist more often makes decisions regarding the type of intervention and the timing of interventions, patients also learn to use the technique and will begin to call for replay sequences and freeze-frame images. In practice the use of two to three freeze-frame interventions in any one session is enough to provide effective input, without excessively interrupting the flow of the session.

Even though the therapist is more often the one to stop the action, the way in which he introduces the material is crucial in determining the quality of the exchanges. The most effective intervention, in my experience, is one which selects a moment but highlights it for *mutual* examination. In not making a definite interpretive statement, the therapist promotes more participation by the patients and encourages the development of mutual work towards better understanding of feelings and behavior. Video imagery is powerful, and its use in a coercive manner can be especially distorting and harmful to the goals of self-development and greater social and contextual awareness. In essence, then, the freeze-frame is used as an index for exploration, and later as a metaphor for the awareness and understanding gained.

In the remaining sections, clinical examples of this technique will be given, with emphasis on the factors influencing the therapist's choice, the reactions of the patients, and the apparent effects of the interventions.

INITIAL FAMILY SESSION

The following descriptions are based on an initial simulated family session, taped to demonstrate the use of video interventions and edited as a 27-minute color film, *Family Circle.** Emphasis will be placed on the freeze-frame sequences. The family was introduced to the video equipment, and an explanation was given that periodically some of the tape would be replayed in order to clarify or explore some particular moments in the session. Participants, as always, were asked to sign releases for the taping, which included permission to use the material for teaching with professional groups.

The presenting problem in the family was the depression of the mother. The particular episode of depression seemed related to the imminent departure of the couple's only daughter, who was shortly leaving for college. The father's parents had agreed to pay for the tuition but recently had added some "strings" to the offer. This put the father in a position between his wife and his own parents, since the wife now objected to the whole arrangement. In the session the father and mother and their daughter, as well as the paternal grandparents, were present. The therapist sat across from the family and utilized a single camera with zoom lens and a one-half inch reel-to-reel VTR.

The session opened by the father stating the problem, and as he talked the therapist noted that his mother and his father both shifted in their seats. This sequence was shortly replayed on video, and the action was frozen on the three of them. This allowed the seating to be emphasized, and it was seen that the father had sat on one end of the line, his mother, the grandmother, to his immediate left, with his father, the grandfather, next. This left the granddaughter between her grandfather and her own mother, who was on the other extreme end of the family group. The

---

* Information about this film may be obtained by writing to the author at 500 East 77th Street, New York, N. Y. 10021.

freeze-frame clearly showed the threesome of the father's original family. A following freeze-frame of the grandfather and the granddaughter showed an inclination of body posture in which the grandfather, although having his arm around his own wife on one side, was leaning sharply towards his granddaughter on the other side. The recognition of this "in-between" stance led him to later acknowledge that there had always been a closeness he felt towards his granddaughter.

The next freeze-frame caught the depressed mother at the far end of the line, and her loneliness and isolation were evident. Up to this point the freeze-frame interventions had been used essentially to emphasize the seating of the family, underlining the alliances which were evidenced, with the resulting isolation and exclusion of the mother.

As the session proceeded, the mother spoke of her loneliness, and the daughter's eyes glanced to the left, towards her mother. This glance of the eye was replayed and frozen on the screen. In response to that image, the daughter said that she had not been aware of how her mother had been feeling and reached over and took her mother's hand. The session continued, and later the therapist made a structural intervention which flowed from the video image of the separation of the nuclear family, with the father at one end and the grandparents in between the father and his wife and daughter. The father was asked to stand, and all members of the family were asked to move down one seat, with the father taking his new place at the other end of the line, now beside his wife. As he took this new place, the therapist noted that almost at the same moment the father crossed his legs towards his wife, while the daughter crossed her legs towards her mother. This sequence was replayed and frozen. The freeze-frame showed the mother literally surrounded by her husband and daughter, closed between the parentheses of their crossed legs. She acknowledged how good it felt to be together, and the father commented how pleased he was that his wife could see that he cared.

As the session continued, the focus moved to the grandmother who now looked somewhat out-of-place in her distant position at the other far end of the line, now that her son had moved next to his wife. As the grandmother responded to her feelings of being taken advantage of, her own husband, the grandfather, was seen by the therapist to make a pursed movement with his lips. On replay this constricted movement of his mouth was frozen, and he was asked to comment. This facilitated a discussion of some of his distaste for his own wife's reactions, and a few moments later another freeze-frame showed a similar narrowing and pursing of her lips. The video replay thus facilitated a focus on the interaction of separate family subgroups, the father-mother-daughter nuclear group, and the grandparent couple. The freeze-frame served to focus the structure and also facilitated experimentation with a different structure. In the newer configurations, the still frames emphasized the feeling of warmth and increased closeness between husband and wife, and the frustration of the father at the mother's not realizing how he did care for her. On the other hand, the freeze-frame helped discern conflict between the grandparent couple and encouraged a more open acknowledgement of the frictions between them. The session ended by a final freeze-frame capturing the grandmother's tongue licking her lips, just as she said that perhaps she would have to look at things in a new way. This vivid image acted as the metaphor described earlier in raising the possibility that new ways could hold the possibility of a new taste for life.

In this particular demonstration the freeze-frame was used more often than ordinary in order to demonstrate various possibilities in the method. As noted before, two or three interventions in any one session seem optimal. This allows the video impact to carry its message, but also permits the participants to elaborate and make further applications together.

COUPLE THERAPY

In the previous clinical example, three generations of a family were seen in an initial session. One of the therapeutic tasks was to restructure the family so that the generations became more identifiable, and eventually the clinical focus became more directed towards two couples, the parent couple, and the grandparent couple.

In the present clinical situation a marital couple was seen alone. The session was taped and edited as a 35-minute film entitled, *Freeze-Frame Video.** The couple and their two children had been in treatment with other therapists over a period of years. Many different approaches, from family therapy to individual analysis, had been used. The family had seen me several times around behavior problems in their two girls, one of whom had just entered her teens. In this present, eighth session the focus had been already moved to the marital pair, and the goal was to establish a more immediate and direct type of communication between the two partners and also among the partners and the therapist.

Marital couples often encounter difficulties in their relationship through communication problems which lead to repetitive sequential behaviors. These frequently escalate to violence or distant impasse. Couples also commonly demonstrate an unawareness both of their own

---

* Information about this film may be obtained by writing to the author at 500 East 77th Street, New York, N. Y. 10021.

feelings, and the way these feelings are represented in their nonverbal behavior towards their partners. Videotape playback is useful both to identify and to interrupt repetitive, stereotyped behavioral sequences and also to highlight by freeze-framing a particularly significant moment or image which can be used to foster greater awareness and communication.

As before, the therapist sat with a camera at one side and the videotape recorder (VTR) at the other side. The session began with the couple sitting together, side by side. The wife sighed; both gazed at each other; next, the woman laughed, whereupon the husband turned, gestured with his hand and said, "Ladies first!" Following this, however, he turned immediately and began to speak in a lecturing style. The first video intervention was a replay of this sequence to demonstrate the way in which the husband and wife participated in his beginning to lecture, a mode of interaction that was common and which was deplored by both. The videoreplay succeeded in identifying the sequence and in interrupting it. This introduction served as a basis for the next intervention which involved the use of a freeze-frame technique.

The therapist commented that perhaps the couple would like to rearrange their seating, since intimate communication involved comfortableness in the distance between them. They took a new position and resumed conversation. The therapist noted, however, that their seated stance towards one another was very stilted, and an angular distance was uncomfortably maintained. This picture was still-framed, and the couple began to discuss their reactions and feelings and consequently moved to a more comfortable distance from one another. Without this videoplayback, the likelihood is that the uncomfortably stilted and close position might have been maintained much longer and would have interfered with the exchange. The freeze-frame made possible an awareness which also demonstrated that corrective action could be taken in the situation.

In a further portion of the session, the wife initiated a use of video replay herself. During the sequence she glanced at the live television monitor and noticed a "grim" expression on her face. During replay she recalled this, and the "grim picture" was thereupon frozen on the screen. She associated that this must be the look that her husband didn't like, and she allowed as how she could understand his reaction. The therapist then ran the tape forward and shortly came to a place where he froze the picture at the wife's smile. The husband noted that this was the kind of expression he wished he could have more often from her. In this way a metaphor was created for shorthanding a quality of relating between the marital pair. The "grim look" and the "smile" came to signify two important modes in this couple's communication patterns. In effect then, the freeze-frames of the "grim look" and of the "smile" introduced an opportunity for the couple to talk more directly to each other about their feelings. He expressed a desire for more smiles in their exchanges, and she acknowledged a new awareness of the way in which her "grim look" could adversely affect her husband. Thus, the goal of encouraging more direct and open communication was facilitated.

In a subsequent segment of the session, the therapist noted that the husband's expression seemed removed and distant. That image was frozen on the screen, and the husband was invited to look at the picture and to describe what he felt that man on the screen might be experiencing. This method of direct image confrontation allows a person to create some distance from the immediate situation, and it frequently supports the revelation of otherwise concealed attitudes and emotions. The patient said, "There is a sad man." He went on to describe why the man was sad, and began to reveal feelings that the wife and the therapist were ganging up on him and that he felt isolated and pushed out. The inclusion of the therapist directly into the dynamics of the session by this intervention with freeze-frame illustrates another powerful way in which the video replay can be integrated into the flow of the therapeutic interaction. By his direct expression and challenge, the husband was able to take himself out of the isolated position, and the therapist was able to change his own position from an alliance with the wife, a position usually taken in that family by the children.

In discussing her feelings after the session, the wife noted that she had not experienced the video as an interference in the session. She also noted that she had learned about her "grim look," and that she had appreciated being able to realize more about her husband's sadness.

DISCUSSION

On the basis of clinical experience it seems evident that the freeze-frame technique has immediate impact. It has usefulness in disrupting repetitive sequences. It is of value in determining cueing and alliances and in demonstrating these to patients. It is helpful in capturing small gestures and expressions and using these to stimulate association and to clarify feelings. It is also of use in identifying ambivalence demonstrated in contradictory body postures where, for example, the gaze is directed one way while the torso leans another.

The value of the method has also been shown in the development of metaphors which become a part of patients' communication shorthand and which persist as visual images with an eduring and vivid quality. In the clinical examples, couples and families were described, but the method can be used with individuals and with heterogeneous groups.

In conclusion, the freeze-frame technique is one of many video methods which can add to our therapeutic repertoire, and when used without coercive intent, can encourage joint inquiry into other perspectives of human behavior and communication.

21
THE USE OF VIDEOTAPE IN FAMILY THERAPY WITH SPECIAL RELATION TO THE THERAPEUTIC IMPASSE

Carl A. Whitaker, M.D.

Milton Berger and others in this volume have described the use of video in psychotherapy. I would like to emphasize that in family therapy the use of the videotape is more important than in the individual therapy or even in couples therapy or group therapy. The family system operates with greater power than either a group of strangers or an individual or a couple. The two generation unit carries an identification with such interpersonal supplementation and amplification that any therapeutic effort is often relatively impotent. Even if there are two therapists, the family may include from three to 10 or 15. Furthermore, families, in living together, have developed a coalition against the outside world which, in addition to their biological identification, makes their techniques for handling interference well developed, expertly integrated and always alert. The family rituals and myths of the family have been refined and developed for generations and, therefore, the exactness of their operation has become covert and precisely calibrated.

A therapist, or therapeutic team, though strengthened by his own professional training, his own therapy and by the freedom accorded him by the focusing power of his role function, is still a smaller system. On threat of change, the family may summate their affects until the therapist becomes extruded as described by Lyman Wynne. That "rubber fence" is powerful. The same family in a different situation may reduce the therapist to a tepid "blob of gluck" by their warmth. Sometimes and with even less effort they invade his person with their own dedication to chaos until the therapist castrates himself with his own razor.

Prevention of such therapeutic impotence is obviously the best pattern. It can often be abetted by an implicit or explicit contract which helps establish the therapeutic relationship as a time-limited, "as if" arrangement. The family are, thereby, free to use the symbolic experience of

253

psychotherapy to play at change and, thereby, suffer less anxiety. Prevention may also be aided by avoiding family splits into protherapy/antitherapy or his and her family subgroups. Delaying the first appointment until all the group have agreed to go ahead obviously helps. Carefully protecting their rights to terminate with or without a reason and at any time also assures them that any change must be authorized by the entire system. This also defines the function of the therapist as coach or assistant in the process of change. He must not become a member of the family except temporarily and with limited objectives. Furthermore, he must carefully protect his maneuverability. A better insurance against the failure of the change effort is the utilizing of a larger system when endeavoring to help change the family system. Co-therapy is the best such arrangement thus far developed. When there are two therapists, the family can actually face a more equal setting. One patient said it graphically: "I can handle one of you guys all right, but having two of you is like having the whole world in." The co-therapy also provides an answer to Milt Miller's famous question, "Who is the 'they'?"

If co-therapy is not possible, for whatever reason, it can be approximated by using a consultant to the relationship. The second interview consultation visit by a colleague establishes a time and method for shifting perspective and thus forming two realities. The greater objectivity of the outsider may be reassuring, comforting or confirming, but at least provides dual perception. The consultant also offers the implicit value of triangulation. Teaming, the function of arbitration, provocation and split transference may be useful and at least help to keep the therapeutic relationship flexible and open to input from different levels of communication by each of the two therapy subsystems.

If a consultation is not available or even if it is, videotape may serve as an effective feedback system. As in any administrative decision, the earlier video is begun the less it interferes with the need for intimacy and bilateral trust. The first interview's value is obvious after very little experience with it. Decisions about playback within that interview, family review after the appointment or before the second appointment should be guarded. However, as the therapy becomes established, the family may elect to review parts or all of that first session or subsequent ones. This experience helps them develop objectivity and an overview of their interaction patterns. Their veto rights should be protected to avoid excess anxiety summation. However, even repeated replay may be useful since it stimulates a distancing perspective in the family members and furnishes exciting data for interaction between them and a better sense of the family as a whole.

Example

A. Jim, I didn't notice yesterday how hurt you were by my innocent comment. Do I do that to you often?

B. Daddy, I didn't tell you how mad I got when you wouldn't answer my question. It made me feel like I was six instead of 18. Won't you ever give me credit for being a voting adult?

C. Mother: Did you all notice that we never let anyone finish his sentence? We interrupted everyone, even Granddad. No wonder we're all so irritable.

Tangential to the assets of feedback is the unique assets of the family's expanding initiative. The initial impulse to change is often converted into a challenge to the therapist—"O.K., we've failed to fix it, now you do your thing, you're the expert." Such a battle will end usually in defeat of the therapist. The only "out" is for the therapist to team with the family and to position himself so that the family carry the initiative for change. They deserve the continued freedom to take their family life-style and even symptom recurrence back into their own hands. The therapist does well to be highly suspicious of his own super-mother impulses. If he cares enough to limit his "take over," the family may reunite and effect a flight into health with amazing casualness.

However, it does frequently happen that the therapy moves smoothly with the formation of a therapeutic family-therapist suprasystem until a significant change occurs. The stress thus induced may be excessive and then develops one of the two stalemating processes: One of these is a therapist incorporating intimacy, while the other is a covert hostile dependent withdrawal. If a consultant, professional or nonprofessional, has been involved, he/she may be invited to revisit.

If neither is possible, videotape and replay may serve to break up the impasse. Comparison or reviewing previous tapes may then serve as a binocular vision assist. That cyclops eye seeks with a scary depth, so again the family's anxiety should be titrated with care. Even more vital, the therapist must face with the family his partial responsibility for the stalemate. The family's impulse for healing and growth is a constant. The therapist's functional adequacy is the variable.

Said one school principal father: "My God, Doc, we were all crazy. We came because Henry was called schizophrenic, but that damn machine— I looked as crazy as Henry. I should never have told you guys I was homicidal during my freshman year at college. I looked violent when I just recounted it. But worse than that it tipped mother into re-opening her old suicidal impulses. Even Joan confessed her delusions about the Catholics being after her when she hid in her room for two weeks last fall."

One husband said he was very impressed and very upset by the video. He saw himself behind a tremendous wall of formality and he didn't look at his wife during the entire hour. "I seemed artificial to myself. I got a new sense of how delusional I was about myself. As a lawyer I seem good and competent, as a person I wasn't who I was in that hour at all. I wasn't letting anything come out of me. In the TV I really scared myself." The wife, picking up, said, "I'm anxious about us and I'm also aware of my lack of feeling." Husband went on, "I sense that if I let my wall down, I'll be taken over and then I guess I'd be eaten up or I'll force them to take me over. It's like my folks. They phoned last evening and I was that way with them. They see my formality as competence and I hadn't known what was really there before this videotape. Now I see my role reversal with my mother from mother-son to father-daughter, and I have never gotten a peer relationship. My Dad, I see now, had done the same thing and here I'd prided myself all this time on not being like him."

THE MACHINE AS CONSULTANT AND AS CO-THERAPIST

The machine has separate functions—I am most concerned with its function as consultant to the family as the patient. I, of course, like to use it as consultant to me, the therapist who is participating, and thus becomes part of that larger family we call the therapeutic family. But I also use it as an extension of me, the manipulator. The machine has the capacity to increase the feedback to me so I become objective about my own subjectivity. One can be objective but in that role one is distant and cold. I want no part of that. One can be subjective, but then I tend to be weak, distorted and less useful. Below the level of these two it is possible to be objective about one's subjectivity and that is what this machine offers me.

The machine also could be a consultant to me as teacher in designing that suprasystem which is the therapeutic family. As teacher, it also helps supervise me, the therapist.

Nor should one underestimate the machine as a co-therapist. It can divert me from my frequent preoccupation with mothering the family. This dissociating allows me to watch what is going on while backing away to think about the process itself. Finally, as a co-therapist, the machine can be a reality tester. Many times this reality testing makes it possible for the therapist to be playful, rather than stay preoccupied with his own internal responses or his intellectual reverberations.

If one of the objectives of psychotherapy is meta-communicating and isolating a time and place for meta-communicating, then videotape is a special aid in accomplishing this. Most powerfully, the couple or family are then tempted to stop meta-communicating at home so that the constant process of disappearing into their own heads is interrupted. They may also develop another signal that this, the office, and this, the machine, are the signals for "let's talk about, let's back off and look" or that this, the machine, is the signal, as in Bateson's famous trip to the zoo, that says "this is play." Furthermore, the machine opens the possibility of helping the family arrive at the stage of not talking about the therapy between sessions, thus making them more free to bring their anxiety back to the interview.

I have insisted for many years that no therapist should practice family therapy without a built-in colleague, co-therapist or consultant. The counter-culture components are too dangerous. Mayhap I can change that dictum. Could it be that a live in machine is a tolerable substitute for a "people partner"?

22
THE USE OF VIDEO REPLAY WITH DISTURBED CHILDREN

Philip C. Morse, Ph.D.

In contrast to the relatively large volume of literature on the use of videotape focused feedback with adults, comparatively little has been written on its use with children. A number of questions present themselves to the therapist who is considering the use of videotape with children. Does the impact of videotape and the treatment interventions used differ when video is used with children rather than with adults? For the child or family therapist contemplating the use of videotape, there are some important practical issues that need to be considered in order for the child to derive maximum benefit. For example, how does the therapist discriminate what material should be presented and in a way understandable to the child? What should the length and frequency of replay sessions be? Should special considerations be given to the context of the therapy situations and what variations of the replay can be individually tailored for its specific use in peer groups or family sessions? Do the considerations of where the videotape sessions take place—in the office, school or institution—prescribe particular focus to the videotape treatment?

Research of these and other questions in the therapeutic use of videotape with children is almost nonexistent, and that which has been done has frequently suffered from poor design, inadequate or nonexistent controls, no replications, and no follow-up. In this paper I will briefly look at some current research, including my own research using videotape with emotionally disturbed boys, in order to sensitize the practitioner to both theoretical and practical considerations in videotape use with children. Consideration is to be given to what it is that children respond to in videotape, and for which children it works best.

STIMULUS COMPONENTS OF VIDEOTAPE

The videotape stimulus components were separated out and examined by Bugental, Kaswan, and Love (1) in order to assess what it is children

258

actually respond to on the videotape. Using videotape messages as stimuli, they examined how contradictory information in verbal and nonverbal channels (e.g., criticism accompanied by a smile) is differentially combined and interpreted by adults and children. Children between the ages of five and 12, as well as their parents, served as subjects. A set of staged videotaped messages served as experimental stimuli. They contained conflicting inputs (friendly and unfriendly) in verbal (content), vocal (tone), and visual (facial expression) channels. Each subject saw and rated four scenes representing one combination of channel imputs, for example, a positive content, positive tone, and negative visual scene. Results indicated that children disregard the visual component of a message if it is not supported by cues from the vocal (tone) or verbal (content) channels. Specifically, children responded more negatively than adults to simultaneously experienced positive facial expression, negative content, and negative voice tone when enacted by a woman. No such difference was found, however, for adult and child ratings of such multilevel, contradictory, simultaneous messages received from males. This suggests that when a woman's smile is the only friendly component of a message, it has a stronger positive meaning to adults than to children.

When children are confronted with conflicting information, the audio component has greater impact than does the visual component. Positive input in one channel will be discounted if the other channel is negative so the child will resolve the incongruity by assuming the worst, and interpreting the message as being unfriendly or disapproving. Adults, in contrast, are more influenced by the visual component.

While the stimulus components of the videotape and the manner in which adults and children react differentially to them are being examined, a more practical issue arises as to what are the identifiable characteristics of children who benefit or fail to benefit from videotape replays.

SUBJECT CHARACTERISTICS INFLUENCING THE IMPACT OF
VIDEOTAPE WITH CHILDREN

Age

Age of subject has been considered a factor influencing the individual's response to videotape. Well designed research assessing the influence of videotape across the life span has yet to be done. Clinical observation by some have suggested that children may benefit less than adolescents and adults from videotaped feedback. Bahnson (2) used focused feedback with 32 hemophilic patients over a one-year period. The data of his study were limited to the patients' spontaneous reaction to the first two self-confrontation sessions, and were presented in a case-study format. Bahnson's dynamic formulation of children's responses is as follows: He speculates that 8- to 12-year-old children were narcissistically preoccupied with themselves and did not separate "phenomenologically" from the film image, perceiving it instead as an extension of a barrierless self. The videotape, for those children, served more to materialize an infantile wish for omnipotence, and exhibitionism, and, in some cases, stimulated the splitting off of the "bad" or damaged self from the intact observing self.

The implication of Bahnson's thesis is that it is only when adulthood is reached and the individual has achieved sufficient ego integrity that the observing capacity of the ego is differentiated enough to make the self confrontation constructive in correcting unacceptable behaviors and achieving consonance between the ideal and consciously perceived self. Bahnson writes, "where low ego strength and brittle defenses against primary material were the rule, the self-confrontation served as a club that splintered the brittle controls." The ensuing confrontation with apparently unsuccessfully controlled drives which they saw expressed in their own behavior increased their panic and served to fragment their defenses even further. In the case of these subjects, there was a lack of diffrentiation between early and late formation of the self-images and self-confrontations further fused and confused these levels for them.

Bahnson questions the usefulness of videotape with children, yet lends little empirical support to his findings.

Diagnosis

Type and severity of psychopathology warrant consideration in determining whether or not videotape should be used, and which particular format of use is most conducive to treatment.

Research with children has demonstrated success with emotionally disturbed children (3), anorexic children (4) and juvenile delinquents (5, 6). Borderline and psychotic children in the previously cited study by Bahnson (2) have been thought to be poor risks for videotape. Morse (7), however, found evidence contradicting Bahnson. Two borderline schizophrenic children were exposed to focused feedback. Both had low ego strength and brittle defenses against primary process material as evaluated by the intake psychologist. The markedly different ways that they reacted to seeing themselves on the television monitor would suggest that factors other than psychopathology and ego intactness influenced their reaction to the videotape. One of the borderline children (A) upon seeing himself for the first time on the monitor yelled "that's me," and then threw a hammer at the monitor. The other borderline child

(B) reacted positively and became involved in the videotape treatment. The borderline child with high cognitive development (B) benefited while the borderline child with low cognitive development did not.

The current source of research data is contradictory and no controlled study has evaluated the effectiveness of focused feedback across diagnostic categories with children. As will be discussed later, consideration of diagnostic categories and, more specifically, of ego deficits may be most helpful in designing uses of the videotape in treatment.

Cognitive Development

Understanding the child's level of cognitive development may be critical in determining whether videotape shall be used or not. A crucial developmental period for normal children and frequently later for disturbed children is 8 and 9 years of age when the child goes through a period which Piagetians label as "decentering," i.e. the child learns to suspend his highly personalized view of the world and take on the perspective of another person. Selman (8) describes this stage as one in which the child first becomes aware that people think and feel differently because they have their own unique motives and values. The child is able to see his own behavior from outside himself as well as from the point of view of another. Various authors have suggested that delays in the capacity to take the perspective of another person may seriously interfere with the development of social competence and, therefore, lead to psychopathology (5, 6, 9, 10, 11). The therapeutic importance of the child's advancing to a less egocentric view of his world is that it allows input into his cognitive field to allow for corrections of any distorted view he has of himself or others. The questions arise:

1. Are children who are unable to take the perspective of another person able to benefit from seeing themselves on videotape?

2. Could the deficit in being unable to take the perspective of another person be remediated by using videotape self-image confrontations, thereby advancing the child's cognitive development and reducing the risk of psychopathology.

Answer in part to the first question was found by this author in a pilot study (7). It was found that children who were less egocentric and had a higher level of cognitive development as measured by Piagetian tasks benefited from the videotape by developing better interprsonal skills, while children of lower cognitive development who are more egocentric did not benefit.

In answer to the second question, the direction of research suggests that videotape can accelerate the child's ability to take the perspective of another person.

A recent study by Chandler, Greenspan, and Barenboim (12) evaluated the social role taking and referential communication skills of 125 institutionalized, emotionally disturbed children between 9 and 14 years of age. The children were randomly assigned to one of three treatment groups for a 10-week training period: 1) videofilms and drama were used for teaching social role taking; 2) communication games graded in difficulty were used to develop preferential communical skills; 3) pretest and posttest measures, as well as a 12-month follow-up, were obtained of the untreated control group. The institutionalized children revealed delays in moving beyond age inappropriate, egocentric thinking when compared to a normal control group. The children who were in the role taking and referential communication groups improved in their ability to take the point of view of another person. Improvement in referential communication was achieved only with the second group, where there was actual practice in translating knowledge about roles.

THE EFFECTIVENESS OF VIDEOTAPE FOCUSED FEEDBACK ON THE
DEVELOPMENT OF INTERPERSONAL SKILLS WITH
EMOTIONALLY DISTURBED BOYS

Logistics

Focused feedback videotaping techniques were examined to evaluate their effect on the development of interpersonal competency of emotionally disturbed 8- and 9-year-old boys in a summer camp setting. Following each of 18 cabin group meetings, 10 children in one cabin individually received videotaped focused feedback of the meetings, while 10 children in the control cabin did not. The purpose of the therapy was to help the children in their interpersonal competency skills, focusing on their capacity to receive information from peers and the environment without denying, distorting, or projecting onto others. Therapy was geared toward helping the children discriminate and label feelings and to communicate more effectively to others. Treatment efficiency was evaluated by pretest, posttest and other measures designed to track the behavior of the videotape group members during the treatment phase.

The tapes were filmed during daily group therapy sessions in the cabins. This presented some technical problems of sound and lighting which were corrected with the use of spotlights suspended from the cabin rafters, four microphones, and a microphone mixer. For purposes of our research it was necessary to keep the wide angle lens opening and the camera stationary at the end of the cabin to assure that all campers were in the visual field at all times, so that standardized scoring procedures could be followed. For therapy purposes this technical arrangement of equipment was less than satisfactory. The use of videotape for treatment purposes could have been improved with the use of a zoom lens, additional mobile cameras and encouraging the children to tape their own meetings. This would have permitted more comprehensive tracking of the children's behavior and allowed for a more personalized impact in the focused feedback sessions. It took four days for the children to get used to the camera's presence in the room and it was necessary to assign one person to protect the equipment from damage by the children.

Cabin group meetings were both structured and unstructured. The unstructured meetings focused on crises which arose over the course of the summer such as sexual and aggressive acting out. Structured sessions focused on special topics such as homesickness, night-time fears, making friends, leaving camp, etc. A story telling technique was used in which conflicts and their resolution were included in the script of the story. Following the stories the children were asked to identify which one of the characters they identified with and spoke about various solutions to the problems contained in the story.

Focused Feedback

The focused feedback technique introduced by Stoller (13, 14, see Chapter 18) was used with the children in individual sessions for a 15-minute period from one to six hours after the group meetings. The tapes were reviewed prior to these playback sessions to select segments for replay and interventions pertinent to the child's needs and difficulties. The novelty of viewing quickly wore off and it was often necessary to build in a reward system with candy to assure ongoing involvement. Alternate day replays were more effective in maintaining their attention and lengthening their interest span.

Making an edited tape for each child of his progress in mastering certain tasks and social interactions over the camp season proved quite effective. This technique helped the child identify cues leading up to frustrating or satisfying situations and to learn appropriate alternative responses, thus helping the child to monitor his own behavior and therefore to gain a greater sense of competency. These personal tapes provided excellent opportunities for the therapist to coordinate treatment in light of the child's specific ego deficits. With impulsive acting-out children it was best to include segments of events leading up to the acting out. After each sequence the tape was stopped and the child was asked to recall what he had been thinking and feeling at the time of that acting out. The pauses during replay allowed the child to label the internal and external precipitants and allowed discussion and suggestion of alternative and more adaptive modes of dealing with this reaction.

Measurement and Results

In my own research (7), behavioral scoring of the videotapes, behavior checklists, and standardized inventories were used to evaluate reality testing frustration tolerance, and the development of self-esteem during a six-week camp experience with an experimental and control group each composed of 10 latency age boys. Positive interpersonal communications scored from the videotapes included children's statements of their own thoughts and feelings, statements about other children in the group, and general statements of information.

Target problems interfering with social competency which were scored included self-deprecating responses, withdrawal, competing gross motor behavior, such as rocking, which interfered with attention, and disruptive behavior such as scapegoating, testing or fighting. Behavior checklists were completed by the counselors for all children each day of the experiment. The following categories were scored; sharing, listening, cleaning cabin, talking things out when upset, helping cabinmates, appropriate mealtime behavior (i.e., the ability to sit through a meal without fighting), getting to activities on time, no teasing, no hitting, no stealing, no temper tantrums, no leaving group without permission, and no "backing off" from group (withdrawal). Self-esteem was measured by the Index of Adjustment and Values, as modified by Koocher (15). Level of egocentricity was measured by the Self Focus Sentence Completion developed by Exner (16). Accuracy of interpersonal perception was measured by a procedure described by Tagiuri (17). Level of cognitive development was assessed using various Piagetian tasks.

Results demonstrated that videotape focused feedback has a specific facilitating effect on the children's capacity to label their own thoughts and feelings as well as on their ability to adequately communicate their perceptions to others. Independently of the focused-feedback treatment the therapeutic camp experience had a positive effect on interpersonal competency behaviors. Boys in both videotape and control groups showed statistically significant increases in self-directed participating and 60-second attention, as well as decreases on 60-second withdrawal and disruptive behavior across pretest and posttest measures. Videotape and control groups were clearly discriminated on behaviors rated on the Behavior

Checklists. The videotaped children demonstrated increases in talking when upset, listening, helping cabinmates, and good mealtime behavior, in contrast to decrements in these behaviors seen in the control group.

Furthermore, the videotaped children shared more, teased less, stayed with their group longer and developed greater cohesivness in comparison to the control group which received no videotape playback.

CASE STUDIES

Three clinical vignettes will illustrate the use of videotape focused feedback with children in a group setting. Discussion will attempt to show the technique and how it can be used to disrupt feedback systems maintaining disturbances in reality testing, frustration tolerance and self-esteem. Special attention will be paid to the facilitation effect videotape has in the development of interpersonal skills.

Case 1—Reality Testing: "The Bat Killer Barks No More"

During a group meeting in which children were sharing their night fears and how they cope with them, Kevin peered through his coke bottle with his thick glasses and in a voice which sounded like gravel told of his daytime terror of frequently seeing a bat swoop down on him to suck blood out of his neck. This hallucination was symbolically descriptive of this 9-year-old's view of the world as evil and himself as perpetually vulnerable to attack. His fearfulness and unwillingness to accept others' attempts to help him often resulted in his yelling at the top of his lungs "you're just trying to cut me off," as he proceeded to kick and bite his fellow campers and counselors. When his biting was controlled he would curl up in the lap of the counselor and motion to be patted as if atoning for his loss of control.

This segment of tape of the events leading up to Kevin's statement "you're cutting me off" and the group meeting on children's fears was replayed in short segments to him over a two-week period. He experienced intense anxiety upon the initial showings but upon the fourth and fifth exposure became less anxious and began listening to the other children on the tape trying to help him. Each point of distortion was studied and clarified before proceeding to the next sequence of interactions. This view of the other children coming to his aid was discordant with his previous perception of their trying to maim him. The videotape provided both a focus for attention and a mechanism for Kevin to check out the external reality. Kevin became moderately depressed after viewing more tape, ashamed at the way he looked. After repeated showings he became more able to label his feelings of rage which previously contributed to his fragmentation. He subsequently had less of a need to project the rage and thereby disturb his reality-testing capacity.

An interesting ending to Kevin's bat terrors came when he accepted the recommendation of other boys in the cabin who suggested: "Kevin, anytime you see the bat, just close your eyes and spray the bat with Raid. It will kill him." The following day when questioned why he was late to a group meeting, Kevin replied he had taken his buddies' idea and it worked. With a glimmer in his eye he stated he was late because he sprayed for a long time just to make sure it was dead. Kevin reported no further recurrences of his hallucination.

The videotape served as a tool, and the therapeutic group the context through which some of the autistic and fantastic ideas he held about himself and his world were corrected. As Kevin's body boundaries became more defined, he was able to move from his non-human environment of dogs and bats to being a little boy who was not quite as afraid of dying.

Case 2—Frustration Tolerance

How to make it through a complete hockey game without losing control by smashing a stick on the head of another player or running away and sobbing was a problem Ted experienced in competitive group sports. He had little capacity to delay gratification and had not mastered what Sullivan called "social subordination" and "social accommodation." If Ted didn't get the position he wanted or had to follow a rule, he became enraged. Ted operated under the principle that the world was his oyster, and if he didn't get his way, a trantrum invariably resulted.

Ted's behavior was videotaped during 12 games and a playback session followed each game to view the tape. His behavior was broken down into stages leading up to his temper outbursts. This procedure enabled him to lead up to his having tantrums and provided a context to reinforce his subordinating his needs to the common goal of the group. The videotape playback provided Ted with a concrete medium for internalizing elements of the experiences of expanded observation of ego functioning and greater frustration tolerance. Playback sessions tracking his behavior during the games were initiated with the therapist focusing on the modulation and control of his anger. After the initiation of these sessions a pattern developed in which Ted would begin to get into a fight but would stop after glancing over at the camera. Ted's looking at the camera during the game seemed to inhibit his acting out. It was as though he was anticipating the pain which would follow his viewing his tantrum later. He seemed to be developing his own internal camera.

The videotape provided an avenue to reenact the affective states, and to delay gratification function. The tape could be stopped so that conflict situations could be introduced at increments so as not be overload Ted's affective system, sending him into a rage unavailable to treatment. Playing the tape with Ted was like setting small fires and putting them out. He developed better controls such that the fears of being consumed by the flames of his own rage became less terrifying to him.

Case 3—Self Esteem: Videotape as a Method of Implosion

Fred was a 9-year-old boy who had been raped by his uncle and subsequently was unable to go to school or tolerate any group setting. He had a devastated self-image, viewing himself as disgusting and the world as hurtful. Any feedback he received that was dissonant with his own self-hatred was answered by his ritualistically placing a pillow, hands or some other object over his ears and calling himself a shithead. Two formidable obstacles hindered any alteration of Fred's negative self-image. First there was a stimulus barrier in which his loud self-recriminations drowned out positive feedback he received from others. Secondly, Fred lacked a sense of himself as continuous in time with a past, present and future. Consequently he continually functioned at a deficit, with no sense of a building of past positive human interactions, a reservoir of a "good me."

An implosion method was successfully used in interrupting this circuit of self-damnation. A portion of tape selected for use was one in which Fred's cabinmates complimented him on his being an excellent swimmer and "good guy." After the initial violent reaction, Fred was exposed to minute segments of the tape and only for as long as it was not too painful for him to hear compliments paid him. He was able to successfully complete the viewing of the tape. His behavior dramatically changed with his acceptance of people getting closer to him as well as his actively seeking support from them.

SUMMARY

Videotaped focused feedback is useful in treating children with problems related to impulse control, reality testing, and low self-esteem. The observation, clarification, and labeling of appropriate and inappropriate feelings and actions help children gain greater mastery and control over their own behavior and a more realistic view of themselves and the outside world.

Anecdotal reports from clinicians and teachers indicate that most of the children in the experimental group have maintained their improvement for over a year following their camp experience with video self-confrontation.

REFERENCES

1. Bugental, D. E., Kaswan, J. W., and Love, L. R.: Perception of Contradictory Meanings Conveyed by Verbal and Nonverbal Channels. *Journal of Personality and Social Psychology*, 16:647-655, 1970.
2. Bahnson, C. B.: Body and Self-Images Associated with Audio-Visual Self-Confrontation. *The Journal of Nervous and Mental Disease*, 148:262-280, 1969.
3. Kaswan, J., and Love, L.: Confrontation As a Method of Psychological Intervention. *Journal of Nervous and Mental Disease*, 118:224-237, 1969.
4. Gottheil, E., Backup, C. E., and Cornelison, F. S.: Denial and Self-Image Confrontation in a Case of Anorexia Nervosa. *The Journal of Nervous and Mental Disease*, 148:238-250, 1969.
5. Chandler, M. J.: Egocentrism and Antisocial Behavior: The Assessment and Training of Social Perspective-Taking Skills. *Developmental Psychology*, 1973.
6. Chandler, M. J.: Egocentrism in Normal and Pathological Childhood Development. In F. Monks, W. Hartup, and J. DeWitt (Eds.), *Determinants of Behavioral Development*. New York: Academic Press, 1972, 569-575.
7. Morse, P.: The Effects of Videotaped *Focus Feedback* on Competency of Emotionally Disturbed Boys. Unpublished doctoral dissertation, Long Island University, 1976.
8. Selman, R. L.: Stages of Role-Taking and Moral Judgment as Guides to Social Intervention. In T. Lickona (Ed.), *Man and Morality*. New York: Holt, Rinehart, & Winston, 1974.
9. Anthony, E. J.: An Experimental Approach to the Psychopathology of Childhood Sleep Disturbances. *Brit. J. of Med. Psychol.*, 32:19-37, 1959.
10. Feffer, H.: A Developmental Analysis of Interpersonal Behavior. *Psychological Review*, 77:197-215, 1970.
11. Sarbin, T. R.: Role Theory. In G. Lindsley (Ed.), *Handbook of Social Psychology*. Cambridge, Mass.: Addison-Wesley, 1954.
12. Chandler, M. J., Greenspan, S., and Barenboim, C.: The Assessment and Training of Role-Taking and Referential Communication Skills in Institutionalized Emotionally Disturbed Children. Submitted for publication, 1974.
13. Stoller, F. H.: Focused Feedback with Videotape: Extending the Group's Functions. In G. Gazda (Ed.), *Innovations to Group Psychotherapy*. Springfield, Ill.: Charles C Thomas, 1968.
14. Stoller, F. H. Videotape Feedback in the Group Setting. *Journal of Nervous and Mental Disease*, 148:457-466, 1969.
15. Koocher, G. P.: Swimming, Competence, and Personality Change. *Journal of Personality and Social Psychology*, 18:275-278, 1971.
16. Exner, Jr., J. E.: The Self Focus Sentence Completion: A Study of Egocentricity. *Journal of Personality Assessment*, 37:437-455, 1973.
17. Tagiuri, R.: Social Preference and Its Perception. In R. Tagiuri and L. Petrullo (Eds.), *Person Perception and Interpersonal Behavior*. Stanford, Calif.: Stanford Univ. Press, 1958.

23

MULTI-IMAGE IMMEDIATE IMPACT VIDEO SELF-CONFRONTATION AS AN ADJUNCT IN THE GROWTH OF SELF

Milton M. Berger, M.D.

This is a report on a technique, multi-image immediate impact video self-confrontation, that I have used in psychotherapy to stimulate the emergence of repressed free associations related to self-images and various other messages incorporated early in life. The technique, which I accidentally discovered in 1972, leads to significant clarifications and insight into the here-and-now self of patients and thus serves as an adjunct in a psychoanalytic, exploratory, uncovering approach aimed at the growth of a healthier self. It was through serendipity, a longstanding interest in intrapsychic and interpersonal communication systems, and some years of experience with the use of video equipment in psychotherapy that I learned how to regularly produce a number of clear and distorted self-images in tandem for self-image confrontation.

Many workers in psychiatry, including Freud, Adler, Jung, Sullivan, Horney, Fromm-Reichmann, Kubie, Spitz, Lewin, and Ives-Hendricks, focused their attention on the development of aspects of self, self-concepts, idealized self-image, potential self, actualized self, real self, and fulfilled self. H. S. Sullivan very succinctly stated that the repeated, reflected images of ourselves that we receive from others early in life determine our self-image and self-concept (1). Among the many methods used to elicit these repressed memories, messages, and incorporated images of self and others and to bring about abreactive or cathartic discharge of the energies associated with them have been: the free association method of Freud, Jung and others; the increasingly more sophisticated tech-

---

*An earlier version of this paper was presented as "Video as an Adjunct in the Growth of Self," at the October 25, 1972 scientific meeting of the Association for the Advancement of Psychoanalysis, Carnegie International Center, New York City.

niques of dream analysis; the use of conscious fantasies in which the patient is directed to take the analyst with him on a trip back into another time and place of his life such as when he was five or seven years old; the gestalt technique of giving a voice to people and things with whom there is unfinished business such as a father or mother or sibling who died when the patient was three or four years old; the use of the Rorschach test or of art, poetry, music or smells to stimulate recall of early memories and experiences; the use of hypnosis with and without drugs to have a person go back into his time-space historical continuum and to function as he did when he was an infant or child; and, more recently, the controlled use of psychedelic drugs to stimulate the emergence of powerful actual and distorted memories. All these have been done with cooperative, motivated patients who trusted their therapists and were willingly engaged in the process of undermining and working through unconscious resistance and transference forces which blocked them from being in touch with the many self-aspects and self-concepts which comprise their total self which is in fluid motion and not static or rigid.

I am reporting my experience with another method to bring a patient who has a positive transference relationship to his or her therapist into touch with deeply registered, repressed identifications, introjections and incorporations of values, attitudes, behaviors and emotional patterns which are daily influencing self-images, self-concepts and feelings and attitudes towards self and others.

The basic equipment initially required for this technique is: one video-tape recorder, two mobile cameras with zoom lenses, two monitors, one split-screen special-effects generator, and one or more microphones. I focus one camera on the patient's face as he faces me or looks in another direction. With the split-screen special effects generator and one camera with zoom lens, I enlarge the picture of his face or part of his face and place it to one side of the monitors so it occupies about one-third to one-quarter of the monitor area. I now point the second camera at the picture on the monitor and immediately the monitor is filled with repeated images of the face on the monitor. These multiple images move in series to either right or left and becoming increasingly blurred the greater their distance is from the original image which remains a clear representation presented through the lens of the first camera. The images created can go from two to six to 10 to infinity and this effect is created by the turning of the focus slowly on camera number two. Moving this focus back and forth brings forth images and effects which will almost always intrigue the patient or therapist enough to want the focal action stopped for a more intensive and longer-lasting view of what is on the monitor. Opening or closing the lens aperture fades or wipes out certain images. The patient can either see and react spontaneously to the closed-circuit multi-images as they are being created or he can react to the multi-images during the replay of the taped interaction or he can react both times and the differences in his reactions and free-associations can be noted and worked with. He can be encouraged to ventilate his reactions to experiencing himself, that is his picture(s) on the monitor, being wiped out or distorted.

After using the technique for some time I discovered, again by accident, that if the patient was seated in front of a live monitor when I was recording with a live camera, duplicate images showed up in the background and so I began to use and refine this experience until I am now skillful at creating the multi-images with just one camera and without the aid of a special effects generator and with only one monitor. This makes the technique available for use by any therapist with basic video equipment who would like to expand his or her repertoire. The patient may be sitting up or lying on the couch in traditional psychoanalytic fashion or in interaction with psychotherapy group members or family during this videotaping for instant replay.

The first reaction to experiencing the many clear and unclear or distorted images of self which are initially created and appear in tandem-series is one of interest, excitement and even "Wow," as the patient experiences the visual impact of what he has previously known only cognitively or experientially or not at all. It brings home to each of us that we are composed of many selves or aspects of self.

Horney repeatedly stated in her work that man uses his idealized image of self to deny, obscure or block his more actual or true images and moments of being (2). The compulsive loyalty to rigidly shaped images, each living in compartments alongside each other as if it were a person's only true self, have led neurotic individuals to denials, blind-spots, profound inner conflicts, self-doubts and much pain.

In his writings Jung refers to powerful intrapsychic "constellations" or "complexes" which tend to split and "detach themselves from consciousness to such an extent that they not only appear foreign but also lead an autonomous life of their own" (3). These energies gathered into complexes not only go out of control of consciousness but may become "autonomous partial systems" which function like small personalities within the total personality. In itself, this is not necessarily an abnormal condition. Such psychic splits are actually necessary if the individual is to specialize the direction of his energies to accomplish some particular work. These autonomous complexes described by Jung seem then to be analogous to what I and others refer to as "inner selves." These inner selves provide the flavor, the unique mixture and distinctiveness of an individual's personality. These autonomous complexes or inner selves are noted and commented on in everyday life when a parent or uncle or close family friend says to a young man with a lot of fire and spirit, "You're a chip off the old block, just like your father."

In my work with multi-image immediate impact video self-confrontations using closed-circuit video and instant or delayed playback, *what appears to be most significant is not that I concurrently reproduce many images of a person but rather that I reproduce and create through electronic means many increasingly distorted images of a person in tandem, one after the other,* as well as a clear image. It is just these shadowlike presentations of self-images which are not so well-known in consciousness nor *approved of and liked* which stimulate the analysand to bring forth associations to deeper inner selves or complexes which have vexed him for many years, but which remained elusive, inconstant and not palpable enough to be harnessed or controlled as they would intermittently emerge from his deeper caverns of self. The patient often tends to see the emergence of such partial inner selves or self-aspects as the popping up, like a genie, of the "bad self."

Examples of reactions to the multiple image self-confrontation experience follow:

PATIENT 1

Jan, a 27-year-old, alienated, self-effacing sociologist who had been victimized in childhood, reacted with antipathy, disgust, pain and sadness to the front images of her face. To the images of her right face, she squealed with delight, pleasure and acceptance. What emerged in her free associations was that in the front images she saw the face of her mother and grandmother in her . . . washed out . . . drained . . . depressed . . . old . . . lifeless . . . really miserable. She saw in her mother's face in herself the injunction, "Don't try to be any different than me 'cause you won't make it anyhow . . . and if you're not going to make it, don't try. So don't ever bother. You'll be a sorry girl." She let out a squeal of anguish and sobbed as she felt the impact of her impoverished mother and grandmother in herself. Then turning to the side and observing her own bright eyes and open, warm smile she said, "But I didn't let them beat me down completely, did I? I must have a lot of fighting spunk in me which saved me. But I do feel bad for them. . . ." I commented quietly, "Yes, you do have a lot of fight and spunk in you and have to continue to separate from them so you can live your own life without being resigned and depressed."

PATIENT 2

Trudy, a 25-year-old, self-effacing elementary school secretary, quietly and reflectively studied her multiple self-images on the monitor during a group session. She said softly, "The image on the left is clear—that is probably how I seem to others. I don't see myself that way. I see myself like the third image in, which is blurred and hazy." When questioned as to what was the threat in seeing herself clearly, she responded, "Then I would have to be responsible for myself." This remark startled all of us but gave us a clear insight into the tenacity of Trudy's dependency and immaturity patterns which seemed so contradictory to her awareness, resources and potentialities. Two months later she entered her group meeting with the announcement, "Hey group! You know what? I'm number two." Seeing the perplexed look on our faces she quickly added, "Don't you remember the pictures on the monitor? I was number three then but I'm feeling more number two now and I like being more responsible for myself."

PATIENT 3

An alienated 32-year-old divorced account executive asked, "Is it possible to be possessed? I see my mother's face in my face on the monitor. I suddenly realize she never let me be myself. As a child I always wondered what was wrong with me because I felt confused and didn't know where and who I was."

PATIENT 4

Mr. R., a 40-year-old detached and alienated executive with few memories up to age 12, said, "As I look at the images getting smaller and smaller, it's as if I'm going back into my childhood . . . to being nothing."

PATIENT 5

Miss L., a 30-year-old opera singer concluding four years of successful psychotherapy, remarked, "I see the clear image as the me I am now and the ones coming up blurred as the ones of my future as I continue to develop my potential."

PATIENT 6

Mr. A., a successful interior designer aged 35, commented on his dislike of video because he often saw the right side of his face, which he disliked. He felt it was feminine and was the "sissy" in him remaining from having grown up as a "mommy's boy." Moments later he recalled with insight and relief the fact that it was his right testicle that had never descended.

PATIENT 7

An attractive 31-year-old industrial counselor volunteered for the opportunity to observe herself in a multi-image playback during a group seminar on the use of video in counseling and psychotherapy. She had previously seen her image on television on one occasion in a department store and had felt amused. Sitting quietly, she watched the formation of the multiple images of herself on the monitor with great interest. Here is the verbatim dialogue between us:

> *Therapist*: "Have you ever been in a place like Coney Island fun house which has mirrors to distort your images?"
> *Patient*: "Yes, as a child."
> *Therapist*: "I hope these images won't be too upsetting to you."
> (Perhaps I intuited what was to come)

About six to 10 distorted images were produced. I played back the tape and asked her to react to what she saw during the playback and to share her reactions with us. There was a long silence. I repeated my question.

> *Patient*: "I see a person with very big eyes and a very long nose."
> *Therapist*: "Does this remind you of anyone from your childhood?"
> *Patient*: "I think of Pinocchio."
> *Therapist*: "Anyone else? From your childhood perhaps?"
> *Patient*: "Alice in Wonderland and Pinocchio."
> *Therapist*: "Do those stories have special meaning for you? What comes to your mind when you think of Pinocchio? What is your remembrance of the story of Pinocchio?"
> *Patient*: "He was very threatened."
> *Therapist*: "Did you have trouble with anyone threatening you when you were growing up?"
> *Patient*: "Yes, I was telling many lies."
> *Therapist*: "And how were you punished or threatened? Were you very fearful?"
> *Patient*: "Yes, I was very often threatened by my parents."
> *Therapist*: "Did you live much in imagination as a child to get away from your threatening parents?"

Patient: "Yes, like Alice in Wonderland."
Therapist: "Has what has come out so far intrigued or interested you?"
Patient: "Yes, like I said . . ."
Therapist: "Let's continue with the playback till you tell us to stop." (I roll tape forward a little further)
Patient: "Stop!!!"
Therapist: "Does that stir up anything in you now? See anyone you recognize?"
Patient (her voice raised in excitement now): "I see a girl sitting in a train going in a tunnel."
Therapist: "Can you take us with you on a fantasy trip on the train as you go through the tunnel?"
Patient: "O.K." (said hesitantly and in a quieter voice) "I go back to the moment when I was born and then I see myself building up into my childhood." (long reflective pause) "The third image looks like a witch."
Therapist: "Do you remember whether you felt that way when you told lies or did you wish to be a witch so you could get even with your parents?"
Patient: "Yes, I did! I wished I could kill them off."
Therapist: "You seem to have some unfinished business. Perhaps you'd like to go beyond where you are and to kill off the witch in you. You can give yourself permission to do that if you want to."

She nodded affirmatively but obviously didn't wish to pursue the issue further at this time in front of the whole group of seminar participants, so I did not press her to do so. I made the following remarks to the group as she walked back to her seminar seat. "This as you see can be a very powerful experience. Within a short time she went into that painful period of childhood of having to lie to tyrannical parents and to wish she was a witch to be powerful enough to destroy them. And this surely was something she paid a toll for." Turning to her, I continued. "Perhaps it's not accidental that you now, here in this seminar today, wear dress spurs on your lovely boots, as if to protect yourself if necessary from what is threatening in the world around you."

PATIENT 8

At the same seminar, a 54-year-old married psychologist silently studied the video playback showing six images of himself. Responding to the distortions in the third and fourth multi-images of himself, he said with smiling recognition, but not great surprise, "I see my monster. This is the monster I've always known was in me. It is a souvenir I remember from my childhood. I first felt this about myself as a child when I saw the mummy in a movie with Boris Karloff."

As the psychologist was witnessing himself on the playback he reached for a cigarette from the man seated next to him, lit it and began to puff at it rapidly which became a sign to us of his attempt to control his tremendous anxiety as he had not smoked for the previous three hours.

> *Therapist*: "Did you see anything else beside the monster from your childhood? And also when you were a child did you wonder if you might become a monster?"
> *Patient*: "I didn't want to become a monster but I felt I must, I was obliged to. . . ."
> *Therapist*: "Did you have any other reactions to the pictures of yourself you were looking at?"
> *Patient*: "I saw my sadness."
> *Therapist*: "In which image?"
> *Patient*: "In the second image."

The distortions of the video image allowed him to get in touch with the inner distortions of his childhood. We get in touch with actual introjections of reality or our childhood distortions of reality or a mixture of both.

The artistry lies in the ability of the video user to use the distortions to give something new or extra to the patient to work on. This subject was asked how he felt about coming in touch with his monster. He said he felt incomplete. I then held a discussion with my co-therapist, Lynne F. Berger, about whether we had enough time to work with him in a gestalt fashion for him to talk to and try to kill off the monster in him. My co-therapist however felt it might be more feasible in the limited time of the workshop to encourage him to confront and make friends with his monster. After a minute of silent reflection, during which he looked at the image of himself on the monitor, he said, "I need you. You were useful to me. . . . It's O.K."

All this occurred in early December, 1975. In response to a written inquiry from me in February, 1976, two months later, about any after effect of the experience on him, he wrote:

"I still see the images on the monitor from time to time and when I do I feel like I'm no longer disturbed by the monster in me. He's become more of a private part of me I feel friendly towards."

DISCUSSION

Forty long-term patients I have seen in individual and group psychotherapy in private practice, most of whom had a diagnosis of character neurosis, have had one or more 10- to 45-minute experiences with the type of multi-image confrontation described here. One 49-year-old woman, depressed and emotionally impoverished, with lifelong suicidal tendencies, stated that she had no response to seeing herself. All the other patients had free associations that were highly significant in terms of what became available for working through or for the ongoing assessment of progress in therapy. There were no immediate or delayed harmful effects, although 70% (28 patients) spontaneously referred to memories of the experience in the following weeks. The multi-image experience served as a marker or milestone in the way it became imprinted, and patients referred back to it at unpredictable moments.

In demonstrating the technique to colleagues in seminars conducted in this country and abroad, interesting responses have always come forth as in examples 7 and 8.

Lewin succinctly stated, "Psychoanalytic technique has various ways of assisting an analysand to recall forgotten events" (4). The technique of multi-image immediate impact self-confrontation expedites recall of events and associations which can lead to catharsis, insight and the giving up of psycho socio-sexual fixations manifested in one of the past images of self, which retard growth and maturation and which are no longer valid.

Through electronic means a therapist thus has an ability to magnify, focus on and distort aspects of a patient's body just as people do to themselves with their inner "eye" and "I." He can then play back the recording made moments before for a more total seeing and experiencing and free associating to what is triggered off. There is both an enlarged objective observing ego at work and a subjective, recognizing, identifying self who feels "at home" with those images or pictures or aspects of self which are now emerging on the monitors.

The type of encounter with self-image(s) and with self-identity and self-concepts triggered by the multi-image immediate impact video self-confrontation technique I am reporting on at this time has been described by patients experiencing it as "surrealistic," "objectifying," "reflection in action," "really taking a look at myself."

CONCLUSIONS

The multi-image method described here is another step in the long evolution of techniques developed to serve as adjuncts in expediting the recall of events and thought-feeling associations that can lead to catharsis, insight, and the surrender of psychosocial self-images or emotional fixations that retard growth and maturation. The technique is not presented as a form of therapy per se or as a substitute for psychotherapy. It is necessary to review and consider revision of theories of the self that regard man from a rigid viewpoint. Although there is continuity in the structural core of each person, the self is not a concrete self but is experienced as being composed of multiple layers or cores within cores (5). A maturing person is composed of many co-existing selves or self-aspects, changing and in flux from moment to moment, yet always having a unifying matrix of a physical body mass, name, gender, life history, incorporated cultural time-binding practices, language, values, and emotional reaction patterns. Each person is unique in his process of creatively synthesizing clear and distorted past and present images that are introjected and identified with as they are amalgamated into his own growing self (6).

Simultaneously experienced, multiple impact multi-images of self presented for introspective exploration and awareness can lead to a person's acceptance of the fact that his self is fluid and in process and that his multiple self-concepts, self-aspects and self-functionings do coexist in and alongside each other in conflict, contradiction, harmony or paradoxically. Energies potentially available to the total self of each person can be more constructively and creatively used for the benefit and growth of self and others and a person can achieve a deeper sense of self-acceptance without guilt as he realizes and assumes full responsibility for concurrent or alternatingly experienced different aspects of self without necessarily feeling he is split, schizophrenic or fragmented.

REFERENCES

1. Sullivan, H. S.: *The Interpersonal Theory of Psychiatry.* New York: W. W. Norton, 1953.
2. Horney, K.: *Neurosis and Human Growth.* New York: W. W. Norton, 1950.
3. Progoff, I.: *Jung's Psychology and Its Social Meaning.* New York: Grove Press, 1953.
4. Lewin, B. D.: *The Image and the Past.* New York: International Universities Press, 1970.
5. Bahnson, C. B.: Body and Self—Images Associated with Audiovisual Self-Confrontation. In R. H. Geertsma (Ed.), *Studies in Self-Cognition: Techniques of Videotape Self-Observation in the Behavioral Sciences.* Baltimore, Md.: Williams and Wilkins Co., 1969.
6. Berger, M. M.: A Preliminary Report on Multi-Image Immediate Impact Video Self-Confrontation. *Amer. J. Psychiatry*, 130, 1973.

24

VIDEOTAPE SELF-CONFRONTATION AFTER NARCOTHERAPY
A Brief Report on the Videoscan Technique

Richard J. Metzner, M.D.

Although many people have been helped by the videotape approaches described elsewhere in this book, there are some individuals with neurotic, psychosomatic, or characterological problems who may benefit from a psychotherapeutic method that combines videotape self-confrontation (VSC) with one of the oldest approaches in modern psychiatry: narcotherapy. The *videoscan* (videotape self-confrontation after narcotherapy) technique involves the videotaping of a patient while he or she is being interviewed under the influence of an hypnotic drug such as sodium amobarbital (Amytal) or sodium thiopenthal (Pentothal). During this interview the patient is typically able to remember, feel, and discuss psychological material that is not readily available during interviews without the medication. Sometimes patients re-live traumatic events which they have previously been unable to remember (abreaction). More often they simply become less inhibited in dealing with painful or emotionally-charged issues.

After the medication has worn off, patients usually forget much of what occurred during the narcotherapy session. VSC enables patients to learn for themselves, without having to depend upon the therapist's word, what took place during the interview. Thus, for the first time, patients can bear witness to ideas and behavior that may only emerge under the influence of the drug. They are then helped to integrate such material into consciousness by systematically "scanning" the contents of the videotape under the guidance of the therapist.

The mechanisms by which such a process might promote therapeutic improvement can be understood within the framework of psychodynamic, social learning, and psychotherapy research perspectives.

The first experimental uses of intravenous sodium Amytal in psychiatry were reported by Bleckwenn in 1930 (1) and Lindemann in 1932 (2). Horsley introduced the term "narcoanalysis" in 1936 (3) to describe the process of conducting psychiatric interviews with the patient under the influence of such medication. However, it was the work of Drs. Roy Grinker, Sr., and John Speigel during World War II (4) that focused professional attention on the powerful potential benefits of narcotherapy. They successfully treated hundreds of cases of combat neurosis with a supportive, psychodynamically-oriented method of brief psychotherapy which they called "narcosynthesis."

After World War II this method was applied enthusiastically by psychiatrists working with civilian populations, and initial reports were optimistic (5, 6). By the 1950s, however, narcosynthesis had become far more popular as a dramatic device in the movies than as a therapeutic tool in psychiatric settings (7). Clinicians had become disillusioned with their failure to obtain the legendary abreactions seen commonly during wartime, and patients rarely remembered or felt enlightened by the Amytal experience (8).

Since many psychiatrists found that, sooner or later, they could uncover the same material through non-pharmacological methods such as insight-oriented psychotherapy or psychoanalysis, and since civilian treatment did not usually present the urgent temporal pressures of military combat, most clinicians finally abandoned the technique. Those who continued to use it have tended to restrict its use to diagnostic interviewing ("narcodiagnosis") (9), and to the treatment of the infrequently encountered acute traumatic neuroses (10).

We have found no previous reports in the literature describing the use of VSC after narcotherapy. This chapter is intended to acquaint the reader with the methods we have used, our initial results, and possible mechanisms of action. Because of the uncommon but potential complications of both VSC (11) and narcotherapy (9), we recommend that the videoscan technique be attempted only with great care and only by psychiatrists who have thoroughly familiarized themselves with the methods that comprise it.

Our approach was to divide the videoscan procedure into five phases: 1) preparation, 2) administration, 3) professional review, 4) playback or "scan," and 5) synthesis.

TABLE 1

Indications for Videoscan

A. maladaptive neurotic, psychosomatic, and characterological symptoms such as amnesia, fugue states, conversion reactions, multiple personality, depression, anxiety states, bronchial asthma, alcoholism, etc.

B. unresolved diagnostic questions relating to the presence of repressed or inhibited psychological contents

C. resistance to traditional psychiatric treatment approaches such as insight-oriented psychotherapy or hypnotherapy

D. legitimate need on the part of the patient for more rapid alleviation of symptoms than had been provided by previous therapies

TABLE 2

Contraindications for Videoscan

A. psychotic or paranoid trends

B. history of barbiturate hypersensitivity, porphyria, or chronic cardiac, renal or hepatic disease

C. acute systemic illness

1. *Preparation*

This phase involved evaluating the patient for indications and contraindications (Tables 1 and 2), establishing a therapeutic relationship, obtaining written informed consent, and presenting pre-instructions. It also included preparation of medications (Table 3) and equipment (Table 4), and arranging the treatment setting.

By the time we had determined whether or not the videoscan was indicated, we had generally spent enough time talking with the patient to have established a positive therapeutic relationship. Having developed this foundation, we asked for written consent from the patient to pursue the rest of the procedure. For educational purposes, we included an optional statement which gave us permission to use the videotapes for professional training purposes. After the patient signed the consent form, a two-hour appointment for the Amytal interview was scheduled, and pre-instructions were given. The patient was asked to avoid meals, alcohol, or psychoactive drugs during the six hours preceding the videoscan, and

TABLE 3

Medications and Materials

three 250 mgm ampoules of Amytal sodium (dry powder)
15cc of sterile water (for preparing a 5% solution of Amytal)
20cc disposable syringe
disposable needle (for making the Amytal solution)
butterfly infusion set
tourniquet, alcohol wipes, adhesive tape, and band-aids
Ambu (respirator) bag
injectable caffeine and sodium benzoate
additional disposable syringes and needles

TABLE 4

Video Equipment and Supplies

half-inch monochrome reel-to-reel videotape recorder (VTR)
video camera with viewfinder, zoom lens, and tripod
11-inch video monitor
two lavalier microphones
audio mixer
take-up reel
two 60-minute rolls of blank videotape
assorted cables and cords
bottle of tape head cleaning solution with applicators

not to eat or drink anything at all during the three hours prior to the procedure. Outpatients were asked to make arrangements for a responsible person to drive them home afterwards.

To assure that the treatment settings were conducive to the procedure, we usually selected facilities that were quiet, private, and convenient. For outpatients, we used our private office. For inpatients, we utilized either a treatment room or the patient's own room at the hospital. In most cases the therapist transported, connected, and pretested the equipment himself. In a few instances, when the procedure was to be recorded for teaching purposes, hospital audiovisual personnel assisted with the preparation and operation of equipment (12).

Generally, all video equipment was placed out in the open in these settings except for the VTR, which was located in a closet or adjacent room to reduce the ambient noise level in the treatment area. Two other settings used were the videotaping room at a university psychiatric facility and the television studio at a VA psychiatric hospital. These latter locations were employed to permit the preparation of teaching videotapes using multi-camera television systems.

2. Administration

This part of the procedure consisted of starting the videotape recorder, administering the Amytal, conducting the interview, and transferring the patient into the care of a responsible person afterwards.

Before administering the medication, we spent a brief period of time reestablishing the patient's sense of relationship with the therapist by allowing him to discuss his anxiety about the situation or any other feelings that he might have. Having done so, the 5% solution of sodium Amytal was slowly injected at a rate not exceeding 50 mgm (1cc)/minute. We asked the patient to count backwards from 100 and waited for the onset of slurred speech and/or counting errors. At that point we stopped injecting the medication but made an effort to maintain the patient at this level of subnarcosis through the periodic re-injection of additional 1cc doses.

In order to elicit useful material during the interview we drew upon information gathered during our evaluation to steer the patient into areas likely to be productive. Using such techniques as age-regression (13), hypnodrama (14), and guided fantasy (15), we attempted to maximize the patient's affective and anamnestic verbal behavior.

3. Professional Review

Having obtained what in many cases represented very potent and potentially valuable psychotherapeutic material on videotape, we then went over the recording in order to become familiar with its contents and to plan the nature and timing of our confrontations. We wrote down the number showing on the index counter of the VTR at various critical points so that we could find these points easily during the playback phase. We also determined during this process whether to avoid playing certain segments that might be counterproductive to the patient's treatment. The decisions were made either by the therapist alone or collaboratively, after showing the tape to colleagues and other members of the treatment team who might be familiar with the patient.

4. *Playback or "Scan"*

At least 24 hours after the Amytal interview when the patient was free of the influence of medication, the first playback session was held. The patient was told that as the tape was playing he should feel free to ask the therapist to stop it whenever he wanted so that he could verbalize his reactions. He was informed that the therapist would do the same. The procedure usually took place in the same setting as was used for the Amytal interview, except that now, instead of reclining, the patient was sitting next to the therapist in front of the television monitor. In a few cases the entire tape was reviewed in one long sitting, but, typically, two to four 45-minute sessions were utilized to permit a detailed systematic review of the material. To maximize the educational potential of the method, we frequently played important segments more than once, trying to optimize the patient's learning through repetitive exposure. This technique was used particularly when the verbal or nonverbal information to be communicated was either too subtle or too affect-laden to be fully comprehensible in one viewing.

5. *Synthesis*

The goal of the final phase of the procedure was to promote cognitive and affective integration of the material revealed by the videoscan. In essence, this phase was simply the pursuit of further psychotherapy using the experiences and symbols which had emerged during the videoscan to expedite the work. Patients were encouraged to "take ownership" of the various ideas and feelings which they had discovered and to recognize that these parts of themselves no longer needed to be feared or denied. Therapy then focused on encouraging the patient to suggest and experiment with new coping strategies and behavioral alternatives. We took the stance that patients should be justly proud of themselves for having had the courage to "look inside," and we supported all efforts at converting their dependency on the therapist and the treatment into increasing autonomy and self-sufficiency. In the event that the patient showed partial improvement but evidenced continued blocking of certain psychological contents, a repeat of the videoscan procedure was performed, followed by resumption of these efforts towards integration and autonomy.

RESULTS

Between October, 1975 and March, 1977 we performed 11 videoscan procedures on eight cases (Table 5). Six of the patients have subsequently improved with respect to target symptoms and general status. Two have

TABLE 5 — Results of Videoscans (V's)

PATIENT ( ) = No. of V's	AGE	SEX	Months in PSYCHOTHERAPY Before V	After V	Primary DIAGNOSIS	TARGET SYMPTOMS Before V's	STATUS SINCE V's (0-worse, 1-unchanged, 2-improved)
#1 (2)	36	F	12	5	Hysterical Neurosis	1. Amnesia	2
						2. Multiple Personality	2
						3. Depression	2
						4. Nightmares	2
						5. Psychogenic Abdominal Pain	2
						6. Migraine Headaches	1
						7. Marital Maladjustment	2
#2 (2)	31	F	6	6	Depressive Neurosis	1. Depression	2
						2. Alcoholism	2
						3. Marital Maladjustment	1
						4. Obesity	2
#3 (1)	33	M	1	3	Hysterical Neurosis	1. Amnesic Episodes	2
						2. Occupational Disability	2
#4 (1)	55	F	1	1	Hysterical Neurosis	1. Hysterical Seizures	2
#5 (2)	28	F	1	8	Depressive Neurosis	1. Suicidal Behavior	2
						2. Depression	1
						3. Occupational Disability	2
						4. Bronchial Asthma	2
						5. Marital Maladjustment	1
#6 (1)	32	M	16	1*	Anxiety ("success") Neurosis	1. Occupational Dysfunction	1
						2. Sexual Dysfunction	1
						3. Marital Maladjustment	1
#7 (1)	38	F	20	6	Anxiety Neurosis	1. Anxiety	2
						2. Marital Maladjustment	2
						3. Maternal Dysfunction	2
#8 (1)	42	F	1	1	Tardive Dyskinesia, Masked**	1. Movement Disorder	1
						2. Depression	1

* Premature termination: "financial problems."
** Referred with diagnosis of "conversion hysteria." Videoscan helped establish correct diagnosis.

remained the same. None has become worse or experienced any complications from the procedure. A brief description of three cases will illustrate the kinds of problems and responses which were encountered.

Patient #1

A 36-year-old Philippine-American housewife had been in psychotherapy for one year and was resisting all conventional approaches to treating her chronic anxiety attacks, depressive episodes, psychogenic abdominal symptoms, nightmares, and unpredictable personality changes. She was amnesic for all events that had occurred during the first seven years of her life and became agitated and physically ill whenever those events were explored. Upon receiving Amytal, she regressed to the age of four and recounted a series of traumatic events that took place in the Philippines during World War II. The most critical of these memories was the witnessing of her father's execution by Japanese soldiers. After the Amytal interview she again became amnesic but was able to remember and abreact her long-repressed grief when she saw the videotape playback. All her symptoms subsequently improved except her personality shifts, which worsened after she returned to her former job as a waitress. A second Amytal interview exposed the continuing presence of an alternate personality into whom the patient had split off most of her aggression, hostility, and self-hatred. After the patient had faced her alternate self on the video monitor, she became more able to assimilate these long dissociated elements of her personality into a more integrated self. Following the two videoscans and a total of two and a half years of intensive psychotherapy, this patient now reports considerable improvement in all her symptoms and a healthier relationship with her husband and children. She recently manifested her subjective improvement by enrolling in a local college to begin pursuing, for the first time, several areas of long-standing vocational and avocational interest.

Patient #2

This 31-year-old unhappily married, overweight airline stewardess was in psychotherapy because of chronic depression, multiple suicide attempts, and habitual excessive drinking. She was started on disulfiram (Antabuse) but, despite her avowed wish for help, she continued to display denial of her symptoms and resistance to treatment in the form of stopping her Antabuse, frequent missed appointments, and drinking prior to those she kept. After six months of making no progress in therapy, she had an alcohol-Antabuse reaction on the job and was temporarily distraught enough to accept a brief psychiatric hospitalization. In the hospital her first videoscan was performed. While watching the replay, she wept as she heard herself describing painful events about which she had previously denied having any feelings. After discharge she stopped resisting treatment and avoided drinking for nearly six months. Her self-esteem was eroded, however, by her husband's continued criticism and sexual disinterest and her failure to lose weight. Following a drinking episode and minor car accident, a second videoscan was performed. During the playback, she was struck, among other things, by her incessant requests for more Amytal, though she was obviously intoxicated by the drug. She became motivated after that experience to regain a self-control and determination that she said she had lost as a result of her marriage. She proceeded to lose 30 pounds, to stop drinking, and was able to terminate psychotherapy about six months later, feeling considerably better about herself. She has controlled her drinking for over a year now, appears much more self-confident, and states that she intends to hold onto her belief in herself regardless of whether or not the marriage survives.

Patient #3

A 33-year-old demolitions specialist had experienced a six-month fugue state upon returning home from Vietnam. He sought treatment at a VA Hospital and was reportedly given a conventional Amytal interview about which he could later recall nothing. For the next three years he was subject to brief continuing amnesic episodes in which he would find himself unaware of what he had been doing for the past several hours or days. After behaving in an uncharacteristically violent manner during one of these episodes, he came to another VA Hospital for help. Following a negative neurological examination and three weeks of psychotherapy, his psychiatrist referred him for a videoscan. During the administration phase of the procedure with his psychiatrist observing, he abreacted a number of traumatic childhood and military experiences which were thematically connected. After reviewing the tape without the patient present, the primary psychiatrist, the psychiatrist conducting the videoscan, and the psychiatrist-in-chief of the patient's ward collaboratively developed a treatment strategy. The primary therapist and videoscan consultant then proceeded to the playback phase together with the patient who initially remembered nothing of the interview but, upon seeing the tape, was able to recognize the major conflicts that had caused his fugue state and his subsequent amnesias. After a brief synthesis phase, conducted by his primary therapist, he was discharged from the hospital with a significant reduction in his symptoms. Three months later, the patient's improvement has continued as he pursues further psychotherapy and is attempting to get off disability status and start his own business.

DISCUSSION

This preliminary investigation raises far more questions than it answers about the videoscan technique. The small sample size, the limited length of follow-up, the use of the same therapist to perform all of the videoscans, and the lack of systematic controls to determine how much of the improvement that occurred was a function of the procedure itself —all of these are methodological problems which will have to be addressed by future investigation. Nevertheless, the fact that a number of patients who were not responding to other treatment approaches improved after this technique was employed suggests the possible usefulness of this method as an adjunct in the management of certain cases.

What are some of the mechanisms by which the videoscan might promote the attainment of therapeutic goals? While a psychodynamic framework has been useful in presenting our material and viewing our results thus far, we have also found that social learning and psychotherapy research perspectives can contribute to our understanding of the phenomena described.

Psychodynamic Considerations

From a psychodynamic perspective the most important factors about the videoscan procedure may be its abilities to promote the catharsis of repressed material, accelerate the development of insight into such materials, and facilitate the establishing of a positive transference. In connection with the latter function, it might be added that by contributing to the patient's fantasies of dominance, seduction, or nurturance by the therapist, this technique may have a disproportionate impact on transference in comparison with more conventional psychotherapeutic approaches. Such an effect might theoretically account for progress during the later phases of treatment (16).

Social Learning Perspectives

In examining what took place during the sessions from a social learning viewpoint, we noted that, along with abreactions, there were two other typical responses which we have called *co-reactions* and *counter-reactions*. Co-reactions consisted of the patient's empathizing with previously blocked verbal or affective behaviors which he or she saw on the videotape, and then being able to perform those behaviors without the medication. Patient #1 might be said to have experienced a co-reaction when she was finally able to grieve over the death of her father following the modeling of such behavior by her age-regressed self on the television monitor. This process is similar to that which goes on commonly in group therapy, where patients who initially have difficulty getting in touch with their own feelings are helped to do so by identifying with or modeling group members who can speak more freely. The disinhibited patient on the screen may be an especially effective model for the patient since it has been shown that the more features held in common by model and subject, the more likely the subject is to adopt the behavior of the model (17). Obviously, this process must be a selective one since not all disinhibited behaviors manifested by the patient under medication will be useful later. Here, reinforcement by the therapist probably plays a significant role in guiding the patient's learning.

Counter-reaction is the opposite process, through which the patient eliminates maladaptive behaviors as a result of seeing them on the television screen. When Patient #2 observed her persistent requests for more Amytal, she experienced a counter-reaction which may have contributed to her later avoidance of alcohol. The mixed results in other studies which have systematically exposed alcoholics to their own drunken behavior (18) suggest that counter-reactions probably have limited effectiveness in patients with marginal self-esteem unless accompanied by co-reactions and other encouraging experiences. The frequency and impact of both counter-reactions and co-reactions may be enhanced during the videoscan as compared with conventional videotape treatment by the fact that the medication catalyses social behaviors which the patient would otherwise have a low probability of emitting in the therapeutic setting. VSC then enables the patient to review those behaviors as well as those that might have occurred naturally, and make discriminations about their adaptiveness with the help of intermittent cues from the therapist.

Psychotherapy Research Perspectives

Another perspective that would account for the impact of the videoscan procedure is that which has been outlined by Jerome D. Frank (19), following many years of rigorous research into the parameters associated with psychotherapeutic effectiveness. He defines six therapeutic functions that are performed by virtually all successful psychotherapies:

1. strengthening and maintaining the therapeutic relationship;
2. inspiring and maintaining the patient's hope for help;
3. provision of opportunity for cognitive and experiential learning;
4. eliciting emotional arousal;
5. enhancement of the sense of mastery;
6. solidifying therapeutic gains.

In this context, the videoscan procedure might be viewed as a contemporary ritual which employs the "magic" of strong medications and electronic media feedback to strengthen the patient's faith in the therapeutic relationship. In doing so, it mobilizes a new hopefulness which previous demoralization and lack of progress may have diminished. The use of intravenous barbiturates in combination with VSC probably increases the opportunity for cognitive and experiential learning as well as for emotional arousal. After completing the invariably anxiety-provoking procedure, the patient frequently experiences an enhanced sense of mastery. The synthesis phase then enables the patient to continue working with the therapist towards the solidifying of therapeutic gains. The apparent value of the videoscan, thus, seems to derive, in part, from the fact that it incorporates, in theory, many of the features which have proven beneficial in other psychotherapies. Whether or not it provides these benefits in fact will only be determined as we gather data about the results achieved by other therapists using this approach, and from future studies of our own.

CONCLUSION

We believe that our work suggests that narcosynthesis is still a viable psychotherapeutic adjunct in selected cases. By combining the ability of certain medications to elicit repressed or inhibited psychological events with the capacity of VSC to transcend state-dependency and show those events to the patient when he has returned to a mental state wherein he can make use of them, the videoscan procedure seems to overcome some of the inherent problems in conventional narcotherapy and to increase the range of problems which can be usefully addressed by VSC. Although future studies will be necessary to confirm these findings, it appears that the videoscan can assist psychiatrists operating from many different theoretical perspectives in promoting treatment goals with a variety of patients in many therapeutic settings. Although we believe that long-term psychotherapy contributed significantly to the results achieved with several of our cases, we are intrigued with the possibility of decreasing both the duration and expense of psychiatric treatment by the judicious application of the videoscan technique.

REFERENCES

1. Bleckwenn, W. J.: Narcosis as Therapy in Neuropsychiatric Conditions. *JAMA*, 95:1168-71, 1930.
2. Lindemann, E.: Psychological Changes in Normal and Abnormal Individuals Under the Influence of Sodium Amytal. *Am. J. Psychiat.*, 11:1083-91, 1932.
3. Horsley, J. S.: Narcoanalysis. *Lancet*, 1:55, 1936.
4. Grinker, R. R., Sr., and Spiegel, J. P.: *Men Under Stress*. Blakiston, Philadelphia, 1945.
5. Burnett, W. E.: A Critique of Intravenous Barbiturate Usage in Psychiatric Practice. *Psychiat. Quart.*, 22:45-63, 1948.
6. New, J. J., and Kelly, A. R., Jr.: Narcosynthesis in Civilian Practice. *South. Med. J.*, 40:349-55, 1947.
7. Schneider, I.: Images of the Mind: Psychiatry in the Commercial Film. *Amer. J. of Psychiat.*, 134 (6):613-620, 1977.
8. Paerregaard, G.: The Value of Narcoanalysis as Shown by a Re-examination. *Acta Psychiat. and Neurolog. Scandin.*, Supplem. 100, 258-264, 1950.
9. Hoch, P. H., nd Polatin, P.: Narcosynthesis, Narcodiagnosis, and Narcotherapy. In G. Bychowski, and J. L. Despert (Eds.), *Specialized Techniques in Psychotherapy*. New York: Basic Books, 1952.
10. Sargant, W., and Slater, E.: *An Introduction to Physical Methods of Treatment in Psychiatry*, Fifth Edition. New York: Science House, 1972.
11. Bahnson, C. B.: Body and Self-Images Associated with Audiovisual Self-confrontation. *J. Nerv. Ment. Dis.*, 148 (3):262-80, 1969.
12. Metzner, R. J., and Bittker, T. W.: Videotape Production by Medical Educators: Some Practical Considerations. *J. Med. Educ.*, 48:743-51, 1973.
13. Cheek, D. B., and LeCron, L. M.: *Clinical Hypnotherapy*. New York: Grune and Stratton, 1968.
14. Enneis, J. M.: The Hypnodramatic Technique. *Group Psychotherapy*, 3 (1):11-54, 1950.
15. Leuher, H.: Guided Affective Imagery. *Am. J. of Psychother.*, 23 (1):4-22, 1969.
16. Kubie, L. S., and Margolin, S.: The Therapeutic Role of Drugs in the Process of Repression, Dissociation and Synthesis. *Psychosom. Med.*, 7:147-151, 1945.
17. Bandura, A.: *Agression: A Social Learning Analysis*. Englewood Cliffs, N.J.: Prentice-Hall, 1973.
18. Schaefer, H. H., Sobell, M. B., and Mills, K. C.: Some Sobering Data on the Use of Self-confrontation with Alcoholics. *Behav. Ther.*, 2:28-39, 1971.
19. Frank, J. D.: Psychotherapy: The Restoration of Morale. *Am. J. Psychiat.*, 131:271-4, 1974.

SECTION IV
Legal, Moral and Ethical Considerations

EDITOR'S INTRODUCTION

In this brief section an attempt has been made to elucidate what are perhaps some of the most significant aspects of the doctor-patient relationship insofar as it applies to the use of videotape.

Since this book was initially published in 1970, the major area of legal concern for those using videotapes in psychiatry continues to be that of "informed consent." Attorneys, such as Patricia Wald, who has been a key figure in the Mental Health Law Project,* have been questioning increasingly whether "informed consent" can exist in a coercive setting. If the information given to a patient about a procedure or medication is only enough to be a gesture, then, according to Attorney Wald, it is not enough.

In my experience it is best to give hospitalized inpatients and/or members of their families an opportunity to slowly read the videotape permission form and to ask them if they have any questions concerning it. The usual anxiety-loaded question is, "How do I know this won't be used on network television?" I respond truthfully and completely by pointing out that the permission form states the videotape is to be used only for medical and psychiatric education and that does not mean we could use it for public dissemination or broadcast. If the patient or his family is not completely satisfied I will offer to write in on the permission form the specific words they would like. e.g., "No part of this videotape being made on (date) can be used on commercial television broadcasts at any time." They are usually satisfied with that added statement and then cooperate voluntarily with participation in the interview which will

---

* The Mental Health Law Project grew out of the Center for Law and Social Policy, an American Civil Liberties Union-supported organization, and was founded in 1972 by attorneys Charles Halpern, Bruce Ennis, Paul Friedman, who still serves as managing attorney, and Patricia Wald, who has recently been appointed by President Carter as Assistant Attorney General for Legislation. Her interest and competency as a lawyer in the field of mental health public interest law were established through her work as Director of Litigation of the Mental Health Law Project in Washington, D.C.

be videotaped by cameras and cameramen completely out in the open in our video studio. Quite often we show part of the taped interview to the patient and family immediately after the interview or arrange for them to see a playback at a later time with their therapist to obtain the potential therapeutic benefits of video replay.

In my private practice setting I function as cameraman as well as psychotherapist. I have found it of value to ask the patient *while the tape is still recording* for permission to use the whole tape or parts of it for educational purposes with colleagues at meetings. This makes available for future replay not only the sound and words of the patient giving verbal permission to use the tape, but also shows the behavioral, attitudinal, and contextual background and interaction of the moment in which permission is asked for and granted. It is still advisable to obtain written permission as well as having this video record. The nature and degree of competency of the patient are visible to the viewer and also enough non-verbal metacommunicational data to determine whether the act is made with free will or whether more or less pressure is being exerted to get the patient to agree to sign the permission form.

In an important legal case, referred to in the *Rutgers Law Review* in 1975,* between a patient and a psychiatrist over whether the psychiatrist had legal consent to publish the patient's story, the court ruled for the plaintiff against the psychiatrist. A patient "can waive confidentiality by consenting to disclosure, but such consent must be given explicitly, voluntarily and intelligently, that is, with knowledge of the material to be disclosed." The general standard of consent applicable to and governing HEW-funded human experimentation projects is: "Informed consent means the knowing consent of an individual . . . so situated as to be able to exercise free power of choice without undue inducement or any element of force, fraud, deceit, duress, or other form of constraint or coercion." The court in the case of Roe v. Doe referred to above stated ". . . A doctor who wishes to publish confidential material about his patient and relies on the patient's consent should take care to get that consent in clear, unambiguous written form."

The Roe v. Doe article covers in a detailed and most enlightening fashion a review of legal decisions on such issues as (a) implied contracts, (b) the patient's waiving of the testimonial privilege of confidentiality by raising his mental health as a legal issue in a suit or by consenting to disclosure, in an explicit, voluntary and intelligent manner, that is, with

---

* Roe V. Doe: A Remedy for Disclosure of Psychiatric Confidences. *Rutgers Law Review*, 29:190-209, 1975.

knowledge of the material to be disclosed, (c) disguise of the patient's identity so there would be no cause for injury if no one could recognize the patient, (d) the concept of privacy and the invasion of privacy for commercial purposes, (e) public disclosure of private fact and (f) the issue of prior restraint as a remedy. The conclusion of the article clearly states that "Implicit in any doctor-patient relationship is the understanding that the doctor will act only in the best interests of the patient and will not violate the confidences learned in the course of treatment. Publication, without consent, of a psychiatric history where the patient is inadequately disguised is a violation of the doctor-patient agreement."

In the general practice of medicine, informed consent is seen to be the cause of much dilemma, particularly for surgeons who experience the issue as a "tightrope" at times and even a "descent to absurdity" because there are times it can be cruel to tell a sick person detailed stories of risks and side effects.* The problem arises from the fact that the advice of attorneys as to how much and what kind of information is legally necessary to meet the qualifications of "informed consent" is not necessarily the amount and kind of information which is medically desirable and of benefit for each and every patient. Fortunately, in regards to the issue of informed consent with videotapes in psychiatry we do not have too much difficulty in assuring our patients that this videotaped information is for professional or medical education of professional audiences only and that these audiences know and respect what is considered confidential or privileged information.

I wish to conclude these comments on informed consent with Harry Wilmer's 1970 clear-cut statement for videotape makers which I quote because of its succinctness and continuing applicability.**

> We never make a videotape without the patient's consent and without fully explaining to the patient beforehand what is being done and why. When minors are involved, consent is also obtained from parents or guardians. With informed consent, there is no intrusion of privacy. The only possible breach of confidence would be the misuse of tapes by showing them to persons other than select professional audiences, and no ethical person would permit this.

Stanley Chesley*** advocates the increasing use of the pre-taped video

---

* Denney, M. K.: Informed Consent—Doctor's Friend or Foe? *Modern Medicine,* p. 74-76, August 1, 1976.

** Wilmer, H. A.: Use of the Television Monologue with Adolescent Psychiatric Patients. *Amer. J. Psychiat.,* 126:103, 1970.

*** Chesley, S. M.: The Use of Videotape—The Expert Witness. *J. Amer. Instit. nosis,* 15:161-162, 1974.

deposition brought into civil courts to expedite the backlog of litigation cases often delayed because the case is being heard in a part-time court which makes it difficult for a physician to appear in person because he is in surgery and cannot appear when scheduled. He points out the value of the jury being able to see the face of the witness to judge his demeanor, warmth, objectivity, subjectivity or impersonality rather than, as is usual, just listening to the words in the deposition.

Prior to 1970 the Federal Rules of Civil Procedure left open the possibility of videotape recordings by stating in former Rule 30, "the testimony shall be taken stenographically and transcribed *unless the parties agree otherwise*" (editor's italics). The 1970 amendment provided for "non-Stenographic Recordings" and "The court may upon motion order that the testimony at a deposition be recorded by other than stenographic means, in which event the order shall designate the manner of recording, preserving, and filing the deposition and may include other provisions to assure that the recorded testimony will be accurate and trustworthy. . . ."

Chesley makes a strong plea for the courts and lawyers to "keep abreast of the times" as the cost of videotape is now less than the cost of court stenographers. The editing out of portions of tape deemed objectionable can be done in advance and tapes can be held safely under the auspices of the court so as not to be tampered with.

McGill and Thrasher have written an article entitled "Videotapes: The Reel Thing of the Future" based on their successful experience with its use in courtroom proceedings.* Their views may very well be prophetic in predicting the real shape of things to come in the use of videotapes of psychiatric interviews of defendants by a psychiatrist in cases where the plea of insanity has been made by the defendant's attorney. If the courtroom proceedings and justice system are really aimed towards seeking truth, then the attitudinal, nonverbal, contextual and other data which were the basis for the psychiatrist's opinion at the time of the first interview with the accused are important data to be brought to court to educate the jury and judge concerning the facts which do or do not indicate evidence of psychosis or insanity.

An important point which is worth repeating is that when a videotape of a session is admitted as evidence in a courtroom setting it should initially be shown in its entirety without interruptions. Then it can be shown again, in segments, with comments from the interviewing witness

---

* G. A. McGill and J. W. Thrasher: Videotapes: The Reel Thing of the Future. *Trial Magazine*, September-October, 1975.

or defendant. Once admitted as evidence in a courtroom proceeding, the videotape may be reviewed during cross-examination of the psychiatrist as is any other evidence brought in by the psychiatrist to serve as basis for his opinion(s). The authors state that the use of videotape recordings in courtroom proceedings ". . . can be expected to expand as the recognition grows that they are not merely 'gimmicks' but can be a highly convenient, most effective, and relatively inexpensive method of presenting certain types of evidence. McGill, an attorney, and Thrasher, a psychiatrist, participated in a criminal trial in which videotapes were used in conjunction with psychiatric testimony.

An important, but almost always overlooked area of concern to anyone who collects videotapes of patients in a private practice setting is the issue of "What happens to my tapes of patients if I die?" Because of my age, 59, and because of recently redoing my will, I realized how important it was to arrange for the disposition of one's confidential office tapes in one's will or in a codicil attached to one's will. Despite our concern for posterity or residual narcissism or simple inability to discard things which relate to ourselves, it is vital that we consider what happens to the audiovisual materials which patients allowed us to have in good faith as confidential, and to provide for their disposal upon our death. Who, besides ourselves, is going to take the time to see what we conjecture is so valuable that it should be preserved? Who would preserve it and in what form? And would respect for the patient's confidentiality be properly and professionally exercised?

My considered opinion is that we should state clearly that "Upon the event of my death I hereby direct my executors to destroy the contents of any audio or videotapes which are in my home or in my office and are my possession which contain the voice or picture of any patient currently seen in practice or who has been seen by me in the past." The destruction of the contents of these tapes can be accomplished by subjecting them to a strong electro-magnetic field, thus preserving the tape stock itself for future use (it is recommended you seek consultation on this), or the entire tapes themselves may be destroyed by placing them in an incinerator.

You may wish to direct that any tapes which remain in your office after you die which have already been edited and for which patients have given written permission for use for medical educational purposes can be donated to a medical or psychiatric center with the stipulation that they would be appropriately treated with regard for privacy and confidentiality and used only for professional purposes with the rights of the patients respected in perpetuity.

I feel it is of value for the reader to ask: "Is much of what is considered an invasion of privacy really an invasion of privacy or a disrespect for secrecy with its bedfellow shame which have for so long masqueraded under the rubric of privacy?" With the undermining of many of the so-called elements of privacy in psychiatry through the introduction of group, family and couple therapy; sensitivity, process or training groups; recorded audio or video closed circuit sessions made available for supervision, training and the treatment of other patients; with the increase in socio-cultural confrontatons in society at all levels which are undermining the perpetuation of that kind of privacy which allows for the perpetuation of double-binding and other attitudinal contradictions, it may well be that ethical and moral considerations concerning privacy and privileged communications must also change. This is particularly significant in the sense that when a patient gives up the self-concept of needing secrecy about his private functioning to avoid shame and embarrassment and realizes a new self-concept which makes him a more universal member of the human race, which increases his sense of belonging and decreases his sense of pathological uniqueness, he has gained more from psychotherapy than when privacy as conceived of formerly is adhered to. In group psychotherapy it is not primarily the confessional aspect of revealing one's private matters that is most helpful. What is helpful is to give up the sense of pathological uniqueness bound up with privacy as one finds acceptance among peers and learns how common and public is what was previously considered private. We cannot really be with real people without being real people. The impact of videotape self-confrontation is a powerful influence in helping patients accept the naturalness and universality of their "human nature."

It is of interest to note recent developments in the law as it applies to privacy and privileged communication. A trend-setting law has recently been passed in Colorado which protects patients participating in group psychotherapy by granting them the right of privileged communication as to what transpires in group therapy sessions to the same degree and in the same way that it protects the therapist. Recent changes in our societal mores as well as the inroad and impact of new technological media, particularly in the realm of communication, transmission and storage of information concerning individuals and groups, require that individuals as well as legislatures realistically reappraise concepts and laws concerning privacy and privileged communication.

California psychiatrists seem to be the ones leading the "long, arduous legal battle" to refuse to disclose what the psychiatrist considers to be privileged communications between the psychiatrist and a patient. George

Caesar was jailed for three days in July 1977 for refusing to testify in his one-man test of the limits of privileged communication.* In his own defense, Caesar stated that to testify ". . . would cause affirmative harm to his patient's psychological well being, that he was under an ethical duty attendant upon his calling as a physician not to injure his patient, and that to answer such questions would interfere with the function of healer which society had placed on him, having licensed him to conduct a medical practice in psychotherapy."

Caesar was challenging the constitutionality of Section 1016 of the California Evidence Code, which states that "there is no privilege under this article as to communications relevant to an issue concerning the mental or emotional condition of the patient if such an issue has been tendered by . . . the patient . . ." by filing a lawsuit. He also sought clarification of the 1970 *Lifschutz* decision, which set a precedent in privileged provisions and which Caesar and his attorney Melchior have labeled a "superficially reasonable rule (that) has proven impossible to implement in a manner not overly restrictive of the constitutional privacy in this area. The *Lifschutz* precedent distinguishes between relevant and irrelevant psychiatric testimony and places the burden on the patient to prove the relevance of the information in question."

All of us owe a debt to colleagues like Joseph Lifschutz and George Caesar who have the courage to take a position which does not capitulate but takes a stand against what they consider unjust and tyrannical laws. Caesar's attorney wrote to the presiding judge a long explanation which included: ". . . History is replete with circumstances, on many of which the ink is not dry, where persons have found it necessary in all good conscience to disobey particular laws and to accept their punishment, rather than to adhere to laws which they conscientiously deem to be wrong and unjust. . . ."

Caesar had been supported from the outset by the Northern California Psychiatric Society through its legal defense fund; the American Psychiatric Association joined the case at the Supreme Court level.

David N. Fields has devoted 37 years to finding solutions for the problems presented by the interface between law and psychiatry. His work as President of the Association for Improvement of Mental Hospitals brought him into repeated contact with patients, relatives and others questioning the legal rights of the mentally ill and their capacity for signing valid contracts which includes the releases we request patients

* "Psychiatrist Jailed in Privilege Challenge" was the lead front page article in the *Psychiatric News,* September 2, 1977.

to sign before or after videotaping them. His review of the issues of competency and incompetency and the rights of persons adjudicated to be incompetent in regard to their making a will or entering into a valid contract is eye-opening in its implications. His chapter on legal implications and complications offers sobering information.

The Fellowship Pledge of the American Psychiatric Association includes "A Fellow of the Association promises: to improve the treatment, rehabilitation, and care of the mentally ill, the mentally retarded and the emotionally disturbed; to promote research, professional education in psychiatry and allied fields, and the prevention of psychiatric disabilities; to advance the standards of all psychiatric services and facilities; to foster the cooperation of all who are concerned with the medical, psychological, social, and legal aspects of mental health and illness; and to make psychiatric knowledge available to other practitioners of medicine, to other scientists and to the public . . . (to) faithfully dedicate ourselves above all to the welfare of our patients; to maintain the dignity of our profession and the practice of medicine; to supplement our own judgment with the wisdom and counsel of specialists in fields other than our own; to render assistance willingly to our own colleagues; to be generous in giving professional aid to the unfortunate; to enhance our knowledge by continuing study, by attendance at meetings of our professional brethren, by association with physicians of eminence, and by freely exchanging experience and opinion with our colleagues." Certainly these aspects of the pledge are particularly significant for those who use videotape in various settings. It is as if the professional who uses videotape not only has to be master of the ship which traverses the narrow passage between Scylla and Charybdis, but also has to be walking a tightrope while at the helmsman's bridge. To advance psychiatric or mental hygiene education by the use of videotapes or films in which the therapist appears in person does in fact move him into the public eye. Is it possible to do this only for others and not for self at all? Hopefully a professional so engaged will be motivated by a sense of the needs of the public-at-large and not primarily for self-aggrandizement.

The overlapping considerations concerning the patient's welfare as well as maintaining public confidence in psychiatry are closely related to generally accepted propositions concerning secrecy, privacy and privileged communication, some of which has been touched upon by Modlin in an article entitled "How Private is Privacy?"*

Rosenbaum in his chapter devoted to the issues of privacy and privi-

---

* Modlin, H. C.: How Private Is Privacy? *Psychiatry Digest*, 30:13-17, Feb. 1969.

leged communication has presented the conservatively accepted professional position. He has added new views on the issue of privacy which has become of increasing interest and importance to our United States Congress as well as to the average citizen exposed to more and more electronic recording and retrieval accessibility of his personal life story. (See Chapter 26, this section).

As a video user you are advised to consult your own attorney(s) to obtain up-to-date legal information to guide and protect you and your patients while keeping in mind as a guiding principle the concept that you are supposed to be of help to your patient and do nothing to harm him or her. Will taping and showing a particular tape do harm now or later to this patient? Your answer can be your guide.

The rules of copyright, ownership and distribution and other rights can best be clarified by your attorney or other experienced experts.

25

LEGAL IMPLICATIONS AND COMPLICATIONS—MODEL FORMS FOR SIGNED RELEASES

David Noah Fields, LL.B.

To do complete justice to the subject "Legal Implications and Complications" in making and exhibiting videotapes of psychiatric patients in private practice or mental hospitals would require the examination of a legal literature which is enormous. To analyze all of the problems discussed in the literature and answer the practical questions necessarily encountered in the making and exhibition of videotapes for treatment, training and research would require more space than is available for this entire book. This book would then become a legal treatise for lawyers rather than a tool to be used in the practice of psychiatry. Consequently the writer has endeavored to narrow the area of discussion. Rather than attempt to analyze every problem and answer every question which may be asked, in the following pages an effort has been made to highlight the problems and to alert the reader to the risks involved in the use of videotapes even for the limited purposes of psychiatric training.

The psychiatrist may see his patient as one who is in varying degrees "dysfunctional," to use the simplified classification of Karl Menninger in "The Vital Balance." He may not need, for treatment purposes, to determine whether, as a result of psychosis or other cause, the patient is incompetent.

Lawyers may not follow suit; they must still use the pejorative labels of the past, including sanity, insanity, competency, incompetency, psychotic and non-psychotic. Menninger says: "Patients who consult us because of their sufferings and their distress and their disability have every right to resent being plastered with a damning index tab. Our function is to help these people not to further afflict them" (1).

The lawyer called upon to help the psychiatrist in the development of a training tool, such as videotape, cannot avoid the unfortunate labels if he is to give sound advice to the psychiatrist as teacher and researcher.

COMPETENT PATIENTS

Most of the adult patients seen by psychiatrists in their private practice, unless they specialize in the treatment of psychotics, are competent. As to them, the fact of being in treatment does not establish even a presumptive incompetency. Such patients can consent to the filming and taping of their therapy sessions. Such consents should, however, be explicit and in writing. The use of the film or tape for the limited purpose set forth in the written consent should be accompanied by practicable safeguards to preclude identification and/or avoid patently humiliating or defamatory material.

If written consent is obtained from mentally competent persons and the necessary safeguards adopted, the risk of legal liability to users of the videotapes should be minimal.

INCOMPETENT ADULT PATIENTS

Who are the incompetent adults? Are they patients who are or have been in mental hospitals? Does release from the hospital terminate incompetency? Are there patients who have never been in hospitals who are incompetent? Is commitment to a mental hospital the same thing as an adjudication of incompetency? These and many other questions must necessarily be answered in discussing incompetency, both in general terms and with respect to the use of videotapes of incompetents. The general subject is comprehensively discussed in a report entitled "Mental Impairment and Legal Incompetency" (2). Some of the findings in the report are the following:

Hospitalization and Incompetency

In some jurisdictions appointment of a guardian or committee is not automatic, even when hospitalization results in an automatic finding of incompetency. In such hospitalization proceedings there is no separate determination of the prospective patient's capacity to manage his own affairs.

Although hospitalization and incompetency are merged (one raises the presumption of the other), release from the hospital—even absolute discharge—is not necessarily a restoration to competency. The legislative trend has been toward a complete separation of hospitalization and incompetency. Where such separation has taken place, an adjudication of mental illness is not an adjudication of incompetency. Even where rules on hospitalization and incompetency are determined separately, frequently there is a finding of incompetency with no evidence whatsoever of the person's capacity to manage his own affairs.

The report recommends that if a hospitalized patient is legally competent, he should not be prevented from executing legal instruments. It further recommends that if hospital officials believe that a patient, who is legally competent, is in fact incapable of engaging in a given jural activity, the hospital should notify the person or persons who may appropriately initiate guardianship or committee proceedings.

The report states the following in its discussion of guardianship:

> There is some variation among the states in the generic term for one for whom a guardian or committee may be appointed, though the most frequently used term is incompetent. Other states employ terms like "insane," "mentally ill," "non compos mentis," and "unsound mind" to denominate legal status.

The report recommends that a uniform set of terms be adopted by all the states to denominate the person for whom a guardian may be appointed and to denominate the person who may serve in that capacity.

Again referring to the subject of restoration to competency the report found that restorations very rarely occur in many states and in some almost never, and recommends that the form of restoration proceedings should be essentially the same as guardianship proceedings.

Perhaps the most important finding of all is the one concerning "Ad Hoc Determinations of Incompetency." In this connection the report states: "All but a handful of interviewees feel that there should not be a single criterion of competency applicable to all legal functions, but rather that the criteria should vary depending upon the function to be performed."

As a concomitant of the foregoing finding the report states that no single criterion could sufficiently reflect the different social values in which ad hoc determinations of incompetency may be made. The report goes on to say: "Neither psychiatry nor law can be static. Because these areas of ad hoc determinations involve delicate balancing of correlative rights and duties, it does not seem feasible to define *a priori* statutory standards. Rather, the law should be permitted to evolve through a decisional process, tempered by the expanding knowledge of medicine and the experience of social and commercial practice."

It can be readily seen that legal problems similar to those raised in any proposal for the use of tapes or films of patients may arise in many other situations where the determination of competency or incompetency may be necessary. The use of such films and tapes for training purposes is obviously useful, even though the use may be prohibited or limited in some cases. The law on the subject of incompetency, of course, is not static but it is slow moving. Both the psychiatric and legal professions face the challenge of bringing about more rapid changes in the law so that the status of alleged or actual incompetency will not interfere with useful activities such as psychiatric training.

As indicated, some patients may need hospital care and yet be able to manage their financial and business affairs and enter into valid contractual agreements. Others may have no need of hospital confinement, yet be incapable of managing their own affairs and incapable of entering into valid and enforceable contracts. "The question of an individual's capacity to conduct his affairs is generally determined in an incompetency proceeding. In order to safeguard the assets of a person found to be incompetent, he is prohibited, for example, from writing checks, selling property, and entering into business. Since the incompetent is not able to engage in these transactions, a guardian, committee or conservator is usually appointed to act on his behalf" (3).

Even though adjudicated to be incompetent, a mentally ill person may make a will or enter into a valid contract. To make a valid will he must have testamentary capacity at the time of executing the will. He may enter into a valid marriage during a "lucid interval" (4). If adjudicated to be an incompetent, can he authorize the use of videotapes showing him in treatment in a hospital setting or in other activities where the use of videotape would be embarrassing? Suppose he is incompetent but does not have a committee or guardian? Who can act on his behalf?

The answer to these questions is not easy. There is no direct decisional law on the subject (5). The general law on the right of incompetents to contract varies from state to state.

Hence, one who deals with an adjudicated incompetent patient, irrespective of whether he is confined in a hospital, should proceed with the utmost caution. Even if a hospital director were to permit the making of films or videotapes of hospital patients, their subsequent exhibition might constitute the tort of invasion of privacy or defamation of character or illegal publication of privileged communications or matters. If film on videotapes can be made in a manner which will not reveal the identity of the patient, the risks of exhibiting them may possibly be avoided.

What should be done in dealing with 1) patients who have been legally found to be incompetent but who have not been legally restored to competency even though they have recovered, and 2) patients who have never been adjudicated to be incompetent but who in fact are so mentally ill that they cannot be said to have the capacity to contract? With respect to the recovered patient it would be wise to defer taping their therapy sessions for showing to others until they have procured a judicial ruling that they have been restored to competency. To tape the sessions of non-adjudicated patients, whose illness raises a doubt as to their capacity to enter legally valid contracts, would be extremely risky and should not be undertaken.

Of course there is a riskless method of dealing with adjudicated incompetents, patients who have not been adjudicated but who are too ill to have capacity to contract, hospitalized patients and others whose status is doubtful. The patient, or his committee, or the hospital director may seek prior court authorization of the taping of therapy sessions, hospital interviews or hospital activities in which the patient is involved. If such court authorization is obtained, there should be no risk at all in making and exhibiting the videotapes. Obviously, however, it would be time consuming and expensive to even attempt to obtain judicial approval in numerous cases and there would be no guarantee that courts would approve in all or most of the cases presented. The concept of prior judicial approval, therefore, must be regarded as theoretically possible but highly impractical.

MINORS

Minor patients, like adults, may be competent or incompetent. It is doubtful that competent minors can effectively authorize taping of psychiatric sessions or hospital activities. Minors may disavow their transactions in many situations, provided their attempts to disavow "are used as a shield and not as a sword." Only subsequent litigation and court decision would determine whether a minor had properly disavowed a consent to the use of tapes or films. Clearly there may be an element of risk in using such films. It goes without saying that the risk would be enormously increased if tapes of incompetent minors were used. In institutions consent by the authorities may limit the risk if identification of the patients is avoided.

RETARDATES

Mental defectives (retardates) are one of the groups that the law seeks to protect. There is no sharp line between competent and incompetent retardates. Films and tapes of retardates may involve considerable risk and should not be undertaken without proper authorization. Again, in institutions risk may be limited by obtaining permission from hospital authorities. Even then, tapes should be used only if adequate safeguards are employed to prevent identification.

Normally the capacity of a mentally ill person to contract depends upon whether or not he is competent or incompetent, as discussed in this paper. There is, however, one jural act which a New York statute permits a mentally ill person to perform without regard to whether or not he has legal capacity to contract. The trend in New York, as well as in many other states, is to encourage mentally ill persons to apply for voluntary admission to mental hospitals. Even patients who have been committed as involuntary patients may seek to have their status converted to that of voluntary patient. Since the act of applying for voluntary admission and the agreement of the hospital to accept the patient on that basis results in what is basically a contractual status, the competency of the patient had to be presumed. Otherwise the whole concept of voluntary admissions would be impossible of achievement. As a result Sec. 71 of the New York Mental Hygiene Law, dealing with voluntary admissions, provides in part as follows:

> No requirement shall be made, by rule, regulation or otherwise as a condition to admission and retention pursuant to this section that any person applying for admission shall have the legal capacity to contract.

The above provision was subjected to constitutional attack, but was upheld by the New York Court of Appeals on December 12, 1968 (6). It may well be that other statutes will permit patients to enter jural relations, including the granting of permission for the use of videotapes and films, without regard to the legal capacity of the patient to contract.

The possible legal pitfalls that may be encountered in proposed uses of videotapes are numerous. The pitfalls, however, chiefly arise in connection with incompetents, minors and retardates. At the beginning of this chapter the status of *competent patients* is discussed. Being in treatment does not raise any presumption of incompetency and such patients can give valid consent to the use of tapes in which they are involved. It is appropriate to repeat, however, that such consents should be explicit and in writing and should be accompanied by safeguards to protect the patients. The safeguards will vary according to the use to which the tapes are to be put.

The following sample form was prepared by the author of this chapter for use by Milton Berger in his private practice. It can be used with or without modifications in other settings. *However, no sample form presented here should be used without consultation with and approval from your legal counsel.*

AGREEMENT entered into this   day of
between Dr. MILTON MILES BERGER (hereinafter referred to as the First Party) and   (hereinafter referred to as the Second Party).

WHEREAS, the First Party is desirous of using and exhibiting videotape, kinescope, motion pictures and/or photographs of the Second Party for the purpose of professional education, treatment and research, and

WHEREAS, the Second Party, in consideration of the premises, is desirous of endorsing and supporting the use of such videotape, kinescope, motion pictures and/or photographs for the purpose of professional education, treatment and research,

NOW, THEREFORE, it is agreed by the parties hereto as follows:

1. In consideration of the mutual covenants contained herein the Second Party consents to the use of videotape, kinescope, motion pictures and/or photographs of himself heretofore made or hereinafter to be made by the First Party. Specifically the Second Party refers to videotape, kinescope, motion pictures and/or photographs of himself, alone or with others, taken in the office of the First Party during the course of individual and group treatment by the First Party.

2. The First Party agrees that the said videotape, kinescope, motion pictures and/or photographs will be used solely in the interest of the advancement of mental health programs and only for the purpose of professional education, treatment or research activities connected with such programs, and will not be used for any other purpose.

3. The First Party agrees not to use or permit the use of the name of the Second Party in connection with any direct or indirect use or exhibition of such videotape, kinescope, motion pictures and/or photographs.

3. The Second Party hereby agrees that he will never sue the First Party or the Estate of the First Party and will never attach the assets thereof and further agrees that this covenant may be pleaded as a defense to any action or proceeding which may be instituted by the Second Party against the First Party or his Estate.

IN WITNESS WHEREOF, the parties have duly executed this agreement the day and year first above written.

                          Patient

It has been suggested that optionally the following additional clause may also be useful:

> I agree that the First Party is to be the sole owner of all rights in and to the said videotape, kinescope, motion pictures and/or photographs for all purposes herein set forth.
> I understand that I shall receive no financial compensation for the use of such videotape, kinescope, motion pictures or photographs.

The following release form was used in conjunction with production of the 16 mm. 45-minute sound motion picture film entitled, "The Scream Inside: Emergence Through Group Therapy" prepared from videotapes taken in the office of the author of this volume who conducted a group of volunteer patients from his private practice for the express intent of making this film. Incidentally, as all meetings of the group are on videotape, the actual discussion about the implications of signing the release forms as well as the signing by members during a group meeting is also on videotape.

> For the sum of $1.00, receipt of which is hereby acknowledged, I consent to the use of the Videotapes, Kinescopes, Motion Pictures and Photographs of myself taken during March, April, May and June 1968 in connection with a project for Sandoz Pharmaceuticals.
> These Videotapes, Motion Picture Films and Photographs may be used by Film Communications or Sandoz, and I further assign to Film Communications all of my right, title, and interest in and to the above described Videotapes, Motion Picture Films and Photographs.

> --
> Name
>
> --
> Address
>
> --
>
> --
> Witness

The following consent form is currently in use at the New York State Psychiatric Institute. It specifically releases from liability a hospital, its university-affiliated psychoanalytic institute, and the State Department of Mental Hygiene as well as the Director of the Hospital and the physician in charge of the videotape production unit of the hospital.

I, ..., hereby consent to the taking of any videotape recordings of me and to the reproduction, publication, transmission, broadcast, or exhibition of the same by the Department of Mental Hygiene or in connection with educational programs or activities of that department, and I hereby consent to the release of information concerning my case from the records of the New York State Psychiatric Institute and Columbia PSA Institute and the Department of Mental Hygiene for such purposes, and I hereby release the State of New York, its officers and employees and more particularly, Dr. Lawrence Kolb, M.D., Director of the New York State Psychiatric Institute and Dr. James H. Ryan, M.D., from any liability or claim in connection with the release for publication of information from such records and in connection with the reproduction, display, broadcast, or publication of photographs of me.

I give this consent and release in consideration of and with the full understanding that the use by the Department of Mental Hygiene of my photograph and information from my records will be in the interest of advancement of mental health programs.

....
Witness   Signature

                                 ....
                                 Date

I hereby certify that I have interviewed and examined the above named patient and in my opinion he is mentally competent to execute the foregoing consent and release, and he did so willingly and as his own voluntary act.

                 ....
                 Signature

                 ....
                 Date

                 _____

CONSENT FOR AUDIO AND/OR VISUAL RECORDING
AND PUBLICATION

TO: DEAN AND DIRECTOR
UNIVERSITY OF MISSOURI MEDICAL CENTER

                                 Date: ....

                        Hospital Number: ....

Patient: ....

I Consent that: still photographs   (Mark out
motion picture photographs   those which
closed circuit television   do not apply.)
television recording
artists illustrations and/or
plastic moldings

may be taken of .... or parts of my
(his) (her) body under the following conditions:

1) The items may be made only with the consent of my (his)
(her) attending physician and under the conditions and at such
times as may be approved by him.

2) The item(s) may be made by my (his) (her) attending physician or by a person approved by him.

3) The item(s) may be used for medical school records and if
in the judgement of my (his) (her) attending physician medical
research, education, or science will be benefited by their use, then
said item(s) and information relating to my (his) (her) case may
be assigned, published, shown, copied and republished, either separately or in connection with each other, in professional journals,
professional meetings, or medical books, or used for any other
purpose which they may deem proper in the interest of medical
and lay education, knowledge, or research, provided however, that
it is specifically understood that in any such publication or use
I shall not be identified by name. Permission is further given to
modify, retouch, erase or destroy the aforementioned records as
deemed desirable by a physician on the faculty in cooperation
with my (his) (her) attending physician.

Signed

Signed by parents or guardian

Witnesses: ....
(2 signa-
tures
needed)   ....

- -

Type: Audiotape   .... Still Photograph   .... Further
                   time   number   Descrip-
                                                                tion:

      Illustration .... Motion Picture   ....
                   number   feet

      Plastic Model .... Videotape   ....
                   number   time

Date record made: .... Location of record: ....

- -

Permission is hereby given to erase or destroy the record approved by this permission.

Date: ....

....
Signed by Attending Physician

Irving A. Goldberg, Ph.D.
555 Medical Dental Building
Seattle, Washington

Date: ....

In consideration of one dollar ($1.00), the receipt of which I hereby acknowledge, I, the undersigned, hereby acknowledge that I have participated in videotaped group therapy sessions under the guidance of Dr. Irving A. Goldberg during the period from .... to .... and I have utmost confidence in Dr. Goldberg, and do hereby authorize him to select from these videotaped sessions a particular session (hereinafter referred to as "the session") of his choosing that will be helpful to me and to others, which will be used as a demonstration or teaching presentation to professionals.

I hereby irrevocably grant to you and your successors, licensees, and assigns the right 1) to use the session initially on a live basis, or 2) to broadcast the session initially by means of "recordings" (by any means of recording television programs, whether now or hereafter developed, including but not limited to tape, film, wire, or disc, and which recording you may edit as you see fit). In addition, you shall have the right to use or authorize the use of the session or any portion thereof in any manner on television or in any other manner or media at any time or times throughout the world in perpetuity, subject to the restrictions here and above stated.

I further grant you the right to use my likeness, and/or my voice and historical information concerning me in connection therewith, including but not limited to promotion in printed media, but not for the direct endorsement of any product or service. This agreement is subject to the limitation that my name shall be retained in confidence and not be disclosed to the general public.

I hereby release you and your successor, licensees and assigns from any and all claims which I may at any time have by reason of any use of the session or any recording thereof or the exercise of any of your rights hereunder or arising out of my participation in the session or as a result of any comments concerning me made by any other person appearing in such session.

If I am a minor, this grant and release shall not be valid unless my parent and/or guardian shall execute the representation in the agreement below.

I do further waive any privilege I may have as to confidential communications between myself and Dr. Goldberg or other persons participating in the session, for that particular session.

For payment   Name: ....
received of
$1. (one dollar)   Address: ....

....

REFERENCES

1. Menninger, Karl: *The Vital Balance.* New York: Viking, 1967, p. 47.
2. George Washington University Institute of Law, Psychiatry and Criminology, "Report of Mental Competency," 1968.
3. American Bar Foundation, "The Mentally Disabled and the Law," The University of Chicago Press, p. 218.
4. *De Nardo* v. *De Nardo*, 293 N.Y. 550, 59 N.E. (2) 24 (1955).
5. 2 Williston on Contracts, ‡251 (3d. ed. 1959), 29 Temple L. Rev.—380, 383 (1956), "The Mentally Ill and the Law of Contracts."
6. In re *Buttonow* v. *O'Neill*, 297 N.Y.S. (2) 97, 23 N.Y. (2) 385.

26

THE ISSUES OF PRIVACY AND PRIVILEGED COMMUNICATION

Max Rosenbaum, Ph.D.

Throughout the history of psychotherapy a strange contradiction has existed. A basic tenet of the treatment contract between patient and psychotherapist is the need to safeguard the patient's self-esteem and dignity. This tenet is often overlooked by therapists in their eagerness to help individuals who come for treatment. We find in the literature pontifical statements concerning "unconditional regard" and yet patients are exposed to all kinds of scrutiny without their knowledge, the morality of which is to be highly questioned. It becomes even more bewildering when we read of the intuitive sensitivity of the many highly disturbed individuals, such as the group labeled schizophrenics, and their awareness of nonverbal messages. Yet consider the following: Harry Stack Sullivan, one of America's greatest exponents of the cultural approach to psychoanalysis, questioned treatment concepts as applied to schizophrenics. He pointed out the duplicities of the culture and the schizophrenic's observation of the artificiality of the hospital structure. Sullivan is described as utterly dedicated to his patients. He served at the Sheppard and Enoch Pratt Hospital as Director of Clinical Research in 1925. By 1929 his influence at the hospital was considerable. He established a ward that was only minimally involved with the rigid structure of the hospital. He ran this ward with a great deal of freedom and this ward became a testing ground for many of Sullivan's theories of interpersonal relations. The reader may ask, "What has this to do with privacy and confidentiality?" With all of Sullivan's concern for the male schizophrenics he was treating, as well as his ostensible concern for their human suffering, he introduced one other innovation.

At Sheppard, Sullivan installed a microphone on his desk, concealed by an ornamental device, so that his conversations with the patient could be recorded. At the time of the establishment of the special ward, this material was sound-tracked down to another floor where

315

recordings were made by Sullivan's secretary. Even before the establishment of the special ward, however, Sullivan had transcriptions made of conversations with patients and collected various kinds of documents from the patients ... (1).

The word, in case the reader missed it, is *concealed.* So the contradiction exists between what is professed and what is practiced. The videotape techniques discussed in this volume are not concealed techniques. Therefore the patient is intimately involved with what is going on. The position of this writer is that the patient *must* be aware at all times of the recording technique. If it is a source of concern, then it must be explored as part of the psychotherapeutic process.

Certain ground rules should be stressed. The American Psychiatric Association has published a detailed statement in the *American Journal of Psychiatry* (January 1968 issue) concerning patient confidentiality. The statement maintains that a ". . . Psychiatrist should never reveal, except with proper authorization or, if necessary, under proper legal compulsion (for example, a court order), confidential information disclosed to him in the treatment process by a patient." The patient must give written authorization to the psychiatrist for the release of information and must detail to whom the information is to be given. The psychiatrist is not bound to reveal the information since his duty is to protect the welfare of the patient. This writer notes that it is conceivable that the patient may give written consent without understanding the implications of such consent. His duress may be external or internal intrapsychic pressures, such as a neurotic or psychotic need to please imagined or real people. This point regarding written consent takes us into a no-man's land since the patient may give written consent to have recordings, movies, videotapes, or other methods of recording made of his therapy sessions without real awareness of what he has done. The shifting winds of law may later penalize a therapist who places too much faith in written release forms from a patient. Or he may not give written consent. Problems of exhibitionism enter here. The APA statement on confidentiality notes that there are occasions where information may be revealed without the consent of the patient in order to protect the welfare of the community. An illustration of this may occur when the patient may injure himself or others. In this situation it is wise to contact next-of-kin and obtain authorization. Here again the psychiatrist may have to use his own judgment. Therefore, written records should be kept confidential.

The death of a patient does not end the psychiatrist's obligation to maintain confidentiality. The American Psychiatric Association urges that psychiatric records should *not* be made available to non-medical personnel nor to non-psychiatrist physicians without the specific consent of the psychiatrist who examined and treated the patient. With slight deviations this position concerning confidentiality is similar to the position of the American Psychological Association. It is this author's experience that confidentiality is rarely mantained in public hospital settings. A variety of administrative personnel appear to obtain access to very personal material that patients have divulged under the illusion that the material is confidential. Actually, when a demand for confidential information is made by public courts or officials upon a psychiatrist or psychologist, it is recommended that legal counsel be obtained so that the professional is not vulnerable to a suit for damages. The patient may claim a breach of confidentiality. This writer questions where videotape should be categorized in the area of psychiatric records. The Board of Directors of the American Group Psychotherapy Association in a statement made January 26, 1968 took the following position:

The Board of Directors of the American Group Psychotherapy Association feels that the confidentiality of the patient-therapist relationship takes precedence over everything else. This rule will apply to any and all aspects of the Conference (annual conference of the AGPA), especially including videotape presentations where anything involving the confidentiality of the patient-therapist relationship may be involved. There is no reason why you (the press) can't take pictures of the equipment, no reason why you can't take pictures of the people using it, but you can't take pictures of the material involving patient and therapist.

The situation becomes quite obscure when we consider that training films are made for training of mental health personnel who are not involved in the issue of confidentiality since they as individuals have not been involved in a specific treatment relationship and are not bound to a therapy contract.

There has been increasing pressure on hospitals by television workers so that patients may be involved in broadcasts. One network was preparing a documentary on unemployables and requested the cooperation of a psychiatric hospital. In this case the concern was with the privacy of the patient as well as the patient's family (personal communication). Shostrom (2) strongly defends his position where he presents group therapy sessions on commercial television. This work is largely found on California television. Stoller (3) also supports this position. Prior to the formal publication of the position paper by the American Psychiatric Associa-

tion on privacy and confidentiality, without specific reference to videotape and television, the Southern California Psychiatric Society (4) expressed its concern about the responsibilities of the psychiatrist with
reference to videotapes as well as television viewing.

So far we have not noted the effects of recording upon the patient.
While many therapists feel that there is no effect, this author questions
the assumption. Is there no effect, or no effect that the patient feels free
to express? After all, once he has decided to enter treatment he may be
considered disruptive if he rejects being observed. It is an old truism in
teaching that the most cooperative students are the ones best liked by
educators. Does this apply to psychotherapy? Bales (5) found no differences in group behavior under different observation conditions. Bellak
and Smith (6) described the effects of recording and/or filming of psychotherapy on the patient and the therapist. They presented no definitive
opinion. Cohen and Cohen (7) found no definitive answers in their work
on research in psychotherapy. In 1960 Rosenbaum (8) pointed out the
various ramifications of research in psychotherapy. Among many points,
he noted that when researchers enter into the field of psychotherapy, they
disturb the subtle and yet tremendously important forces at work. Colby
(9) found significant increases in talk about male figures when a male
observer was present. He also found that the presence of an observer
served to raise the total activity of the image system (as measured by the
amount of talk about people).

It is interesting to speculate as to the patient's fantasies about the
television camera in the psychotherapy setting—both with the therapist
operating the equipment and with the trained technician present.
Does this validate Colby's finding? Gottschalk and Auerbach (10) touch
upon the methods of research in psychotherapy and while they do not
specifically cover privacy and confidentiality, the contributors to their
volume, Haggard, Hiken and Isaacs (11), in what may be the first detailed effort in the area of observations of filming and recording, analyzed
the first 40 hours of four cases and one set of eight supervisory sessions.
Three cases were recorded and filmed and the fourth was a "control"
case the data from which were obtained from the therapist's extensive
written notes. Their comments add little to the specific issue of privacy,
but they do note the impact of observations. Lamb and Mahl (12) in
their work contribute little to clarifying the problem of privacy and confidentiality where sound recordings are used. Shakow (13), Roose (14),
and Sternberg, Chapman and Shakow (15) have concerned themselves
with psychotherapy research and privacy. Again, their work appears to

contribute little. Recently the observations appear to have become more sophisticated. Soskin and John (16) used a wireless radio transmitter to collect data naturally. They used this technique as a data-collecting medium using two husband-wife pairs in a vacation setting initially unfamiliar to the subjects. They gained the impression that the subjects did accept and habituate to the continuous recording of their personal lives. Moos (17) studied psychiatric patients on a psychiatric inpatient ward. He used a wireless radio transmitter. He observed 16 patients and questioned whether patients would behave differently when they had the microphone on than when they did not. The evidence was based on patients observed during both group therapy and community meetings. The general effect of the microphone was to constrain the individual from moving about. The major exception to this is in group therapy where talking was considered the most important activity. Roberts and Renzaglia (18) studied the influence of tape recording on counseling. They found differences in clients' positive and negative self statements under three different observation conditions. It is important to note that in the latter study there were no differences in the quality of talk and the ratio of client-counselor talk under the three conditions. They studied eight counseling trainees each of whom discussed adjustment problems for at least three sessions with two different clients under each of the following conditions: tape recorder visible and running, microphone only, not recorded (but actually running). Purcell and Brady (19) described their work with a miniature radio transmitter as the patient's "adaptation to the invasion of privacy." Among all of the authors mentioned to this point, they are most honest in describing their work as an "invasion of privacy." Purcell and Brady used a transmitter to monitor the vocal behavior of 13 young adolescents in a cottage environment for one hour a day on 10 different days. They found that the adolescents appeared to behave naturally after two to four days of experience (at only one hour per day) with a microphone transmitter. Whether research conducted with adolescents may be applicable to adults or children is to be questioned.

Rosenbaum (20) has pointed out the impact of the social revolution in the treatment of adolescents. Certainly they are very conscious of privacy of treatment and what they view as the establishment's effort to manipulate them. Argyris (21) touches upon this in some comments about rigorous research. Students in courses are often resentful of the experiments they are asked to cooperate with. In many cases they expressed their pent-up feelings by "beating the researcher" in such a way that he never found out. This is an activity frequently observed among frustrated employees. Could this have relevance with regard to videotaping of patients in groups, especially with structured short-term groups where hostility to the therapist may rarely come to the surface?

The theoretic issues involved in videotaping are rarely faced. Does videotaping indicate that correct cognitive maps for the patient are generated as well as the proper psychological set? Is the psychological set impaired by the patient's perception that privacy is tampered with? Videotaping is two-dimensional and may ignore or overlook much that is significant in the emphasis on feedback. Von Neumann (22) pointed out the essential difference between the computer and the brain. His thesis is that a crucial difference between the computer and the brain is the brain's capacity to be accurate with a lot of noise going on in its circuits. The brain can operate relatively accurately with a calculus that, for the computer, is relatively sloppy. Human problem solving is in a realm of overlapping, redundant concepts. Does the videotape capture the redundancy? How does the invasion of privacy tamper with human problem solving? Or does it?

There are many contradictions and confusions evident in the use of videotape. Stoller (23) has developed the concept of "focused feedback" (see Chapter 18, this volume) in the use of videotape in group therapy. He warned that if used indiscriminately and without some control by the therapist, videotape feedback can overwhelm the group. Yet there seems to be a surprising lack of concern about how public television viewing of group therapy may overwhelm the audience—much less the patients in the group. Shostrom (2) defends his position on presenting group psychotherapy sessions over commercial television with the statement, "I am humanistically oriented and believe that television viewers will not grossly misuse therapeutic data and are potentially able to constructively use what they see and hear. . . ." However, Danet (24, 25) has made a beginning effort to study experimentally the audiovisual feedback in group therapy. He videotaped two outpatient student psychotherapy groups under identical conditions, with only one receiving playback. The majority of data strongly suggested the hypothesis that the playback served to disrupt the experimental group's functioning when compared with the control group which received none. Incidental to this, the group members were unanimous in their favorable reaction to participating in both groups. This chapter will not concern itself with the central issue of confrontation as a therapeutic technique since this is also debatable if it reinforces resistance mechanisms. (See Chapter 2.)

Videotaping is essentially concerned with learning concepts. What we face here is the transfer of learning. The patient who is videotaped is confronted with a cognitive experience that will hopefully reach the emotional or conative area. The integration of these hoped-for learning experiences by the patient apparently justifies the use of videotaping. Certainly there is an invasion of privacy. The therapist has every right to justify this invasion if he believes that it will be beneficial to the patient. But the patient believes in a set of cultural norms which for the most part values the concept of privacy and confidentiality. The therapist, encouraging the patient to cooperate in videotaping, offers the reward of "cure" or, at a minimum, some emotional relief in exchange for the patient adopting the therapist's value system with reference to privacy. At this point he must have significant regard for the therapist and assurance that he will not be hurt by the therapist's technique. If the therapist has complete control over the videotape it would appear that he can offer the patient assurance. If the therapist is in turn surrounded by a setting, e.g., hospital, clinic, which restrains him, he must share with the patient the restrictions on privacy and confidentiality, otherwise he takes liberties with his patient. Some therapists at this time question whether the culture supports the "old norm" of privacy. This is an empirical question which systematic research should answer but, in this writer's opinion, answers will elude us in the near future. Psychotherapists who use videotape are in the avant-garde. They may not sense the conservative patterns of the U.S.A., especially if they practice in larger urban settings. Over the past five years there have been many protests lodged against psychological testing as an invasion of privacy. These protests have even reached the halls of Congress. The signs are clear. The 1965 Congressional inquiry into psychological testing revealed a nation-wide reaction to the accumulation of dossiers of computerized test results from the scores of many thousands of Americans. Videotaping could easily be caught up in the same kind of national inquiry. All of these conditions must be carefully assessed as we consider privacy and confidentiality and the impact upon each specific patient.

All of this has been an effort to present a sober appraisal of the complex issues involved in videotaping. It is an exciting technique which offers great promise for psychotherapy. It must be used with discretion and care. None of the cautions should deter the reader from an engagement with a new approach to psychotherapy. The other chapters in this volume present an informed and enthusiastic approach. The ethical issue must be determined by each therapist who uses the technique. He owes this to himself as well as to each patient who is videotaped.

AN OVERVIEW

Freud wrote almost nothing on privacy and psychoanalysis. He as well as his early students assumed that the medical patient's communications were held in confidence and the same situation should apply to the patient in psychoanalysis. Early pioneers generally ignored the area. Representatives of the "cultural approach" to psychoanalysis touched upon the area of confidentiality insofar as this related to sharing information with a referring physician or members of a patient's family. Lawrence Kubie (26) was very specific in his point of view. He stated: "Of all physicians, the psychoanalyst has the least right to talk about his patients, even to his colleagues, without protecting meticulously the identities of these patients. A good analyst is close-mouthed."

Haggard, Hiken and Isaacs (11) stated: "When the therapy is conducted under conditions in which several persons have access to the private (and hence privileged) disclosures or other communications of the patient, it is essential that all such persons adhere strictly to the rule of confidentiality regarding whatever transpires within the therapy."

Voice recordings, used for some years in psychotherapy treatment as well as research, up to this point have not aroused as much concern as filming or videotaping of psychotherapy. This is primarily because sound recording can be masked, deleted, etc. However, the recording of sound and image exposes the patient rather completely.

What safeguards may the responsible person take when using videotape in psychotherapy? The American Medical Association Law Department has developed sample forms and made recommendations about procedures which make certain that: "A patient has the same right of privacy as any other individual has" (27). Further guidelines have been developed by the World Medical Association (28) because of the concentration camp "medical experiments" during the Second World War. In 1964 the Declaration of Helsinki was established and this applies to workers in medical research and human experimentation. This Declaration calls upon "scientifically qualified" persons to "remain the protector of the life and health" of the patient or experimental subject. Therefore, the responsible professional person who is in charge of videotaping, as well as all technicians, editors, projectionists and transcribing secretaries, must be fully aware of the confidential nature of the videotape. There should be a constant emphasis on the need to safeguard the integrity of the patient.

REFERENCES

1. Sullivan, H. S.: *Schizophrenia as a Human Process,* with Introduction and Commentaries by Helen Swick Perry. New York: W. W. Norton & Co., Inc., 1962, p. 21.
2. Shostrom, E. L.: Replies to Danet, Lubin and Hurvitz. *American Psychologist,* 23:760-761, 1968.
3. Stoller, F. H.: Group Psychotherapy on Television: An Innovation with Hospitalized Patients. *American Psychologist,* 22:158-162, 1967.
4. Southern California Psychiatric Society: The Responsibilities of the Psychiatrist. *Southern California Psychiatric Society News,* 14:1-3, 1967.
5. Bales, R. F.: *Interaction Process Analysis.* Cambridge: Addison-Wesley, 1950.
6. Bellak, L., and Smith, M. B.: An Experimental Exploration of the Psychoanalytic Process: Exemplification of a Method. *Psychoanalytic Quarterly,* 25:385-414, 1956.
7. Cohen, R. A., and Cohen, M. D.: Research in Psychotherapy: A Preliminary Report. *Psychiatry,* 24:46-61, 1961.
8. Rosenbaum, M.: Obstacles to Research in Psychotherapy. *Psychoanalysis and Psychoanalytic Review,* 47:97-105, 1960.
9. Colby, K. M.: Experiment on the Effects of an Observer's Presence on the Imago System During Psychoanalytic Free-Association. *Behavioral Science,* 5:216-232, 1960.
10. Gottschalk, L. A., and Auerbach, A. H.: *Methods of Research in Psychotherapy.* New York: Appleton-Century-Crofts, 1966.
11. Haggard, E. A., Hiken, J. R., and Isaacs, K. S.: Some Effects of Recording and Filming on the Psychotherapeutic Process. *Psychiatry,* 28:169-191, 1965.
12. Lamb, R., and Mahl, G. F.: Manifest Reactions of Patients and Interviewers to the Use of Sound Recording in the Psychiatric Interview. *American Journal of Psychiatry,* 112:731-737, 1956.
13. Shakow, D.: The Recorded Psychoanalytic Interview as an Objective Approach to Research in Psychoanalysis. *Psychoanalytic Quarterly,* 29:82-97, 1960.
14. Roose, L. J.: The Influence of Psychosomatic Research on the Psychoanalytic Process. *American Psychoanalytic Assoc. Journal,* 8:317-334, 1960.
15. Sternberg, R. S., Chapman, J., and Shakow, D.: Psychotherapy Research and the Problems of Intrusions on Privacy. *Psychiatry,* 21:195-203, 1958.
16. Soskin, W. F., and John, V. P.: The Study of Spontaneous Talk. In R. G. Barker (Ed.), *The Stream of Behavior.* New York: Appleton-Century-Crofts, 1963.
17. Moos, R. H.: Behavioral Effects of Being Observed: Reactions to a Wireless Radio Transmitter. *Journal of Consulting and Clinical Psychology,* 32:383-388, 1968.
18. Roberts, R., and Renzaglia, G.: The Influence of Tape Recording on Counseling. *Journal of Counseling Psychology,* 12:10-16, 1965.
19. Purcell, K., and Brady, K.: Adaptation to the Invasion of Privacy: Monitoring Behavior with a Miniature Radio Transmitter. *Merrill-Palmer Quarterly,* 12:242-254, 1966.
20. Rosenbaum, M.: Group Psychotherapy with Adolescents. In B. Wolman (Ed.), *Manual of Child Psychopathology.* New York: McGraw-Hill, 1972.
21. Argyris, C.: Some Unintended Consequences of Rigorous Research. *Psychological Bulletin,* 70 (3):185-197, 1968.
22. Von Neumann, J.: *The Computer and the Brain.* New Haven: Yale University Press, 1958.
23. Stoller, F. H.: Focused Feedback with Videotape: Extending the Group's Function. In G. M. Gazda (Ed.), *Basic Innovations in Group Therapy and Counseling.* Springfield, Ill.: Charles C Thomas, 1967.
24. Danet, B. K.: Self-Confrontation by Videotape in Group Psychotherapy. Unpublished dissertation, University of Minnesota, 1967.

25. Danet, B. K.: Self-Confrontation in Psychotherapy Reviewed: Videotape Playback as a Clinical and Research Tool. *American Journal of Psychotherapy*, 22:245-257, 1968.
26. Kubie, L. S.: *Practical and Theoretical Aspects of Psychoanalysis.* New York: International Universities Press, 1950, p. 102.
27. American Medical Association Law Department, 1961. *Medico-legal Forms with Legal Analysis.* American Medical Association, Chicago.
28. Human Experimentation: Code of Ethics of World Medical Association. *British Medical Journal*, 18 July, 1964.

ADDENDUM

Since the original writing of my chapter for the first edition of this book, the legal and social climate concerning confidentiality, has become quite troubled. It is important that the clinician who uses videotape techniques be thoroughly conversant with the legalisms surrounding confidentiality. The recent *Tarasoff* (1, 2) decision, upheld by the California Supreme Court, clearly states that psychotherapists in the state of California *must* warn the authorities or the intended victim if a serious criminal threat is made during the course of psychotherapy. Psychotherapists have expressed astonishment at this judicial decision but it is a clear and unambiguous statement.

At this writing, it is speculative as to how many states will follow the lead of the state of California. Yet almost a decade ago, there was an article in the professional literature warning of the possibility of a "future-crime" exception to client-attorney privilege and noting that it would probably be extended to patient-psychotherapist privilege. There is the very real possibility that confidentiality will not exist, at least the way the patient may understand privileged communication.

The situation becomes even more confusing as we consider privileged communication in group psychotherapy. At this point, members of the group are third parties, not part of the hoped for patient-psychotherapist privileged communication. In other ways of stating the problem, the patient has waived privileged communication by permitting a fellow group member to hear the confidence which would on other occasions be expressed in individual psychotherapy. There is the very real possibility that unless privileged communication is extended to the group, a patient will refuse to participate in group therapy. The situation will become especially critical when patients inquire as to how a videotape will be used—by whom and for what purpose.

It is not inconceivable that unscrupulous individuals will attempt to incorporate videotape material into data bank material. In essence, there is definite need for the psychotherapist to stipulate the need for as well as benefit of videotape. More important, the patient should be clear as to how the videotape material is to be used and who will retain ultimate ownership/control of the tapes. Unless this is done, the psychotherapist may become the target of legal action and this may also involve other patients, if the videotape is that of a group.

REFERENCES

1. *Tarasoff* v. *Regents of the University of California,* 13 Cal. 2d 177, 529 P.2d 553, 118 Cal. Rptr. 129 (1974).
2. Shah, S.: Privileged Communications, Confidentiality, and Privacy. *Professional Psychology,* 1:56-69, 1969.

SECTION V
Technical and Artistic Considerations

EDITOR'S INTRODUCTION

In Chapter 27 of this section, Wilmer, who is one of our most creative and imaginative workers, has touched upon the artistic as well as the technical aspects of videotape in psychiatric teaching. The artistic and creative potential of video is being continuously expanded. In its fall 1969 issue, *Art in America* published an exciting article entitled "TV— The Next Medium" and quoted Andy Warhol as saying, "It's the new everything." Whereas our interest as psychiatrists lies in exposing distortions of reality, Warhol's interest is paradoxically in the creative process available with the range of color and image distortion possibilities in the videotape medium.

I am intrigued with the fact that my interest in multiple image immediate impact self-confrontations with exposure of the patient to himself simultaneously on four monitors with two different views from two different cameras* is paralleled by the interest of sculptors like Les Levine whose "Contact: A Cybernetic Sculpture" was completed in 1969 for the lobby of the New Gulf and Western headquarters building in New York City. The eight-foot high television sculpture has identical "seeing" sides facing in two directions, each side having nine monitors and four TV cameras equipped with different lenses and set at different angles. The screens of each monitor are covered by different colored acrylic sheets. As the spectator stands before Contact, he sees images of himself in close-up, mid-range and long-range focus and material programmed through a slide scanner; the images jump from monitor to monitor in random sequence. The sculpture is encased in stainless steel with reflective plastic bubbles covering each "seeing" side. "Contact is a system that synthesizes man with his technology," says Levine. "In this system the people are the 'software.'"

Just as a program titled "The Medium Is the Medium" which was broadcast nationally in March, 1969, symbolized the erasure of all lines

---

* A colleague who came to my office for a workshop became acutely anxious at felt this way before." A six-year-old girl joyfully exclaimed, "Look, Mommy. there are so many of me!"

between painting, sculpture, the performing arts and technology,* so will the use of video reduce those barriers which have kept in a mystical fashion the psychiatrist and his way of functioning aloof from the public-at-large. This should reduce the aura of mystique which surrounds the psychiatrist and his work.

Scheflen, one of the foremost researchers of communicated behaviors which serve to establish, maintain and regulate human relationships, has classified** those factors which influence the choice of audiovisual media. He and Brosin, Birdwhistell, Condon, Loeb, Freedman and Cherney, amongst others,‡ have for some time been recording in detail the multiple behaviors which in natural context are involved in interpersonal influencing. These workers are stimulating the invention of technological instruments to measure the units, process and systems involved whether they be vocal, visual or behavioral. He emphasizes that although the availability of compatible equipment in many institutions makes motion picture film more usable for the study of the structural units of the stream of communicational behavior,† the video recording is less expensive and easier to make and has far greater flexibility for the general uses of the clinician in treatment and training. The capacity of the video recorder for instant playback and review, as well as the possibility of recording multiple camera images on single tape and the potential of the video camera for closed circuit television, makes it more than a formidable competitor to motion pictures. However we do not have to think of an either/or approach, but rather to review which technological resource will best suit our needs for research, training and/or treatment in our particular setting. Their value as data collection devices is increased if both types of equipment are combined and video data transferred to film or vice versa.

The chapter by Corbitt covers the what and how of the basic equipment required in various settings for using video for training, treatment and the preparation of audiovisual materials for presentation to professional audiences.

In the following chapter, I have tried to cover some of the rudiments

---

* Margolies, J. S.: TV—The Next Medium. *Art in America,* 57:48-55, 1969.

** Scheflen, A. E.: On the Choices of Audiovisual Media. In *Videotape Techniques in Psychiatric Training and Treatment,* First Edition.

‡ See "The Sound Camera—Breakthrough in Research, Training, Therapy" in the *Roche Report, Frontiers of Hospital Psychiatry,* Vol. 6, No. 11, June 1, 1969.

† Scheflen, A. E., Stream and Structure of Behavior (1965). *Behavioral Studies Monograph No. 1,* Eastern Pennsylvania Psychiatric Institute, Philadelphia, Pennsylvania.

involved in appraisal of videotapes. You have to have a capacity for toughness, specific objectives and a clear sense of whom you are making your tape for if you are going to be able to adequately critique your own production. I have prepared a series of questions for your own rough appraisal and also included a copy of the film certification appraisal form utilized by the Department of Audiovisual Communication of the British Medical Association. The film appraisal can be modified for use with videotapes.

27
TELEVISION: TECHNICAL AND ARTISTIC ASPECTS OF VIDEOTAPE IN PSYCHIATRIC TEACHING

Harry A. Wilmer, M.D., Ph.D.

The psychiatric literature about television is practically devoid of illustrations of what television productions look like. Moreover, the techniques of videotaping are rarely described, so that it is usually impossible to know who or what appeared on the screen, or whether it was a planned program of camera work or a random, improvised account. This author has advocated the open, undisguised camera in psychiatric videotape teaching (1), describing practical and theoretical aspects,* its use for studying phenomena in group psychotherapy (2) and individual psychotherapy (3). This paper is on the practical and theoretical aspects of camera angles, sequential programmed techniques and the technical and artistic qualities of the production. It provides a graphic illustration of exactly what is shown on the monitor.

RECORDING EQUIPMENT

The availability of high-quality portable videotape equipment offers unique practical opportunities for television teaching, supervision, research and treatment. Elaborate studio television facilities provide the challenge of creating psychiatric videotapes of unusual technical and artistic quality.

The Office of Television Research of the University of California has broadcast-quality studio equipment and trained personnel for sophisticated videotaping. In addition, there is portable videotape equipment for recording and replay anywhere in or away from the University.

Reprinted from *The Journal of Nervous and Mental Disease*, 144:207-223, 1967. Copyright © 1967 by The Williams & Wilkins Co. This research was supported by the General Research Support Grant, National Institute of Mental Health.

* Unpublished manuscript.

Television cameras at the San Francisco General Hospital can broadcast on an ultrahigh frequency channel to the medical school for videotaping and teaching.

Television videotaping has unique advantages over one-way mirror observation, audiotapes and closed-circuit television in that the participants can see themselves in the immediate replay. This graphic record can be repeatedly examined to study in depth the complexity of human behavioral relationships. The advantages of videotape over the motion picture film are that it is less expensive, does not require time delay for developing, and permits several cameras to be used simultaneously. Portions of videotapes can be recorded ("dubbed") on other tapes and saved for later use, so that the original tapes can be reused. Kinescopic 16mm sound films can be made from the videotapes for ordinary motion picture projectors.*

INTERVIEW VIDEOTAPE TECHNIQUES

With the portable videotape equipment in a small television studio it is possible to get a variety of camera angles and zoom angle shots with undisguised cameras and cameramen in view. The teacher either operates the videotape monitor or the camera, in order to experiment with sequential patterns of videotaping and camera angles. The camera work thereby becomes a graphic and dramatic commentary on the supervision of the interview. It is possible to teach camera technicians the psychological subtleties of such recording. The psychiatrist can also learn from cameramen and directors the intricacies of their craft.

In supervising residents, the following television technique is used: A videotape is made of 10 to 15 minutes of a psychiatric interview between a resident and a patient. Immediately after the interview, the resident and patient are shown the replay of the videotape on a monitor in the television studio. The resident holds a manual remote control box, which permits him to stop the videotape on a single picture for discussion and start it again. He can signal to have the tape replayed. On the premise that the patient often has much to contribute to the understanding of what happened, the resident is encouraged to use the replay time of 45 minutes for mutual exploration of the clinical transaction with the patient. At a later time, the tape is again replayed before the resident and his teacher, after which the videotape is erased for reuse. Any portion

---

* Three kinescopic films, each 30 minutes in length, have been completed and edited. These are the first in a series on community psychiatry to be entitled, "The Offender." San Quentin Prisoners participated in one film; San Francisco Policemen in the second, and parole agents in the third.

that would serve as unusually good teaching information is dubbed onto a second tape and saved.

Because of the vast amount of information on videotape, only short vignettes are recorded. Often five to 10 minutes are adequate for detailed analysis with the patient and, subsequently, with the teacher. Videotapes of more than 20 minutes tend to be overwhelming for routine teaching and are used only for research purposes. Clinical experience with this technique has shown that the patient and the student are eager participants; it seems that the immediate replay is the key to their motivation. Patients are generally not disturbed by the open camera unless it is moved close to them. For the most part they become quickly absorbed in the interview and disregard the machinery. There is some distortion of the interview by the very nature of the mechanical process of videotaping, but this is in the direction of bringing into focus certain personality characteristics relative to exhibitionism, voyeurism and counterphobic reactions. What is particularly anxiety-provoking is that a record is being made over which the resident has no control. The interview is not subject to his corrections, retrospective memory, or conscious or unconscious distortions during supervision.

The videotape is a live documentary sound motion picture, which demands skills in direction and camera work to enhance the artistic, dramatic impact, the visual cue discrimination, and memory recall. From previous experience with extensive motion pictures made of a therapeutic community (4) and from the experience with writers, directors, and cameramen in making a commercial television dramatic documentary of that same therapeutic community* a program of camera direction has evolved.

Videotaping interviews in our television research studios allows us to use two or three cameras, six technicians and a director, all experienced over many years with television work. There is great flexibility of camera experimentation in the studio. The purpose is to produce interesting, artistic productions with the camera guiding the viewer through the evolving natural drama of the psychiatric interview.

A PROGRAM FOR VIDEOTAPING INTERVIEWS

The skills demanded of the director for coordinating a videotape production in the studio with two or three cameras can be grasped from a diagram of the people and machines involved (Figure 1). Decisions must be made quickly, with an intuitive sense of artistry. The team should resemble the surgical theater with its quiet, quickly responsive, mutual

---

* Further information can be obtained directly from the author.

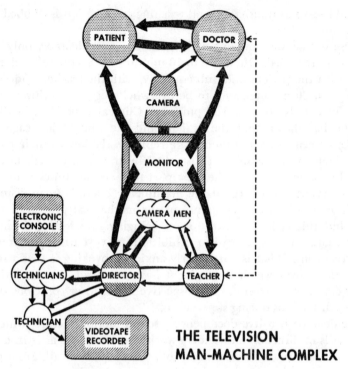

THE TELEVISION
MAN-MACHINE COMPLEX

Fig. 1. The television man-machine complex.

intent on the serious work at hand. Yet there are moments of relief, for not only are we viewing the human tragedy but also the human comedy.

A standard plan of sequential camera angles has been programmed to orient the viewer:

1) A wide-angle shot shows the entire bodies of both participants and the room furnishings. Residents are asked what furnishings they prefer (a desk or table or just two chairs) and how they wish them arranged. After this opening shot, the camera lens zooms in "tightening" on the upper portions of the individuals.

2) A second camera focuses on the full face of the patient, the primary object of interest.

3) A picture of the full face of the residents follows. These last two pictures show how each subject looks to the other.

4) There is now one camera behind each individual. Although they are not necessarily close, by zoom lens they can bring the subjects as close as the director wishes. For a variable period of time, depending on the

nature of the evolving transaction, these two camera shots alternate, first from the perspective of the doctor, and second, from that of the patient —the patient again being first established as the primary object. The camera is now telling the story from the point of view of each participant.

When two cameras are being used the participants are not aware of which camera is recording or what special effects are being used.

The cameraman shooting over the shoulders of the individuals is directed to include in these pictures a portion of the head of the person from whose perspective he is photographing. The purpose of this is to photographically reinforce the impression of a relationship, to portray the image of seeing oneself as another sees one. When one sees oneself all alone on the screen all the time, the narcissistic investment vitiates the purpose of videotaping, namely to see ourselves as others see us. The solitary face on the screen is a familiar image to the viewer, one that he knows from any mirror, but the inclusion of the part of the other "mirror" person is a totally new psychological experience.

5) A split-screen effect with the two faces side by side is recorded. To convey the image of one person as the primary object, being seen by the other, we first use a full face of the patient, and a side view of the doctor looking at the patient. Then this is reversed. The impression is of one person looking at another who is looking at the viewer. If split-screen effects are used with two full-face pictures looking at the camera, the viewer is confronted with a decision as to which of the two faces looking directly at him he will look back at.

6) Various zoom lens closeups are made, depending on what the teacher wishes to emphasize (the hands, the feet, or any portion of the body or face, particularly the eyes).

Closeup pictures of the eyes of each person are followed by a horizontal split-screen effect with the patient's eyes above, and the doctor's eyes below.

When individuals move their heads, the camera moves slightly to keep their eyes in the picture as much as possible. Hence we see head movement as well as eye movement. Eyes are the most expressive portion of the face, as all artists, photographers and lovers know, and their reciprocal interactional relationship is dramatized in this split-screen picture. This gives us a striking picture of eye contact, eye movements, and, more than that, it shows the variations in pupil size which reflect attitude and emotion (5, 6, 7). Eye movement and pupillary dilation and constriction also are clues to the transference relationship. By studying videotapes frame by frame, it is possible to measure pupillary changes.

7) The final picture is of the two persons again. Gradually the camera "dollies" back so that, at the end of the videotaping, the entire bodies of both participants are shown exactly as they were at the beginning of the interview.

While this sequential pattern of camera angles forms the basic program of the camera work, it is interspersed with closeup shots of significant movements, and occasionally a "two shot" of both participants in full view to remind the viewer of the total relationship. The program is a guideline around which the director can build the dramatic documentary.

The "stare" of the paranoid schizophrenic patient, which may be the most significant facial clue for the clinician's intuitive diagnostic impression, can be clearly demonstrated. The fixed stare is revealed as holding steadily with quick side excursions, periodic reconnaissance of the environment, returning to keep an eye on the therapist. It is as if he must be certain of the therapist's unwavering attention and presence and constantly alert to any possible changes in the periphery. Because the peripheral environment is not shown, and because of the dramatic light and dark contrast of the pupil and sclera, eye movements are conspicuous. To illustrate this, there was one patient who, when questioned about her heart, showed a quick wide nystagmus which was noted only on the videotape replay. On further questioning it was found that she was often preoccupied by obsessive fears of a heart attack. Patients commonly "roll their eyes up and back" when they are thinking back on their life or searching their memories; others reveal characteristic eye movement patterns when discussing the same issues, e.g., Quentin convicted as a thief had repeated quick wide eye excursions up and to the side. Perhaps he was always "on the look-out." This striking repetitive behavior was not noted until the videotape was reviewed. The eye movements of the therapist are of equal importance. Some therapists telegraph their intention of speaking by characteristic premonitory eye movements, which sensitive patients probably detect subliminally. Some interviewers have roving eyes, some mostly downcast, others more or less fixed, with patterns of quick side or upward glances. It usually is possible to relate eye movements to the momentary elements of the interview.

One of the characteristics of a good interviewer seems to be a constant slow weaving eye movement as he continually scans the patient. Awareness of what the eyes say is usually a part of preconscious thinking. It is instructive to bring this to consciousness, and it is fascinating and useful to speculate on its unconscious significance.

Psychoanalysts may spend years analyzing a patient without ever seeing his eyes during the analytic hours. It is a curious matter to speculate upon the fact that Freud, who could not bear to look at his patients or be looked at for long periods, discovered the Oedipus Complex, and that Oedipus, upon the discovery of his crime, blinded himself. Perhaps psychoanalytic insights will broaden to include eyesights with the newer ego psychology of psychoanalysis.

When a 50-minute interview is videotaped, effective teaching use can be made by selecting short segments (five minutes or less) for detailed study by a small class. For example, the first five minutes may be examined to make predictive inferences as to the subsequent material. Subsequent five-minute random segments might then be replayed for evaluation and further predictions. An alternate method is to stop the playback after significant statements, selected in advance, to teach the timing and formulation of interpretations, predictions and alternate hypothetical inferences. Long tapes are stopped three to five minutes before the end for discussion of "the closure phenomena" and to make predictions about how the session will end. The same techniques apply in studying videotapes of entire group psychotherapy sessions.

VIDEOTAPING GROUPS

Videotapes of group psychotherapy and small group seminars can be effective in teaching group dynamics. The videotape of a group is replayed to the group immediately after the session, just as the interview is, and for the same reasons.

Videotaping of groups has not been widely used, and some have found it confusing. Whether or not it facilitates understanding, observation, and decision-making depends entirely upon having clear purposes and suitable methods of videotaping. Videotaped group sessions for 45-60 minutes are too long for ordinary teaching. Videotaping the group's first 10 minutes is adequate, and 20 minutes seems to be the maximum, if the tape is going to be replayed and understood by members.

Videotaping groups cannot recreate the total group process and atmosphere because of the large numbers of people, the small size of the television screen, and the low definition of the picture. The view from the lens cannot encompass the entire circle at any one time, to see the faces of all participants. If one accepts the principle that videotape is useful for highlighting selected elements of the group process, it can be an invaluable tool. The use of the split-screen with half of the group on the upper and half on the lower portion of the screen allows one to watch all the participants at one time, but the reduction obscures details and the splitting undermines the feeling of circular encompassment.

One may videotape a small portion with one camera, moving about and showing the faces of a part of the group, and still keep the entire group on camera. With multiple cameras one may focus on the speaker with one camera and keep another on reacting members, showing alternating closeup shots of portions of the group. It is possible to superimpose shots of one member of the group over a portion of the rest of the group so that one can see his full face and still note a number of the other group members. This technique graphically reproduces one of the cognitive perceptual mechanisms of the therapist—seeing and hearing one person clearly and simultaneously attentive to the others. We have videotaped groups of as many as 30 members in a large room at San Quentin Prison with quite satisfactory results for viewing. The perception of a human participant observer resembles camera work. The camera follows the teacher's direction and therefore illustrates how the group was seen through his eyes. Once a week for one year, a small group psychotherapy session of psychiatric outpatients led by the teacher was videotaped. The therapy sessions were observed live on closed-circuit television by a group of six psychiatric residents. After the group therapy session was over, the residents came into the studio for a post-group critique with the therapist. This discussion was videotaped. Residents reviewed their discussion videotape before watching the next group session.

This is a technique of metagroup psychology. The residents focused their learning experience, on their group-about-a-group, referring to the original group therapy videotape for a clarification of any point in question. To avoid the pitfall of residents waiting at the start for the therapist "to explain it all" or the temptation of the therapist to dominate the beginning and set themes, one resident was asked to begin the discussion by briefly recounting his observations and opinions. So that each resident was prepared to summarize the group session at the beginning of the videotape, the residents were given numbers, and the cameraman drew a number just before the videotaping began. Edited portions of these sequential videotapes of group psychotherapy and post-group discussions were used for instruction in group dynamic seminars of the following year.

For instance, the difference between the "convex" and the "concave" therapist, as David Shakow observed in a personal communication, was demonstrated. The group therapist who sits in a hunched-over position (concave) generally assumes a more passive role, is more quiet and hesitant in his formulations, it was observed. The "convex" therapist is more outgoing and aggressive and his formulations apt to be more crisp and verbose than the therapist bending the other way. The "upright" therapist assumes a more moderate clinical position between the "convex" and the "concave" therapists.

A METHOD OF SENSITIVITY GROUP TEACHING

A group of six members meets with a leader three hours one afternoon a week for ten weeks. In the first session they screen a videotape, from the library of tapes, of a psychotherapy session. It is interrupted and discussed, portions replayed, and single frames studied. The next five sessions begin with videotaping an unstructured discussion of ten minutes followed by immediate replay for analysis by the group and the leader. This critique, lasting 50 minutes, is also videotaped.

The group sits in a "U" shape, and is first established on one camera. One by one, each participant is then shown in a full-face portrait by a second camera. The entire group picture of the first camera is shown between each succeeding member. The pictures slowly fade in and out. Cameras and cameramen move quietly around the group.

Next one camera follows the speakers, and the other camera is free to show all or part of the group or to focus on one reacting group member, as the director chooses. Closeup shots of any unusual movement are also made. Finally the camera ends on the entire group, a picture which was interspersed during the entire videotaping.

Directors become so sensitive to the nonverbal gestures by which individuals reveal their intention to speak that the closeup camera often has a person on the screen just before or at the moment he speaks. The dramatic impact of the final production often conveys the group drama almost as if the director had a prepared script.

During the replay discussion a monitor is placed in the open end of the group. On another monitor, in the control room, the videotape is replayed before another camera. By use of a split-screen the original group videotape is inserted into the lower right-hand quadrant of the videotape. The second videotape picture shows a group within a group. Because of the small dimensions of the insert, closeup pictures are seen more clearly. We may see a portion of the group watching the insert or one person watching himself.

As the group watches the original videotape playback, the studio microphones are turned off, so that the sound quality of the new videotape is the same as the original tape. Any member of the reviewing group can signal the director to stop the replay by raising his hand. He may request to see portions of it played again or held on a single frame for discussion. The eye movements of the individuals watching the replay generally show intense interest in all members. Some members seem to watch others more intently than themselves, often closing their eyes or looking away from the screen when their own image is on it.

During discussion of replay, the studio microphones are switched on and the still picture at the point they are discussing is held in the corner of the new recorded picture. The group leader paces the replay discussion so that the entire 10-minute first group is completed within 50 minutes. After that the group remains in the studio for an uninterrupted replay of the 50-minute videotape. With the necessary delays, this technique requires three hours for each training session.

The final videotape effect is of the participants viewing themselves as they watch their first videotape. From a theoretical and practical point of view, this is a fascinating phenomenon. Its emotional impact stems from the novel effect on the group members who see themselves acting, then reacting, and finally reacting to the reacting. Thus they experience three levels of self and group participation: 1) original group; 2) group discussion as they watch the original group; and 3) re-experience of both groups by viewing the final tape.

After these six sessions, the next four sessions are spent in reviewing, in sequence, the videotapes of the groups. Group members are usually amazed at how vividly they re-experience the group feeling; their memories of the groups having blurred, they are often astonished at what they see and hear.

The group interaction of the final replays is the fourth exposure of the group to themselves in action and has powerful teaching impact, for they now have some distance and are not concerned with any more videotaping. The videotape is reinforcing, clarifying, and correcting impressions and distortions by solid information feedback to the viewers. This self-study in depth is a form of sensitivity supervision, or more correctly, *sensitivity-revision*. It can be used in modified form for interviews or small group seminars. It has the unique effect of holding life still, so that one may look closely at segments of a human drama again and again.

FEEDING LIGHT SIGNALS INTO VIDEOTAPE

It is desirable to have videotape methods for recording the unspoken thoughts of the psychiatrist. While these are ordinarily reconstructed in retrospect, there are always the problems of distortion by unconscious and conscious resistance.

Instant cues of the therapist's thinking can be recorded on the video-tape by the use of light signals or handwritten notes. A light signal system was built, which would allow the interviewer to pull one or two levers activating light signals mounted on a large board behind the patient. Then the videotape may be made either showing the total scene or use of split-screen effect placing the two figures side by side. The light board may be set in another room before a camera and the light signals superimposed on the picture of the participants.

The control box with levers is beside the doctor and below the desk top. The lever is connected with a rheostat. The further down the lever is pulled, the brighter the light becomes, until at maximum position it triggers a switch which causes the light to blink. The light is covered with red plastic to prevent glaring on the camera.

We have used light signals to indicate the time, intensity, and duration of a doctor's "inner dialogue." In general only one lever is used, because of the difficulty of mastering the technique.

SILENCE, BEHAVIOR AND INNER DIALOGUE

Thinking is symbolized in external speech, but a form of preparatory internal speech precedes it. Such internal speech is defined here as the preverbal, internalized precursor of vocal speech. It often takes the form of a fantasied, incredibly quick and condensed "conversation." As a guide to what, when and how to speak, it takes place as the therapist is listening for cues as to whether to correct, rephrase or reject his contemplated speech. Interviewers reveal various patterns of meditative silence and contemplative inner dialogue.

The light signal gives a gross demonstration of how an individual uses his silence in relation to speech. When the patient sees the videotape replay, the silence of the psychiatrist begins to take on new meanings. The patient and doctor learn more about listening to one another, and that silent listening involves highly active mental work.

The second light may be used to signal cues of patient behavior such as significant metaphors (phrases such as "you know" [1]), halting or blocked speech, unusually strong affect, transference, counter-transference, fantasy, intellectualizations and symbolic gestures. For purposes of simplicity only one behavior clue is used per session.

FEEDING WRITTEN MESSAGES INTO THE VIDEOTAPE

Note-taking is distracting, dividing attention between the "here and now" and the "record." Each time the patient sees the doctor write he is aware that something noteworthy has been observed. But what? And for whom? Can the doctor write and listen simultaneously? Yet, in learning interview techniques, it is sometimes useful to take brief notes as an aid to memory.

Once a resident has mastered the basic elements of interviewing, he should give up taking notes except under unusual or special circumstances. One way of emancipation from note-taking is the use of transitional videotape supervision in which abbreviated notes are "taken."

In one videotape method, the interviewer writes with a white charcoal pencil on a large pad of black paper held on his lap. A camera behind and at the side of the interviewer focuses on the notes. This picture is superimposed on the portrait of the interview made by one or two other cameras. The interviewer's writing appears instantaneously across the screen. Watching this live, one is struck with the incredible slowness of writing notes (in contrast to the speed of thought) as well as the patient's behavior which the note-taking doctor does not see. The difficulty of performing two complex skills at the same time is obvious: note-writing occurs after thoughts are formulated while the attentive interviewer is already thinking ahead.

In the videotape replay the notes are of interest to the patient and the doctor. They help the patient see the interview as a thoughtful, living relationship. Awareness of the doctor's unspoken observations, reasoning, self-questions and speculations can give a new kind of usable insight to a patient with good ego strength. Replay, thereby, reconstructs and reinforces effective interpretations and illuminates off-target interpretations. The patient becomes a collaborator in the learning experience, adding dignity and importance to his role.

A second method has been developed to eliminate the camera looking into the doctor's lap. With the Victor Electro-Writer, the doctor writes with a pen connected to an electronic transmitter which sends the messages to a receiving unit where they are instantaneously reproduced.* The transmitter is placed on a small table at the doctor's side just out of the patient's sight. The electronic receiver is in another room before a camera. By the use of split-screen effect, the lower portion of the final picture shows the notes as they are being written. The ink-flow pen of this particular receiver is preferable for videotape reproduction to automatic writing equipment with ballpoint pens.

SUMMARY

Several videotape techniques for recording interviews of individual and group psychotherapy sessions are described. A general program of camera

---

* Victor Business Machines Company, Chicago 18, Illinois.

angles and sequential views of clinical transactions, to dramatically convey the evolving nature of the doctor-patient relationship, is given. Special methods of introducing light signals and handwritten notes into the videotape picture are presented. A method for reproducing the original group and the discussion group pictures on the same videotape picture is illustrated.

A teaching-learning method for the use of videotapes in psychiatry involves the recording of very short clinical vignettes, the immediate replay of that videotape to the participants, and supervised review with the teacher.

Portable videotape equipment, as well as elaborate studio equipment, is used. At all times the camera is undisguised and operated in the open with a cameraman. Emphasis is placed on the artistic and dramatic quality of the videotape for teaching and supervision of residents as well as for its clinical therapeutic impact on the patient. The use of video taping techniques of clinical psychiatric practice is a most significant technological advance in psychiatric teaching. It is an adjunct for clinical teaching and a method *par excellence* for objective study of human behavioral relationships (8-14).

REFERENCES

1. Wilmer, H. A.: The Undisguised Camera in Videotape Psychiatric Teaching. *Visual Sonic Med.*, 3:5-11, 1968.
2. Wilmer, H. A.: You Know: The Use of Seemingly Meaningless Injectory Phrases in Group Psychotherapy. *Psychiat. Quart.*, 41:296-323, 1967.
3. Wilmer, H. A.: Murder, You Know. *Psychiat. Quart.*, 43:414-447, 1969.
4. Wilmer, H. A.: *Social Psychiatry in Action*. Springfield, Ill.: Thomas, 1958.
5. Hess, E. H.: Attitude and Pupil Size. *Sci. Amer.*, 212:46-65, 1965.
6. Hess, E. H. and Polt, J. M.: Pupil Size as Related to Interest Value of Visual Stimuli. *Science*, 132:349-350, 1960.
7. Hess, E. H. and Polt, J. M.: Pupil Size in Relation to Mental Activity During Simple Problem Solving. *Science*, 143:1190-1192, 1964.
8. Benchoter, B. A., Eaton, M. T., and Smith, P. L.: Use of Videotapes to Provide Individual Instruction in Technics of Psychotherapy. *J. Med. Educ.*, 40:1159-1161, 1965.
9. Cornelison, F. S., and Tausig, T. N.: A Study of Self-image Experience Using Videotapes at Delaware State Hospital. *Delaware Med. J.*, 37:229-231, 1964.
10. Geertsma, R. H. and Reivich, R. S.: Repetitive Self-observation by Videotape Playback. *J. Nerv. Ment. Dis.*, 141:29-41, 1965.
11. Kagan, N., Krathwohl, D. R., and Miller, R.: Stimulated Recall in Therapy Using Videotapes: A Case Study. *J. Consult. Psychol.*, 10:237-243, 1963.
12. Moore, F. J., Chernell, E., and West, M. J.: Television as a Therapeutic Tool. *Arch. Gen. Psychiat.* (Chicago), 12:217-220, 1965.
13. Schiff, S. B. and Reivich, R. S.: Use of Television as an Aid to Psychotherapy Supervision. *Arch. Gen. Psychiat.* (Chicago), 1:84-88, 1964.
14. Suess, J. F.: Teaching Clinical Psychiatry with Closed Circuit Television and Videotape. *J. Med. Educ.*, 41:483-488, 1966.

28

BASIC VIDEO EQUIPMENT

Patrick M. Corbitt

From its earliest days television has been a fascinating fluid entity—capable at times of eliciting exceptional expenditures of human creativity in the service of its own artistic and technical development. Every author attempting to explicate video's current technical juncture and usefulness in the highly specialized applications of health care treatment and training is indeed facing a significant task.

It is characteristic of the medium to foster daily "breakthroughs"—a smaller, better camera, a more sophisticated editing device, etc. At any one moment the picture of video technology in psychiatry may get a new splash of color, greater detail, another whole dimension—all these the secondary gain of some production or engineering "find" somewhere else in a related field.

Appreciative of these historical and contemporary realities we shall discuss some available basic elements of popular equipment, some applicable configurations, and some projections on technical developments in video technology for the psychiatric setting for the near and not-so-near future.

AVAILABLE BASIC ELEMENTS OF POPULAR EQUIPMENT AND SOME APPLICABLE CONFIGURATIONS

There are several general things that ought to be said at the outset about equipment. Chief among them is that the evaluations of equipment design, performance, and reliability and the resultant shades of praise or deprecation are based on a number of variables:

1. The model and/or "run" of the equipment in question.
2. The competence of the operator.
3. The conduciveness of the environment.
4. The preventive maintenance and/or repair criteria and execution.
5. The prevalence of unrealistic expectations.
6. The thoroughness and fairness of the evaluator.

A comment here about each may serve the potential or present user well.

For example, a new model of a proven videotape recorder will not always be better than its older relative; the new model may need some "shakedown" time to get the "bugs" out. Or it may not be so well made or designed—the first "run" or two may have small errors attributable to production management "wrinkles" at the factory. Even after it is on the market successfully, one finds a bad "batch" or "run" now and again. Responsible manufacturers, fortunately, are usually quick to notify dealers of the serial numbers of problem machines; trade publications* are most responsive to consumer needs and publish the word.

And then there is the question of conflicting reports about even established, generally well-respected video equipment. How can we account for the fact that we not infrequently hear contradictory evaluations about the same piece of equipment? Variables 2. through 5. above help us understand the dynamics. For example, even an excellent device in the hands of the technically inexperienced is fair game for abuse and a subsequently damaged reputation. "So and so had that tape recorder and he didn't like it." Rumors based upon such dubious origins are as rampant in certain video circles as ever they could be. No matter that "So and so" couldn't operate the device properly, didn't take the time to read the instructions or the technical manuals, installed it in a hot, dusty room, poorly maintained it, etc. No . . . it was the device that was "bad." If videotape recorders could talk . . . what another version of this tale we would hear.

To be certain, the majority of equipment does not receive such brutal treatment, but sometimes in the best of homes too much is expected of it. It is most important to select equipment on a realistic cost-effective basis and to appreciate the fact that often less sophisticated equipment has its limitations. One manufacturer once—in advertising its ½″ videotape recorder/reproducer—claimed essentially that it was "all you needed" to get into broadcast. And, although it is true that remarkable things have been done with "smaller format"** equipment, it is simply not a fact that a recorder can do it all—usually an armamentarium of time base correction and related processing equipment is used to air

---

* Some video publications of interest to medical educators and clinicians are listed in the selected bibliography. (See Section VI.)

** As traditionally defined, any recording format whose tape width is less than 2″ was considered an "inferior" format. Today, "smaller" does not carry such pejorative connotations, for, in fact, the 2″ Quad machines are being replaced by 1″ and ¾″ (videocassette) decks of impressive performance capability.

small-format originated programming. Learn what proposed equipment will and will not do. Ask for a demonstration—if you can't get one, refuse to consider the equipment for purchase.

And lastly—is the evaluator being fair? Equally, is he or she thorough? The video business is an extremely complex field and the more circumspect one can be the better. One should always question the sources, ask for second opinions, get through the advertising to the specifications, the carefully observed performance, the service record. Solid, successful, and effective purchases are made when a customer carefully looks at the body of evaluative literature (product test reports, field studies, etc.), considers their source and compares with other available documentation.

That said, understand that the following suggestions and considerations are paid for dearly through years of trial and error and that they are a view shared, at least in large part, by a number of colleagues. What about available, popular equipment and its configurations? We will consider each video element.

Sound

Everywhere one hears or reads that sound is the "forgotten" part of video . . . and so it is. Sadly one often finds the treatment of sound and its cardinal importance hidden away at the end of someone's chapter—tucked between connectors and miscellany. That is not where sound belongs; it must be up front in such a treatment as this. Similarly, it must be a foremost consideration in every telecast or taping.

Before the videotape, there was the audiotape. At worst, if one has excellent sound and the video portion has its problems, the program can be salvaged by:

1. recutting similar or related video;
2. making an audiotape out of the program;
3. making an audiotape with a flyer, booklet, or, through another post-production photographic phase—a sound/slide synchonized program;
4. "living with" the intermittent video problems;
5. transcribing *in toto* the presentation or preparing an outline for study and appropriate action, discarding the original tape.

And, at best, if all's well with the picture, one will have an excellent videotape enhanced by the audio element.

Evaluation of sound quality can often depend on a largely subjective experience . . . albeit well-founded in a familiarity with objective technical parameters. The more one hears good audio and studies its effects on the senses, the better one will recognize its elements and understand their successful combination. Accordingly, then, in an inferior audio track you will be able to analyze those parts of the whole which are contributing to the less-desirable "total effect" and the marginal quality.

The ways to achieve good audio are legion; to varying degrees they depend on the nature of the pick-up, mixing and recording instruments, the tape, the talent, and the setting. No matter what video or audiotape recorder is used, good audio originates long before the video or audio deck records it. And, for that matter, what you hear on the earphones at a mike mixer (sound *en route* to a tape recorder) is not always what you get out of the tape recorder's TV set. Furthermore, televisions are notorious for having small "tinny" speakers. Also, television sets found in treatment and training settings are sometimes placed in a relatively noisy place (near a 1″ videotape recorder can be noisy enough—so one cannot really *hear* the audio).

Appreciating the interdependence of components in an audio system and realizing that there are clear basic rules for getting good sound at each point in the circuit, consider for a moment this evaluation of the nature of video sound . . . and the equipment needed to successfully record and reproduce it. I like a tripartite view of TV audio:

1. what you hear (dominant audio—of a speaker, panel, group, symphony, etc.);
2. what you hear *behind* what you hear (background, "ambient" sounds), and
3. what the tape recorder insists you must hear from itself (tape hiss, wow and flutter, "pops" at edits, etc.).

When we want to record, we want to record someone or something. This is the dominant sound we want to hear in the recording. In order to "pick up" the sound emanating from the subject, several basic audio components are needed:

1. a microphone,
2. a cable from the mike to the recording device,
3. a stand, boom, lanyard, tie or shirt clip to position the mike,
4. possibly a wind screen for the mike.

The microphone is the instrument that converts the physical sound energy to electrical energy . . . the form of energy needed by any passive tape recording device. Microphones are traditionally classified by both the method they use to convert sound energy into electrical energy (their "physical" design) and by the pattern in which they pick up sound (so-called "polar pattern").

It is of importance to the potential user to know something about the generating elements used in the internal physical design of a microphone since it is usually the type of generating element that determines the durability, longevity, fidelity, and cost of the unit.

By internal physical design the microphones more popularly available are classified as:

1. Ceramic/crystal. Utilizing a piezoelectric generating element, this low-fidelity and relatively fragile type is the least desirable of all available microphones for videotape applications. None are recommended . . . and *caveat emptor* of any dealer who tries to sell you one for television.
2. Ribbon. Sometimes called "velocity" microphones, these mikes—although characterized by low distortion and internal noise, wide frequency range, and good sensitivity—are generally far too delicate for mental health treatment and training applications. A good blast of air can easily rip the thin foil that forms both the diaphragm and the voice coil.
3. Condenser. There was a time when the condenser mike was reserved for a careful existence in the recording studio—next to the ribbon type. Not so today. Although still a bit less rugged than the dynamic, there are currently a number of excellent condenser microphones available for videotape studio and field production. One need be careful of extremes in shock, humidity, and temperature, but condenser microphones like the Sennheiser K2U, ME* modular series, Sony ECM-50** as well as the Spectrum SML-15*** lavaliers (and to a lesser degree the sibling ML-10 and ML-5) are currently making a good name for themselves in teleproduction.
4. Dynamic. Rugged and reasonably priced, this excellent high fidelity microphone is the workhorse of video studios and on-location crews. It is admirably suited for the health care setting.

To be sure there are a number of more exotic generating elements but, except for the carbon mike—often used in studio camera operators/director headset intercom systems, most fall outside of our parameters for usefulness.

Of special interest to us is the second—and more functional—classification of microphones—by pick-up pattern. When we speak of the pattern

---

* Available from Sennheiser or authorized dealers.

** Available from Sony dealers.

*** We have found this excellent microphone hard to get but available from Comprehensive, Inc., New York City, and Giffen Video, Staten Island, New York.

in which a microphone "picks up" sound, we need think in terms of solid geometric figures. Most common pick-up patterns used in videotape productions are:

1. Omnidirectional. These microphones pick up sound from all directions (hence the prefix "omni"). It is as if the microphone were at the very center of a sphere with constant pick-up 360° around at all attitudes. Some examples of good omnidirectional mikes are: (a) Electrovoice—RE-55 dynamic,* (b) Electrovoice—635-A dynamic, (c) Sennheiser K2U-ME electret condenser, and (d) Shure SM-61 dynamic.

We should note here that the lavalier or "tie-tack" microphone is an omnidirectional mike at least in the general sense (although some lavaliers are a bit more unidirectional at certain frequencies). Some good lavalier type omnidirectional mikes are: (a) Sony ECM-50 electret condenser,)b) Electrovoice RE-85 dynamic, (c) Electrovoice CO-85 electret condenser, and (d) Electrovoice 647A dynamic.

2. Unidirectional. There are a number of types of unidirectional microphones. But the obvious-sounding prefix "uni" does not mean that the microphone picks up solely in one direction. In fact, there are degrees of "unidirectionality." Here are some:

(a) Cardioid. Here again thinking in solid geometry, the pick-up pattern resembles a slightly laterally compressed apple with the microphone pointing down at the position of the apple's stem. The analogy of the heart-shaped pattern is obvious from the cardioid root; it is apt. Sound pick-up in this type of unidirectional mike is somewhat less at the sides and quite subdued at the rear of the mike. Some popular cardioid mikes are: (a) Sennheiser MKH-435 condenser, (b) Sennheiser K24-ME40 electret condenser, (c) AKG C451E-CK-1 condenser, (d) Electrovoice DS-35 dynamic, (e) Sony ECM-250P electret condenser, (f) Altec-Lansing 689BX.

We should note here that the cardioid mike family has grown so that a number of types of cardioid mikes are currently available. The interested reader is advised to consult the manufacturer for exact details of pick-up patterns and frequency response(s)** of these excellent "hybrid" cardioid mikes: (a) Sennheiser MKH-415 super cardioid condenser, (b) Sennheiser MD-441 super cardioid MD-441 dynamic, (c) Electrovoice RE-16 and RE-15 super cardioid dynamic, (d) Electrovoice 667A cardioid dynamic.

---

* All mikes listed except Spectrum noted above are available from manufacturer or authorized dealers; prices vary on all items. We will always note type of generating element in these descriptions, *e.g. dynamic* omnidirectional.

** Some specialized cardioid mikes highlight or mask different frequencies in the sound spectrum; some are switchselectable, some fixed. The interested user should always thoroughly investigate models for his/her applications.

(b) Ultradirectional. Certain unidirectional microphones have pick-up patterns whose characteristic may be described as conical.* The pattern thrusts outward from the mike head in a cone typified by extreme rejection of all sound not in the plotted pattern. Often called "shotgun" mikes, these instruments isolate the desired sound, pick it up at impressive distances and have an excellent performance record. Some are: (a) Sennheiser MKH-815 shotgun-condenser, (b) Sennheiser K24-ME-80 shot-gun-electret condenser, (c) AKG C-451E CK-9 interface tube-condenser, (d) Electrovoice DL 42 "cardiline"-dynamic. As was the case in "generating elements" above, there are variations on these popular pick-up patterns. One can obtain true bidirectional and polydirectional mikes for various applications—reputable sound engineers can be most helpful here.

Because of their pick-up patterns, omnidirectional, cardioid, and shotgun mikes afford the video user a wide variety of potential solutions to vexing taping problems. For example:

1. Good omnidirectional mikes:
   (a) are often less affected by breath pops than cardioid mikes;
   (b) are generally more rugged than cardioid mikes;
   (c) offer smooth, very wide range;
   (d) with proper mike placement, enable more than two persons to be heard.

On the other hand,

2. Good cardioid and shotgun mikes:
   (a) lessen considerably the pick-up of ambient background noise;
   (b) enable mikes to be placed farther from subject (two or more times the distance of the omnidirectional mike);
   (c) of a certain type increase intelligible frequencies while retaining bass for "depth."

Proper placement of the right microphone(s) by a trained individual after careful acoustic analysis of the environment where sound is to be recorded will result in a good start for effective sound pick-up.

Some important microphone miscellany for videotape use should include that all instruments be of the low impedance type (so-called low-Z). Cables should be "two conductor shielded" to provide hum and noise protection (by the shield). Connectors used in mike wiring should be 3-pin "XLR" type. Microphone windscreens or "puffs" are available to help reduce the undesirable effects of wind and breath extremes.

* The directionality varies at different frequencies, distances, and indeed from instrument to instrument.

There is a wide variety of floor and desk stands and shock mounts available from mike manufacturers. Similarly, a selection of baby and full-size booms can be obtained from such established suppliers as F and B Ceco, Mole-Richardson, Atlas, and Bogen.

A word about "wireless" microphones is in order. Edcor, Vega, Sennheiser—to name three popular manufacturers—all produce fine wireless mikes for applications where cables are a problem. It seems that the Edcor PM-1 mike and ST-3 Sensationer—at about half the cost of the other comparable units—represent the best value. The state-of-the-art today in wireless mikes is such that, once properly set up on established, clear frequencies, they provide trouble-free service for years.

The standard wireless unit consists of a microphone (a number of different types are available), a transmitter, and a receiver. The units are compact, battery-powered where necessary, and a delight to use. Multiple channel receivers are available to permit four or five wireless mikes to be simultaneously operational in the same area.

Use of a microphone mixer is often indicated in treatment or training sessions. In this case, multiple microphones are fed either by individual extension cables, an audio "snake," or a multi-conductor trunk cable to the mixer.

Although there are any number of highly sophisticated mixers available—indeed, the prices start at $1000 and go up to $25,000 to $30,000 or even more—probably the most flexible, inexpensive, and adequate mike mixer available is the Shure M67. Now one can add a number of additional mike or line inputs to the basic mixer by strapping on the 677 add-on mixer. The 677 module has made the basic Shure M67 the instrument of choice. The basic unit can be powered by batteries for field or location mixing. Also popular for mobile applications using up to three mikes (and a high impedance line) is the Transist-O-Sound MA-3C.

Although it is best to correct frequency problems at the source (treat environment, use an appropriate microphone, etc.), from time to time boost or cut of frequencies and general "coloring" of the program sound may be required. And this is one of the features of the expensive audio mixer—elaborate filter capability. Still the Shure Audio Master or Notch Filter can be helpful in treating the program audio. Both should be used carefully and with professional advice.

Names to explore when looking for program sound amplifiers and speakers are: RCA, Altec, Bogen, Electrovoice, Atlas, and JBL. A Bogen CHB-10 and matching 8-ohm speaker will do well for most program monitoring.

Studying and experimenting with these factors of sound pick-up, transmission and mixing with further technical reading will help the interested user develop the ability to consistently obtain better sound for video recordings.

There are proven sound component configurations that can serve as a base for effective audio pick-up in treatment and training settings.

1. The simplest, when one person is the subject, is to "close mike" the individual—that is, to use a Sony ECM-50 or Spectrum SML-15 or similar lavalier/tie-tack mike on the person. One can also use an "off-camera" mike—a super cardioid or shotgun type, for example—out of sight of the camera; properly selected for maximum range/fidelity efficiency this is an excellent second choice. Also, an omnidirectional mike "hand held" at close range will work very nicely, but, unless it can be operated at a maximum of 8-10 inches from the sound source, the user risks picking up unwanted ambient background noise.

2. When two or more persons have to be simultaneously recorded, more elaborate miking procedures have to be employed. In the limited space herein we cannot outline more than the basic techniques—extensions and elaborations of which may be necessary for the large group (large family and group therapy, for example).

   First, one can "close mike" each individual in the group—lots of wires, restricted movement, and a number of individual volume controls on the mike mixer—nevertheless, a reliable way of having complete control over the group/individual sound. Needless to say, the individual at the mike mixer must be very good at his/her job.

   Second, stick mikes (omnidirectionals, for example) can be placed (perhaps on low stands or suspended from the ceiling) between individuals to get sound at a ratio of 1 mike per 2 people. Again, the working distance should be kept as close as possible to avoid unwanted background noises.

   Third, a super cardioid or shotgun mike can be mounted on one or two booms and swing over the group. This is the least desirable way since it requires excellent timing by the boom operators, and the boom can be a significant distraction to the group (booms are large, imposing devices).

   Fourth, on rare occasions in rooms with ideally suited acoustical properties and where near perfect group placement exists, a single, superior-quality omnidirectional mike can be suspended over a group to obtain acceptable sound. But remember that hanging an omnidirectional mike over the average group in the average room is normally a good way to hear a lot of ambient noise and poorly intelligible group participants.

In the placement of multiple omnidirectional or cardioid mikes, one should seek advice from a local technical source since problems such as phase error, shifting, frequency response voids, cancellation and the like can reduce the effectiveness of the instruments, resulting in poor sound.

Light

It used to be true that to make good television pictures one had to have a lot of light. Gone are those days. It is no longer necessary to flood an area with 100-200 foot candles of light to make excellent black and white videotapes—in fact, new, while still expensive, color cameras are capable of producing an impressive color picture at 25-foot candles. We shall discuss these excellent cameras later; now, let us outline the qualities of and instruments needed for good illumination.

Visible light is only a small part of the electromagnetic spectrum. Yet the range of light color quality in the visible spectrum alone is substantial—bound by infrared on one side and ultraviolet on the other. To describe the color property (or "temperature," as it is more properly called) of light, scientists have developed an arbitrary measure known as the Kelvin scale. The lower the degree on the Kelvin scale, the "redder" the quality of the light, the closer to the infrared side of the spectrum. Conversely, the higher the degree Kelvin, the "bluer" the quality of the light, the closer to the ultraviolet. Some examples of common color temperatures are:

Source	Approximate Color Temperature
A candle	1800-1900°K
Quartz T.V. light	3200°K, 3400°K
Fluorescent	range in color temperature from "warm" at 2900°K to "cool" at 4300°K to "daylight" at 6500°K
100-watt incandescent	2850°K
Sunlight	5500°K
Skylight	10,000°K to 20,000°K

We mention color temperature not because it makes all that much difference in today's black and white videotaping, but because many individuals converting to color systems need be reminded that color temperature uniformity is still necessary to assure the successful operation of the popular inexpensive color cameras. Mixing light sources of different color temperatures can lead to color reproduction problems. Using a quartz light for "fill" on a cloudy day, for example, can lead to yellow-brown faces unless proper filtration is added at the quartz light source.

It is good advice to keep a supply of color filter media (obtainable from, among others, Rosco, the industry standard) to assure that all sources of illumination for color taping be matched in color temperature. One can, for example, apply a Rosco filter element to a room window to convert incoming daylight to 3200°K to match the quartz lights if these are used as the main source of illumination. After the taping, the filter media can be easily removed from the window.

Also—and this does not relate to color temperature but to the use of self-adhering media—one can use a neutral density filter to limit the amount of light coming from that window if, in fact, it is too extreme.

And this leads us to another quality of light: intensity. Perhaps the safest rule to follow is that the light be balanced. By balanced we do not especially mean "flat." What we do mean is that we work for a picture in which no bright spots are so "hot" or intense as to cause the camera to "burn," "streak" or "bloom." We want to be able to see detail in the darker spots of the scene. Varying light intensity can create interest in a scene as long as extremes beyond the camera's compensating capability are avoided.

Sometimes intensity is less at fault for bright spots than the unusually high reflectance of the problem object. Highly reflective articles often cause unwanted "specular highlight" in a picture—bright spots that may even damage certain types of camera pick-up tubes. The solution is to remove the object where possible or, at least, to mute it with removable dulling spray.

There are any number of lighting instruments and bulbs as well as a variety of positioning devices to achieve good lighting. The first task, however, is to analyze the existing light to determine if it is technically adequate for the camera.

One measures light either by experience or by light meters or by both. After years of looking, one can guess rather accurately at light intensity, but for most of us a reading in foot candles should be made by a good incident light meter. Some meters capable of such measurements are: 1) Gossen Lune Pro; 2) Sekonic Studio Master; 3) Spectra Professional.*

The details of taking incident light readings are discussed in the manuals accompanying the meter. Once these are learned, one need only be sure the ambient light level of the scene meets or exceeds the camera manufacturer's lighting equipment specification for the camera to be used.

---

* All three meters are available at most large photo shops and lighting sales and rental firms; prices vary.

Often, for example, a bank of modern fluorescent ceiling light is more than adequate for most contemporary black and white and some color cameras.

In certain indoor applications, some additional or quite substantial basic light must be provided. Being careful of color temperature uniformity, the user can increase the ambient light of a scene by using any one of these quartz fill or base luminaires (directly or indirectly aimed at the subject): 1) Lowel Softlight 1500—portable, shadowless light source—very bright (about the equivalent of conventional 2000-watt studio fills); 2) Colortran Minibroad—portable non-focusing fill light—650 watts of illumination; 3) Colortran Multi-broad—a full 1000-watt light for heavy stands or studio pipe grids; 4) Lowel-light—modular, portable 1000-watt fill for a variety of applications; 5) Ianiro Mini-fill 1000—full 1000-watt portable fill lights.

It should be noted that any quartz light is bright. Often bouncing the light off a white ceiling will accomplish the task and avoid bothering the subjects. If lights must be aimed at the subject, the use of "scrims" or diffusers (popularly known as "tough spun") can be helpful in limiting the apparent intensity of the luminaire.

On occasion, particularly in training tapes, the use of a spotlight is required to achieve highlight and modeling. Some popular spots are: 1) Colortran Mini-pro—the workhorse of portable focusing spots; 2) Ianiro Ianebeam 650/1000—650 and 1000 watt versions of the same durable spot; 3) Kliegl Fresnels—any number of focusing spots of all sizes and power; 4) Strand Century Fresnels—as with Kliegel, a wide variety of spot instruments.

Sometimes location shooting requires portable battery-operated lights. In such a circumstance the Sylvania SG-77, SG-65 EXG or Cine 60 "sun guns" are excellent choices. One can use the manufacturer's battery packs (normal or "quick charge") or a power pack from an independent manufacturer such as the 800 NC from Frezzolini.

For most lights listed here, a full complement of gel frames, barndoors, flags, dichroic (daylight conversion) filters, clamps, and stands are available from the manufacturer or large video dealers.

Once basic technical requirements are fulfilled, the user can develop the artistic subtlety necessary for the more sophisticated videotape. As in the discussion of sound there are in lighting accepted basic instrument configurations. Here are some:

1. For lighting the average individual, one can use fill and spot lights to create base, fill, spot, hair and background light.

2. For a panel each participant should have a key and a hair light. The scene receives base lighting, the background appropriate illumination.

Probably the greatest challenge is to achieve interesting visuals through creative lighting. The user can find a number of excellent seminars available to sharpen his/her talents.*

Cameras

While the microphone picks up sound, the video camera responds to reflected light. And as one might imagine, there are a number of kinds of cameras.

The basic principle of any camera is that the lens affixed to its front gathers and focuses the light reflected from the subject onto a target at the end of the pick-up tube located inside the camera behind the lens. The pick-up tube—its photo-electric conductive material in tube target being struck by a regulated flow of electrons from a "gun" at the end of the tube—converts the physical energy to electronic pulses of corresponding nature. The elaborate processes necessary to achieve the electronic likeness of the physical entity being videographed vary in precision and configuration from camera to camera.

There are, however, certain identifiable characteristics of different kinds of cameras. We can consider black and white cameras first. And here there are essentially two types available—described by the kind of pick-up tube used:

1. *Vidicon tube type.* Earlier vidicon tube cameras needed a great deal of light to achieve an acceptable picture. Today, improved ancillary circuitry and advanced "separate-mesh" vidicon tubes have produced cameras that operate well under "normal" light. In many applications the new vidicon tube cameras provide adequate sensitivity, excellent contrast and resolution. Standard among black and white vidicon cameras are: (a) Sony AVC-3260 ($650-$700). A 2:1 sync** vidicon camera—not a particularly advanced design but, nevertheless, the one commonly found camera in the mental health setting.*** (b) Sony AVC-4600 ($800 range).

---

* Los Angeles and New York VideoExpos usually have lighting seminars. Perhaps the best source of lighting knowledge is Imero Fiorentino Associates in New York—this group conducts individual and class lighting instruction throughout the country.

** All cameras utilized today should have 2:1 interlace, RS-170 synchronization for maximum picture stability. There is no longer any need to use the inferior "random" interlace sync. No matter what the pick-up tube, the camera should be driven with RS-170 sync.

*** Camera can be purchased with attaching electronic viewfinder if so desired.

A 650-line resolution camera driven by RS-170 sync—better resolution than many, good sensitivity. (c) RCA-TC-1000 series ($400-$700). A line of high sensitivity cameras capable of RS-170 sync and some up to 800-line resolution. No electronic viewfinder is currently available from RCA for mounting on the camera.* Currently the TC-1005 is the finest non-viewfinder camera available at $575-$600. (d) Panasonic WV 342 P ($650-$700)—Furnished with viewfinder, this camera has 2:1 sync and an excellent performance record.

2. *Low light level tube type.* The first widely available Low light level (LLL) tube was the Plumbicon;** silicon diode type followed. Although these tubes are still in use, perhaps one of the most satisfactory among contemporary LLL tubes is the Newvicon.*** It affords the user excellent sensitivity and resolution with a minimum of blooming or burn.

Almost any camera can be equipped with a LLL tube. The Newvicon is a popular option with portable black and white cameras such as the Panasonic WV 3085 hand held; the results are impressive: usable pictures in what appears to be virtually no appreciable light.

Color cameras, on the other hand, present the psychiatric user with a more difficult set of choices. Color cameras have achieved surprising results from packaged components whose size and price get lower all the time. Though debate continues over the necessity of color in treatment qua treatment, there is growing acceptance of the desirability of color in training programs where pretaped clinical elements are used. Although color cameras can be defined by the type and number of tubes used, perhaps the easiest way for our purposes here is to delineate color cameras by price****/performance features. Following that model we shall briefly outline some of the more established ones:

1. Under $7000:
   (a) Sony DXC 1600. One of the first inexpensive portable color cameras. Has given respectable color pictures of surprising definition and colorimetry under good lighting conditions. This camera has no low light capability and tends to show lag (image retention, ghosting) when illumination falls below manufacturer's specifications. Several versions of this 1600 series camera exist.

---

* Certain models in this RCA series can be considered suitable for low light applications.

** "Plumbicon" is a registered trademark of the N. V. Philips Co.

*** Trademark Panasonic Co.; the Hitachi Saticon is also an excellent low light level tube—quite popular in color cameras.

**** Manufacturer's suggested list prices are used.

(b) Hitachi Denshi FP-3030. One of the "second generation" inexpensive portable color cameras; a truly remarkable performer with good sensitivity, fine colorimetry and thoughtfully designed handling hardware.

(c) JVC GC-4800U. A two-tube, second-generation portable camera with fine performance akin to the FP-3030 mentioned above.

(d) Akai CCS-150S. Offspring of one of the first inexpensive portable color cameras, this camera offers improved performance over its predecessor. One of the smallest and lightest portable color cameras available, it enjoys sufficient illumination and returns acceptable pictures.*

(e) Panasonic WV-2150. This studio camera (complete with CCU) utilizes the Newvicon tube we spoke of earlier—now in a color camera. The camera boasts sensitivity to 25 foot candles with the 6dB gain switch on and an impressive signal to noise ratio of 46dB with 200-foot candle illumination. Still relatively new at this writing, this handy looking studio camera holds much promise.**

(f) JVC NU-1800U. A three-tube color studio camera, JVC claims the color stability, fidelity, and luminance to be better than other cameras in its class. Like the Panasonic WV-2150, the unit holds great promise, although still new and untested at this writing.

(g) Cohu 1400 series. Designed primarily for scientific and microscope work, this simple single-tube unit is available in a "Hetero-Junction Image Tube" for increased sensitivity. The tiny, non-viewfinder camera could very well have significance for a variety of mental health applications, although immediately it has seen little use in that treatment or training field.

2. Over $7000 to about $25,000. The cameras in this category are characterized by the excellent sensitivity and resolution of the new breed of "mid-price" color cameras. Using low light level tubes (the Saticon developed by Hitachi being a popular one), they more than exceed the requirements for treatment settings and perform admirably to give training programs impact and high quality color. Some are:*** (a) Hitachi Denshi FP-1020; (b) Hitachi Denshi SK-80; (c) Asaca ACC 2000; (d) Ikegami ITC-300; (e) Ikegami HL-37 Minimate; (f) GBC CTC-7X; (g) Ikegami HL-33; (h) Hitachi FP-1212 and 1000 series.

---

* At this writing we have insufficient experience with the Magnavox Chromavue 400, Sharp XC 2000, Panasonic WV-2200 or WV-2310 and Asaca ACC-5000 to comment on these inexpensive cameras; the interested reader is advised to encourage "side by side" demonstration of all such cameras before making a decision on which to purchase.
** We should note here that the Panasonic WV-2150 squeaks in under the $7000 limit at $6500 *without* a lens, whereas the other portable cameras above are supplied with a zoom lens.
*** Some of these units creep into this category priced "without lens" so the user is advised to check closely in purchasing.

With the exception of the Thompson CSF Microcam at $30,000, the RCA TK-76 at $35,000, the CEI 280 at $28,000 and 290 at $35,000, and possibly the Sony BVP 100 and Philips LDK-11 at $40,000, the balance of available color cameras are more legendary than economically available to the mental health trainer. But the current trend in developing new and improved, and less expensive ENG* and EFP** cameras continues to be a benefit to the training—if not yet to the clinical—applications of video.

Accessories essential to obtain maximum service from any camera, be it black and white or color, are:

1. *A good lens.* Here the choices are extensive. But beware that the pick-up tubes in cameras vary in size and the types of lenses needed vary with them. If a given camera uses a ⅔" width pick-up tube target, the normal lens used for it will not be appropriate for a camera using a 1" width pick-up tube target. Most lens manufacturers are able to furnish complete charts of proper lenses for popularly available cameras. If one knows the size of the pick-up tube in the camera, then the charts will tell the rest of the lens selection story.

Another lens factor that should be remembered is the "speed" of the lens. Some lenses can allow more light to pass through than others. If a lens can permit a great deal of light to pass, then in low light it will give the pick-up tube more light to "see"; we call it a fast lens. If a lens has poor light transmission properties, we call it a "slow" lens. Such a lens will be no asset (and in fact a liability in many cases) to the camera's pick-up tube under marginal or low light conditions.

Lenses are calibrated in "f-stops."*** The lower the f-stop number, the wider the aperture of the lens diaphragm, the greater the amount of light entering the camera. And the higher the f-stop, the narrower the aperture, the less light can strike the target on the pick-up tube.

A lens with a f 1.4 or f 1.2 maximum aperture is generally considered a fast lens. A f 2.8 lens is a slow lens; a f 3.5, while acceptable in still photography, is a very slow lens for TV. Normal fixed (that is, non-zoom) lenses should be relatively fast lenses, but the zoom lens presents certain inherent design problems that make the inexpensive fabrication of very high speed zoom difficult; a f 1.8 zoom lens is usually about the fastest available.

Some popular video camera lens manufacturers to be consi-

---

* An acronym for Electronic News Gathering portable color camera.
** The same for Electronic Field Production; the term refers to high quality, portable color cameras.
*** A name for the relationship expressed between the focal length of the lens and the diameter of the diaphragm's aperture.

dered before lens selection is final are: (a) Rank-Taylor-Hobson; (b) Schneider; (c) Angenieux; (d) Canon; (e) Fujinon.

The lens can provide the camera operator with a range of views of a given scene. The wide angle lens permits coverage of a large area by the camera; the telephoto, a closer look at a smaller part of the whole picture; a zoom lens, all those interesting places in between.

Clearly the instrument for the clinical or training setting is the zoom lens; prices start at around $550 for a good one.

2. *A tripod.* Proper positioning equipment for the video camera is crucial to smooth camera movement. A reliable camera on a poor tripod is at best useless and at worst a disaster of jitter, slides and bumps in the picture. An operator who tries to hold a "hand held" (i.e., "portapack" type) camera without a good body brace asks for disturbingly shaky video and muscle cramps within five minutes.

On the other hand, the right tripod or body brace with a camera properly mounted and balanced gives the operator with basic skills a full day of satisfactory service and steady shots.

There are a number of tripods available. The lighter cameras do well on a simple all-metal tripod-dolly* with a spring-loaded friction head.** This particular type of head adjusts and locks at any number of positions, and the spring keeps the camera from sudden tips back or tilts down that could cause damage. Sanford Davis and Quick-Set, Inc. both make this type of tripod for about $130-$150.

In more critical applications the use of a special head may be advisable. Perhaps the smoothest available today is the fluid head. Miller, Inc., Vinten, Inc., and O'Connor, Inc. all make excellent fluid action heads for cameras of all sizes and weights. A major supplier for these fine lines is F and B Ceco, New York and California.

Heavy cameras require more substantial positioning equipment than the lightweight tripod-dolly. The selection is enormous and the criteria simple: (a) the weight of the camera; (b) the degree of quality desired; (c) the financial parameters.

Quick-Set, O'Connor, Vinten and Miller all have a full line. Other excellent manufacturers are: ITE (Innovative Television Equipment), Gitzo, and Hervic.

---

* Unfortunately the words tripod and dolly often appear interchangeable when used to describe the three-leg device with wheels on a carriage at its base. But a tripod is a tripod. It does not ordinarily come with wheels; it has feet (hence the name). The wheeled assembly that you can obtain to fasten the tripod so you can roll the camera around on the ensemble is called the dolly. There are tripods that do not have feet but rather a wheel at the base of each leg; such an arrangement is called a trolly.

** The head, mounted at the top of the elevator column, directly supports the camera; all pan and tilt actions are accomplished by moving it left and right or up and down.

A variety of other specialized camera mounts are available—suction cups, hi-hats, spiders, elaborate dollies, and cranes—but one of the most useful devices for clinical and training work is the body or shoulder brace. For the small "portapack" type cameras the Peter Lisand line* or SOS-M-25670** body braces can't be beaten. Models differ and it is best to indicate which camera will be used to assure the best fit. Rock-steady pictures are possible in the hands of a skilled camera operator using this kind of brace.

The Videotape Recorder and the Monitor

The electronic image produced by the camera is the video signal carried through any "closed circuit" or "open circuit" system. We shall now consider two of the elements essential to creating—with the camera and microphone—that system: the videotape recorder/reproducer and the monitor.

Videotape Recorder/Reproducer

The proliferation of videotape recorder/reproducers in this decade is staggering. Perhaps the most convenient way to classify them is their "format." It should be understood that the decision as to which type of tape recorder is "best" to buy is perhaps the most thorny of all questions facing the video user. Before we address that, here is a listing of popular smaller format*** videotape recorder/reproducers:

1. New 1″ Tape Format ($20,000 and up, depending on options): (a) Sony BVH 1000; (b) Sony BVH 500; (c) Ampex VPR-1.
2. ¾″ U-matic Videocassette Format: (a) JVC CR 6060U editor, recorder/reproducer—$1750; (b) JVC CR 6100U recorder/reproducer with tuner and timer—$1745; (c) JVC CR 6300U recorder/reproducer—$1960; (d) Panasonic NV 2110M reproducer only—$1350; (e) Panasonic NV 2121 recorder/reproducer—$1750; (f) Sony VP 2000 reproducer only—$1495; (g) Sony VP 3000 reproducer only—20 minute portable—$1295; (h) Sony VO 2600 recorder/reproducer—$1845; (i) Sony VO 2800 recorder/reproducer—$3395; (j) Sony VO 2850 editor, recorder/reproducer—$6000; (k) Sony VO 3800 portable recorder/reproducer—$3000;

---

* Available from Giffen Video, Staten Island, New York.

** Available from F and B Ceco, New York, New York, Hollywood, California.

*** We have avoided listing available 2″ Quad Commercial Broadcast equipment as well as the Sony and IVC 2″ Helical VTRs because they are of lesser importance to the average psychiatric user.

(l) Nippon Electric Co. VC-7200P reproducer—$1170; (m) Nippon Electric Co. VC 7300P recorder/reproducer—$1570; (n) JVC CR 4400U portable recorder/reproducer—$2700; (c) Teac VT-1000 (virtually the same as the Sony VO 3800)—price not available; (p) Sony BVU 100 Broadcast ¾″ recorder/reproducer—$3500; (q) JVC CR-8300U editor, recorder/reproducer—$5850.

Other specialized time lapse ¾″ videocassette recorders are available from NEC.

3. Black and white ½″ EIA-J Open reel (reel-to-reel) videotape recorder*/reproducer: (a) Sony AV 3650 editor, recorder/reproducer—$1250; (b) Sony AV 3600 recorder/reproducer—$895.
4. Color and Black and White ½″ EIA-J Open Reel (reel-to-reel videotape recorders) : (a) Sony 8650 Editor, recorder/reproducer—$2750; (b) Panasonic NV 3160 Editor, recorder/reproducer—$2295; (c) Panasonic NV 3130 Editor, recorder/reproducer—$1800.
5. Portable Black and White ½″ EIA-J camera/videotape recorder ensembles ("Portapacks"): (a) Sony AV/AVC 3400 Rover II—$1850; (b) Panasonic NV/WV 3085—$1750.
6. Portable Color ½″ EIA-J videotape recorder Sony AV 8400B—$1250.
7. ½″ Cassette or Cartridge color and black and white videotape recorder/producers:** (a) Panasonic NV-5110 color cartridge reproducer only—$1050; (b) Panasonic NV-5120 color cartridge recorder/reproducer—$1350; (c) Panasonic NV-5125 color cartridge recorder/reproducer with off air tuner—$1450; (d) Norelco color VCR N1481 ½″ cartridge recorder/reproducer—$1425; (e) Sanyo VTC-7150X black and white portable ½″ cassette recorder/reproducer and camera ensemble—$1995; (f) Sanyo V-Cord II VTC-8400 ½″ color cassette recorder/reproducer with 2 hour capability—$1200; (g) V-Cord II VTC-8410 ½″color cassette reproducer only with 2 hour capability—$1095; (h) Sanyo V-Cord II VTC-8200 ½″ color cassette recorder/reproducer with 2 hour capability and built-in UHF/VHF antenna inputs and an RF modulator for channel 3 or 4—$1290; (i) Sony Betamax SL-7200 'Beta" format ½″ color cassette recorder/reproducer—$1260; (j) Sony Betamax*** SL-8200 "Beta" format

---

* Other ½″ VTRs are available, but not generally easy to obtain, from other manufacturers such as Hitachi, JVC, and Concord.

** Several of the new format machines have 2 and 4 hour capability; these are noted —otherwise maximum play/record time is 60 minutes.

*** At this writing the Zenith Corp. has announced marketing of a "Beta" format videocassette recorder/reproducer nearly identical to the Sony Betamax.

½″ color cassette recorder/reproducer with 2 hour capability—
$1300; (k) RCA "Selectavision" ½″ color cassette recorder/
reproducer—$995; (l) JVC* "Vidstar" selectavision format ½″
color cassette recorder/reproducer—$1280.

To be sure there are still a number of more exotic recorders not listed
above, but even from this incomplete listing the potential user is stunned
by the choices. It is obvious that anyone preparing to buy a videotape
unit should carefully evaluate his/her needs and the features of the
proposed equipment.

If, for example, a good deal of freeze frame adn frame-by-frame "slow-
motion" analysis is required, then perhaps the open-reel half-inch EIA-J
VTRs** are best; they offer interchangeability and easy access to hand-
shuttle the tape. If true slow-motion (without frame bars***) is necessary
and interchange of tapes with other users is unimportant, then the Sanyo
VTC-7150X ensemble could be the choice.

If a trainer needs a reliable format to exchange or distribute tapes,
the popular U-matic or new ½″ cassette (the "Beta" or "VHS" type)
formats afford simple, full color reliable machines. The cost of the VTR
may be only a part of which format is better; one must consider the cost
of the tape also (the "Beta" format and similar ones being significantly
less expensive).

In video one is never certain of a company's commitment to the long-
term production of a given line. It is better to be conservative, to purchase in an established but continually improving line. To be sure, the
¾″ format appears established, but the lower purchase and operating
costs of the Beta format gives us pause to reflect on what the future
will hold.

It seems safe to assume reasonable longevity for the ¾″ format and,
because of the large consumer market, and in spite of the promised video
disk, a bright future for the Betamax-type "home video" systems. While

---

* An interesting JVC feature is a small color camera to mate with their "Vidstar"
VTR—cost of the basic camera is $1600; fully equipped with electronic viewfinder,
etc., $2100.
** "VTR," meaning Video Tape Recorder, is now used almost interchangeably
with VCR, Video Cassette Recorder (meaning the ¾″ U-matic device and ½″
"Beta"-type cassette recorders).
*** Hand rotating the heads causes "slow motion" but also reveals disturbing frame
bars that roll up the screen at the same time. True slow motion is the "instant replay"
often seen on commercial T.V. sports telecasts; it is "clean" and without visual disturbance.

the quality of certain second generation ¾″ videocassettes recorders makes them usable as professional and medical/industrial mastering instruments, the economic edge of the Selectavision and Betamax VTRs makes them a good possibility for a number of instructional distribution networks and modest clinical applications.

But no matter what the format of the VTR, each deck performs a like role in the system. The videotape recorder is a passive recording device that receives the video signal from the camera and "imprints" it in a magnetic process on tape. Upon replay these electronic images are read by the VTR and displayed on a video monitor, television set, large screen projector—whatever.

The quality of a VTR is usually easy to establish. Two favorite criteria are: resolution and signal-to-noise.

For a given dollar amount look first for the VTR with the best horizontal resolution: 320 lines or better in a monochrome (black and white) picture and 250 lines or better in color are very good VTR; 280 monochrome and 240 color are acceptable.

In the same price category, look next for video signal-to-noise.* A VTR that gives you back a picture with 45 db or better signal-to-noise is doing an excellent job. Forty db is the lowest one should go in color. Essentially the higher the rating, the better (50 db is the practical ceiling). Audio signal-to-noise should be in the same range.

A simple camera/VTR ensemble is the "portapack." An umbilical cable connects the recorder to the camera. It carries sound and picture from the built-in microphone and video pick-up tube in the camera to the VTR. Essentially every single camera system is like it: modifications and variations are not functionally very significant.

One can connect a microphone and camera by their respective cables to virtually any videotape recorder.** Similarly one can connect two videotape recorders together so that "dubbing" or copying from one deck to the other can be accomplished. The process is simply to connect a video cable from the video "out" of one deck to the video "in" of the other. An audio cable is then connected from audio "out" of one deck to the audio "in" of the other. Excellent aids to exact systems interconnection are found in the manufacturer's literature.

---

* That is a rating of the amount of noise or "snow" (seen as specks) in proportion to the amount of signal or picture.

** A videotape reproducer or player only has *no* capability for recording but only for the playback of tapes recorded on its particular format.

Monitoring/viewing Equipment

For replay of tapes or live camera origination, it is most often essential* to connect some sort of monitoring device or viewing equipment to see the product. Today we are fortunate to have a wide variety of excellent black and white and color video monitors and receivers. Large screen video projectors are commonplace where groups watch closed circuit video.

It is impossible to name just a few good black and white monitors. Almost any monitors from major manufacturers** will render years of trouble-free service. In color monitors the Trinitron tube offers an excellent performance value. Once only Sony manufactured TVs with the Trinitron tube but now Videotek, World Video, Inc., Amtron, and Unimedia (and others) have full lines of Trinitron tube televisions.

Some comment about the traditional mix-up over monitors and receivers seems to be in order.

1. A home television is typically a television *receiver.* It can be tuned to receive outside telecasts. It has no provision for displaying anything but a *modulated* television picture that can be *tuned in* to one of its VHF/UHF channels. If one has a videotape recorder with an RF modulator (sometimes called an RF "convertor") for, say, channel 6, then a cable can be connected from the VTR to the VHF antenna terminals on the rear of the TV receiver. The receiver is then tuned to channel 6† and both the video and audio from the videotape can then be viewed.

2. A video monitor is a different kind of viewing instrument. It has *no* provision for displaying a modulated picture for it has no tuners. It is so designed as to display "raw" or "baseband" video—video that is not modulated. This kind of video signal characteristically comes from the video out of a VTR or camera. A monitor can be connected to this source and the picture will be seen from the videotape. Normally a video monitor displays only the picture; but now some monitors do have an audio am-

---

* In certain cameras (such as the portapack) one can view the picture as it is being recorded and see it played back—right in the electronic viewfinder in the camera. Studio cameras show the camera picture as it leaves the instrument *en route* to the VTR; but in nearly all cases we need a television monitor or other viewing device connected in the system to facilitate screening the recorded material or watching the line origination.

** Firms like: Setchell Carlson, Sony, Panasonic, JVC, Hitachi, Electrohome, etc.

† Channel 6 is arbitrary here; it need only be an unused channel in that local area. If *no* commercial station is broadcasting on channel 4 in the area, but one is on channel 6, then an RF modulator for channel 4 (unused) would be provided by the local dealer.

plifier and speaker to receive "raw" audio from the VTR to permit simultaneous picture and sound reproduction.
3. A monitor/receiver combines the features of both the receiver (tuning for UHF/VHF channels) and the sound and picture monitor. It is the most versatile and the best single purchase.

Large screen viewing equipment has matured to the point of respectability with the Advent* Video Beam. These feature-packed devices are monitor-receivers with a 5-foot (at $2500), 6-foot (at $2900) and 7/10-foot (at about $4000) diagnoal size picture. Although delicate, they are reliable, attractively designed instruments with surprising resolution, excellent color, and visual impact. Their place in training is being quickly established. Their major feature is that more individuals can be "up front" and close for a good look at the material on the screen.

Tape

Currently the video and audio media depend almost exclusively on tape. It does not seem that the promised video disc will change that very much for quite some time.

Each of the videotape recorders listed above utilizes some form of magnetic tape; there are any number of videotapes on the market today.

As to formats, commonly available tape comes in varying widths and housings: 1) 1″ wide open reel; 2) ¾″ wide U-matic videocassette; 3) ½″ wide open reel; 4) ½″ wide Beta or VHS format cassette;** 5) ½″ wide cartridge (various subtypes); 6) ¼″ wide open reel (for Akai videotape recorders).

Most modern videotapes will adequately record both color and black and white video signals. Any tape that will not record color successfully is hardly worth a purchase.

Many believe that 3M Scotch has the best all around line for videotape in the industry. Certainly for anyone doing editing with ¾″ U-matic systems, the 3M Master Broadcast Cassette is the tape of choice to withstand high degrees of stress encountered in shuttling during editing. It is also a durable tape with high performance specifications for general taping of important material since it is less susceptible to stretching or tearing than conventional tape.

---

* There are other emerging large screen projectors and seeing is believing. Each should be judged on its relative merits and the user can tell the picture quality just by viewing; the service records should also be reviewed.

** Often the type of ½″ cassette or cartridge is further described by the machine it is used for: e.g., *Betamax* ½″ Cassette.

In addition to 3M, another respected name in tape is Sony. Both manufacturers produce excellent high energy and standard tapes in a number of formats.

Any tape can be damaged or short-lived if normal precautions in handling and storage are not observed:

1. No food and no smoking near tapes.
2. Only handle the end of the tape to avoid natural skin oils collecting on the video heads and subsequently damaging the tape.
3. Avoid heat, dust, moisture and sun *extremes* with tape.
4. Since taped information is stored in magnetic configurations, do not allow a stray magnet near the tape or accidental erasure may occur.
5. If you don't know how, don't attempt to open a cartridge or cassette.
6. Do not leave partially unspooled tape on the machine.
7. Keep VTR heads, guides, drums, etc., clean.
8. Think of a videotape reel as a phonograph record—handle it by the edges and store it upright in its box.
9. Avoid creasing or crimping the tape.

Remember also that, unlike audio recording tape, on videotape the shiny side is the recording side; the dull side is the back.

Graphics

A very exciting device for the fabrication of television and other graphics is the Reynold Leteron lettering machine (the firm is located in California). This device uses tape and punches perfect white (or whatever color) letters out for use on key cards, posters, and the like. The machine comes in either a manual or an electric version and it puts professional-looking television graphics within easy reach of the "average" trainer.

Storage and Moving Equipment

Organization is the key to even the humblest of video installations. Tapes must be carefully labeled, supplies and equipment properly stored, moved and positioned. Here are some tools:

1. The Wilson, Bretford, and Advance Products Companies all have a full line of tape, monitor, and VTR storage racks, rolling tables and carts.
2. The Winsted Corporation, in addition to traditional and "floating aisle" storage shelf systems (whereby one can put a great deal in a little space), has a series of adjustable, modular "editing consoles" for VTR, monitor and related instrument positioning.

These items are space-saving, functional pieces that can be made to fit around corners to do the job of keeping equipment at arm's length.
3. For getting portable ENG or "mini-cam" tape ensembles from here to there: (a) Camera Mart, New York City, has a "Crash Cart." (b) Gruber has a "Wheelit." (c) Giffen Video, Inc., Staten Island, New York, has a collapsing hand truck. (d) Portabrace has a wheel carriage. Each item can be fitted for any number of camera/VTR rigs. They are an invaluable asset.

Test Equipment

Eventually most of us learn at least the basics of equipment "trouble-shooting." Test and measurement tools are a necessary addition to the video system. At first it may be a simple volt-ohm meter, but often the test equipment need grows with the sophistication of both the system and the user.

Perhaps the finest and most established "industry standard" in test equipment is Tektronix, Inc. of Beaverton, Oregon. Television signal measurement and test equipment from this firm is simply the best there is. Other fine lines of TV test equipment are manufactured by Sencore and B & K Electronics.

A full set of hand tools is another useful addition to even the basic video system. Much money could be saved if the new purchaser of video equipment were to insist that the vendor completely familiarize the customer with preventive and simple maintenance.

For electronics hand tools one of the leaders is Jensen Tools & Alloys in Tempe, Arizona. The basic tools needed are: 1) several small files; 2) knife (heavy duty "penknife"); 3) nutdriver set; 4) long-nose and chain-nose pliers; 5) diagonal cutters; 6) electrician's scissors; 7) Phillips and slotted (regular) screwdriver set; 8) soldering gun; 9) solder (electronic), flux; 10) tweezers; 11) wire stripper; 12) allen-hex wrench set; 13) ball-peen hammer; 14) Triplett 310 VOM Meter.

Most basic repair can be done by the user; even those who have not thought of themselves as technicians have learned preventive and basic maintenance. This is a satisfying and economical practice that keeps more equipment "up" and used—not to mention the positive feeling of accomplishment.

Video Equipment Shows

These groups sponsor some of the more popular annual and periodic expositions and shows for the latest video equipment: 1) The National Association of Broadcasters; 2) The National Association of Educational

Broadcasters; 3) The Society of Motion Picture and Television Engineers; 4) Knowledge Industries: New York Video Expo; 5) The Los Angeles Video Show; 6) The International Video Conference and Exhibition (Cannes, France). There is good reason to visit an equipment show: ample opportunity to shop and compare, to use it to see it work.

SOME PROJECTIONS ON TECHNICAL DEVELOPMENTS FOR THE
NEAR AND NOT-SO-NEAR FUTURE

Some parts of the future are with us now. We have rapid access video data systems, high speed duplication equipment, sophisticated computer controlled, time base corrected videotape editing ensembles, and elaborate microwave and laser beam transmission systems.

We know we can expect the further development of fiber optic transmission techniques, the evolution of the video disc as a home and potential medical/industrial program replay medium. The introduction of a practical, good resolution, low cost pocket-size mini-camera seems imminent. Flat screen (non-picture tube) television and holographic movies seem likely to become everyday realities before very long. And certainly the marriage between video and computer technologies is destined to create fascinating progeny.

What all this can mean to the mental health care professions may depend largely on those in the professions. Manufacturers tend to respond to need. It would seem beneficial for the professional to demonstrate the need for video as an adjunct to treatment and training process by actively learning about and carefully integrating developing technologies into the care of the ill. One clear lesson we have learned to date is that any technology—existing or emerging—will serve humanity only as much as we force it to.

29

VIDEOTAPE APPRAISAL

Milton M. Berger, M.D.

In the last decade we have moved from the reluctant acceptance of so-called "home movie" type videotapes to a demand for quality presentations which come closer to, if not exactly approximating, what we technically experience daily on commercial television.

We can now hold a voluntary viewing audience for our video programs only if we pay attention to those technical, production and editing considerations which will affect the television picture quality that finally emerges on the monitor(s) or large-screen and to the sound as well as to the contents.

When an original video recording is made on equipment which is low resolution capacity, then any and every defect in the picture or sound is magnified tremendously when enlarged and projected on a large screen.

In reviewing and evaluating a tape there are a number of areas to be examined and scored on a scale of your own creation. I find it easy to grade the following on a scale of 1 to 5:

I. Does the tape clearly state its content and objectives and does it fulfill those objectives? Does it have academic and other educational value? Are there built in questions and answers?

II. Does the tape maintain viewer interest? and is it aesthetically satisfying?

III. How is the picture quality? Clear or blurred? Are there break-ups or "glitches"? Are special effects used? Are they appropriate? helpful? overdone? Are edits and bridging smooth or jumpy and distracting?

IV. How is the sound? audible? even? sometimes clear and sometimes inaudible? Do I have to strain to hear the dialogue?

V. How about the camera work? Is it steady? jumpy? all over the place? Does the picture fit in with and complement the sound of the speaker or narration or graphics? Are total group, dyads and individual shots

370

interspersed? Any pan shots? speed o.k.? even? Does the context come through?

VI. Are graphics used? enough? too many? Are they on camera long enough? too long? too short? Do individual graphics carry too much data?

VII. Are there credits?

VIII. Could this tape be improved if it were shortened? How?

IX. Would I use this tape for training? If not, why not?

If you intend to prepare videotapes for loan, rental or sales to other professionals and/or institutions it is advisable to include the following data:

1. The title.
2. The producer.
3. Physical description: Length, whether sound or silent, in color or black and white.
4. Contents accompanied by the objectives for the presentation.
5. The audience for whom it is intended.
6. Whether it does or does not contain privileged or confidential information thus restricting its potential audience.
7. Whether supplementary materials such as a guide book, self-assessment quiz or references are available with the videotape.
8. Whether it stands alone or is part of a series.
9. What format it is available in, i.e., video, film, film-strip; which video formats, one-half inch reel to reel, three-quarter inch cassette, one inch reel to reel, two inch or 8, 16 or 35 mm. film?
10. Whether available free on loan, or prices for rental or sale.
11. How to obtain it.

SECTION VI
Bibliographies and Glossaries

An attempt has been made to bring together here as comprehensive a listing of articles in English as possible. Because of the newness of the field, a glossary is also included in this section. It is divided into two parts: the first dealing with professional and theoretical terms, and the second a technical glossary referring to the "hardware" and to production terms.

SELECTED PROFESSIONAL REFERENCES ON VIDEO

ABROMS, G. C. and CHILES, J. A.: A Basic Psychiatry Course for Medical Students. *J. Med. Educ.*, 17:071-978, 1972.

ADLER, L. M., et al.: Changes in Medical Interviewing Style After Instruction with Two Closed-Circuit Television Techniques. *J. Med. Educ.*, 45:21-8, 1970.

AFFLECK, D. C.: Two-Way TV in Group Psychotherapy. *Counc. Med. Telev. Newsl.*, 2:2-3, 1962.

AGNELLO, S. A.: Closed-Circuit TV for Hospitals—Application and Guidelines. *Canadian Hosp.*, 47:31-4, 1970.

ALGER, I. and HOGAN, P.: Use of Videotape Recordings in Conjoint Marital Therapy in Private Practice. *Amer. J. Psychiatry*, 123:1425-1430, 1967.

ALGER, I. and HOGAN, P.: The Impact of Videotape Recording on Involvement in Group Therapy. *J. Psychoanal. Groups*, 2:50-56, 1967.

ALGER, I. and HOGAN, P.: Enduring Effects of Videotape Playback Experience on Family and Marital Relationships. *Amer. J. Orthopsychiat.*, 39:86-98, 1969.

ALGER, I.: Therapeutic Use of Videotape Playback. *J. Nerv. Ment. Dis.*, 148:430-436, 1969.

ALGER, I.: Television Image Confrontation in Group Therapy. In C. J. Sager and H. Kaplan (Eds.), *Progress in Group and Family Therapy*. New York: Brunner/Mazel, 1972.

ALGER, I.: Audio-Visual Techniques in Family Therapy. *Seminars in Psychiatry*, 5: 185-193, 1973.

ALGER, I.: Integrating Immediate Video Playback in Family Therapy. In P. J. Guerin (Ed.), *Family Therapy: Theory and Practice*. New York: Gardner Press, 1976.

ALGER, I.: Motion Pictures and Psychiatry. In B. Wolman (Ed.), *International Encyclopedia of Psychiatry, Psychology, Psychoanalysis and Neurology*. New York: Aesculapius, 1977. Pp. 276-280.

ALGER, I.: Audiovisual Techniques in Psychotherapy. In B. Wolman (Ed.), *International Encyclopedia of Psychiatry, Psychology, Psychoanalysis and Neurology*. New York: Aesculapius, 1977. Pp. 211-212.

ALKER, H. A., TOURANGEAU, R., and STAINES, B.: Facilitating Personality Change with Audiovisual Self-Confrontation and Interviews. *J. Consult. and Clin. Psychol.*, 44:720-728, 1976.

374   *Videotape in Psychiatric Training, Treatment*

ALKIRE, A. and BRUNSE, J.: Impact and Possible Casualty from Videotape Feedback in Marital Therapy. *J. Consult. and Clin. Psychology,* 42:203-210, 1974.

ALPERT, M.: Television Tape for Evaluation of Treatment Response. *Psychosomatics,* 11:467-469, 1970.

ANDERSON, C. M.: In Search of a Visual Rhetoric for Instructional Television. *AV Communication Review,* 20:43-63, 1972.

ANDERSON, C. and SAINATO, H. K.: Use of Videotape Feedback as a Psychotherapeutic Nursing Approach with Long-Term Psychiatric Patients: A Pilot Study. *Nursing Research,* 22:507-515, 1973.

ARCHER, J., et al.: New Method for Education, Treatment, and Research in Human Interaction. *J. of Counsel. Psychology,* 19:275-281, 1972.

ARCHER, J. and KAGAN, N.: Teaching Interpersonal Relationship Skills on Campus: A Pyramid Approach. *J. of Counsel. Psychology,* 20:535-540, 1973.

ARMSTRONG, R. G. Playback Technique in Group Psychotherapy. *Psychiat. Quart.,* XXXVIII, 38:247, 1964.

ARMSTRONG, J. D. and WORSEY, R. C.: The Adding of Visual Information to Previously Recorded Video-Tapes: A Functioning System. *Quart. J. Experimental Psychol.,* 24:361-363, 1972.

ATKIN, CHARLES K.: The Relationship Between Television Violence Viewing Patterns and Aggressive Behavior in Two Samples of Adolescents. *Dissertation Abstracts International,* 32:7021, 1972.

BAHNSON, C. B., IFFARRAGUERRI, A., and CORNELISON, F. S.: Personality and Self Image in Hemophilic Patients. Proceedings of the Fourth World Congr. Psychiatry, Madrid, Spain, 1966. *Excerpta Medica Intern. Congr.* Ser. No. 150, Part IV, 2752-2755, 1968.

BAHNSON, C. B.: Body and Self-Images Associated with Audio-Visual Self Confrontation. *J. Nerv. Ment. Dis.,* 148:262-280, 1969.

BAILEY, K. and SOWDER, T.: Audiotape and Videotape Self-Confrontation in Psychotherapy, *Psychol. Bulletin,* 74:127-137, 1970.

BAKER, T. B., UDIN, H. and VOGLER, R. E.: The Effects of Videotaped Modeling and Self-Confrontation on the Drinking Behavior of Alcoholics. *Int. J. Addict.,* 10:779-93, 1975.

BANDURA, A., ROSS, D. and ROSS, S. A.: Imitation of Film-Mediated Aggressive Models. *J. Abnorm. So. Psychol.,* 66:3-11, 1963.

BARBER, W. H. and LURIE, H. J.: Designing an Experientially Based Continuing Education Program. *Amer. J. Psych.,* 130:1148-1150, 1973.

BARNES, L. H., et al.: Psychiatric Patients and Closed Circuit Television Teaching: A Study of Their Reactions, *Brit. J. Med. Educ.,* 3:58-61, 1969.

BAUM, D. D.: Equivalence of Client Problems Perceived Over Different Media. *J. of Couns. Psychol.,* 21:15-22, 1974.

BEAN, B. W. and DUFF, J. L.: The Effects of Videotape and of Situational and Generalized Focus of Control Upon Hypnotic Susceptibility. *Am. J. Clin. Hypn.,* 18:28-33, 1975.

BECK, T. K.: Videotaped Scenes for Desensitization of Test Anxiety. *J. Behavior Ther. Exper. Psychiat.,* 3:195-197, 1972.

BELMONT, L., BIRCH, H., and BELMONT, I. Auditory-Visual Intersensory Processing and Verbal Mediation. *J. Nerv. Ment. Dis.,* 147:562-569, 1968.

BENSHOTER, R. A., EATON, M. T., and SMITH, P. Use of Video-tape to Provide Individual Instruction in Technics of Psychotherapy. *J. Med. Ed.,* 40:1159-1161, 1965.

BENSCHOTER, R. A., CECIL, L., WITTSON, C. L., and INGHAM, C. G.: Teaching and Consultation by Television, I: Closed Circuit Collaboration. *Ment. Hosp.,* 16:99-100, 1965.

BENSCHOTER, R. A.: Multipurpose Television. *Ann. N. Y. Acad. Sci.,* 142:471-478, 1967.

BENSCHOTER, R. A., et al.: The Use of Closed Circuit TV and Videotape in the Training of Social Group Workers. *Soc. Work Educ. Report.* XV:18, 19, 30, 1967.

BENSCHOTER, R. A.: Defining Our Foundations. *J. Biocommunicat.,* 4:3:2-4, 1977.

BERGER, M. M. The Use of Films for Mental Hygiene Education. *Int. J. Soc. Psychiat.,* 3:109-113, 1957.

BERGER, M. M. and GALLANT, D. M.: The Use of Closed Circuit Television in Teaching of Group Psychotherapy. *Psychosomatics,* 6:16-18, 1965.

BERGER, M. M., SHERMAN, B., SPALDING, J., and WESTLAKE, R.: The Use of Videotape with Psychotherapy Groups in a Community Mental Health Service Program. *Int. J. Group Psychother.,* 18:504-515, 1968.

BERGER, M. M. Therapist Insight Sharpened by Video Technique: Wide Use in Private Practice Predicted. *Psychiat. Progr.* (Eli Lilly), 3:2:3-5, 1968.

BERGER, M. M. Notes on the Communication Process in Group Psychotherapy. *J. Group Psychoanal. and Proc.,* 2:29-36, 1969.

BERGER, M. M. Integrating Videotape into Private Practice. *Voices,* 5:78-85, 1970.

BERGER, M. M. (Ed.): *Videotape Techniques in Psychiatric Training and Treatment,* First Edition. New York: Brunner/Mazel, 1970.

BERGER, M. M.: Self-Confrontation Through Video. *Amer. J. Psychoanal.,* 31:48-58, 1972.

BERGER, M. M.: Review of Research Papers on Videotape. *J. Comparat. Group Studies,* pp. 177-190, May, 1970.

BERGER, M. M.: A Preliminary Report on Multi-Image Immediate Impact Video Self-Confrontation. *Am. J. Psychiat.,* 130:304-306, 1973.

BERGER, M. M.: Video in Group Psychotherapy. In G. Goldman, et al. (Eds.), *Group Process Today.* Springfield, Ill.: Charles C Thomas, 1974, pp. 273-288.

BERGER, M. M., FREIMEIR, R. C., RYAN, J. H., FORREST, D. V., SHAMASKIN, R. B., et al.: Video Psychiatry Comes of Age. *Frontiers of Psychiat.,* Vol. 4 (No. 4), pp. 1, 2, 8, 11, Feb. 15, 1974.

BERGER, M. M.: The "I Can't Believe It" Reaction to Video Self Confrontation. *Current Concepts in Psychiat.,* 3:2-6, 1977.

BERGER, M. M.: The Use of Videotape Techniques in Clinical Practice. *Week. Psychiat. Update Series,* No. 50, Sept. 1977.

BERMAN, A. L. Videotape Self-Confrontation of Schizophrenic Ego and Thought Processes. *J. Consult. and Clin. Psychol.,* 39:78-85, 1972.

BERNAL, M. E., DURYEE, J. S., PRUETT, H. L., and BURNS, B. J.: Behavior Modification and the Brat Syndrome. *J. Consult. Psychol.,* 32:447-455, 1968.

BERNAL, M. E.: Behavioral Feedback in the Modification of Brat Behaviors. *J. Nerv. Ment. Dis.,* 148:375-385, 1969.

BERTOU, P. D.: An Analysis of the Relative Efficacy of Advance Organizers, Post Organizers, Interspersed Questions and Combinations Thereof in Facilitating Learning from Televised Instruction. *Dissertation Abstracts Intern.* 32 (6-A):3084, 1971.

BLANCHERI, R. L. and MERRIL, I. R.: Television in Health Sciences Education: Camera Placement. *Nurs. Res.,* 13:217-221, 1964.

BODIN, A. M.: Videotape Applications in Training Family Therapists. *J. Nerv. Ment. Dis.,* 148:251-261, 1969.

BODIN, A. M. The Use of Videotapes. In A. Ferber, et al. (Eds.), *The Book of Family Therapy.* New York: Science House, 1972.

BORTON, T.: Dual Audio Television. *Harvard Educat. Review,* 41:64-78, 1971.

BOYD, H. S. and SISNEY, V. V.: Immediate Self-Image Confrontation and Changes in Self-Concept. *J. Consult. Psychol.,* 31:291-294, 1967.

BOYD, J. and VADER, E. A.: Captioned Television for the Deaf. *Amer. Annals of the Deaf,* 117:34-37, 1972.

BRAUCHT, G. N.: Immediate Effects of Self-Confrontation on the Self-Concept. *J. Consult. Clin. Psychol.,* 35:95-101, 1970.

BRAYTON, D.: Postgraduate Education in Medicine by Television. *Biomed. Sci. Instr.,* 3:81-88, 1967.

BROOKS, D. D.: Teletherapy Or How to Use Videotape Feedback to Enhance Group Process. *Perspect. Psychiat. Care,* 14:83-87, 1976.

BROSIN, H. R., SCHEFLEN, et al.: The Sound Camera Breakthrough in Research, Training, Therapy. *Roche Report: Frontiers of Clinical Psychiatry,* 6:15-16, 1969.

BUGENTHAL, D. E., LOVE, L. R., KASWAN, J. W. and APRIL, C.: Verbal-Nonberval Conflict in Parental Messages to Normal and Disturbed Children. *J. Abnorm. Psychol.,* 77:6-10, 1971.

BUGENTHAL, D. E., LOVE, L. R., and KASWAN, J. W.: Videotaped Family Interaction: Differences Reflecting Presence and Type of Child Disturbance. *J. Abnorm. Psychol.,* 79:285-290, 1972.

BURR, M. and HAZEN, B.: The Use of Television in the Rehabilitation of Stroke Patients with Perceptual Difficulties. *Australian Occup. Ther. J.,* 19:19-23, 1972.

CALDWELL, K. S.: Guidelines and Principles for the Utilization of Animation in Instructional Films and Videotapes. *Dissertation Abstracts Intern.,* 33 (10-A):5613, 1973.

CALLAWAY, S., BOSSHART, D. A., and O'DONNELL, A. A.: Patient Simulation in Teaching Patient Education Skills to Family Practice Residents. *J. Fam. Pract.,* 4:709, 1977.

CAMPEAU, P. L.: Selective Review of the Results of Research on the Use of Audiovisual Media to Teach Adults. *Av. Communicat. Review,* 22 (1):5-40, 1974.

CARPENTER, K. F. and DROTH, J. A.: Effects of Videotaped Role Playing on Nurses Therapeutic Communication Skills, *J. Contin. Educ. Nurs.,* 7:47-53, 1976.

CARRERE, J.: Le Psycho Cinematographie. Principes et Technique. Application au Traitement des Malades Convalescents de Delirium Tremens. *Ann. Medico Psychol.,* 112:240-245, 1954.

CARRERE, J., CRAIGNOU, C., and POCHARD. D.: Quelques Resultants du Psycho Cinematographie dans la Psychotherapie des Delirium et Subdelirium Tremens Alcoholiques. *Ann. Medico Psychol.,* 113:46-51, 1955.

CASSETA, D. M., et al.: A Program for Enhancing Medical Interviewing Using Videotape Feedback in the Family Practice Residency. *J. Fam. Pract.,* 4:673-677, 1977.

CHANEY, D. C.: Involvement, Realism and the Perception of Aggression in Television Programmes. *Human Relations,* 23:373-381, 1970.

CHESLEY, S. M.: The Use of Videotape—The Expert Witness. *J. Amer. Instit. Hypno.* 15:161-162, 1974.

CHODOFF, P.: Supervision of Psychotherapy with Videotape: Pros and Cons. *Amer. J. Psychiat.,* 128:810-823, 1972.

CLINE, D. W.: Video Tape Documentation of Behavioral Change in Children. *Am. J. Orthopsychiat.,* 42:40-47, 1972.

CLINE, B., and DROFT, G.: The Desensitization of Children to Television Violence. *Proceedings of Annual Convention of Amer. Psycholog. Assoc.,* 7:99-100, 1972.

COLTON, F. V.: Cognitive and Affective Reactions of Kindergarteners to Video Displays. *Child Stud. J.,* 2:63-66, 1972.

COONE, J. G., et al.: Role of the Classroom Instructor in a Televised Introductory Psychology Course. *Psychol. Rep.,* 23:43-47, 1968.

CORNELISON, F. S. and ARSENIAN, J.: A Study of the Response of Psychotic Patients to Photographing Self-Image Experience. *Psychiat. Quart.,* 34:1-8, 1960.

CORNELISON, F. S.: Samples of Psychopathology from Studies of Self-Image Experience. *Dis. of Nerv. Syst.,* 24:133-139, 1963.

CORNELISON, F. S. and TAUSIG, T. N. A Study of the Self-Image Experience Using Videotape at Delaware State Hospital. *Del. Med. J.*, 36:229-, 1964.

CORNELISON, F. S.: Learning About Behavior. A New Technique: Self-Image Experience. *Ment. Hyg.*, 50:584-587, 1966.

COZEAN, C. E. and REIVICH, R.: TV in Psychiatric Nursing Education: A preliminary Report. *Counc. Med. Telev. Newsl.*, 2, 1962.

CZAJKOSKI, E. J.: The Use of Videotape Recordings to Facilitate the Group Therapy Process. *Int. J. Group Psychother.*, 18:516-524, 1968.

DALE, E. and TRZEBIATOWSKI, G.: A Basic Reference Shelf on Audio-Visual Instruction. *Eric.* Stanford, Calif., Series 1, 17 p.., 1968 (Aug.).

D'AMBROT, F.: General Psychology Over Closed-Circuit Television: A Decade of Experience with 20,000 Students. *Av. Communica. Review*, 20:181-193, 1972.

DANET, B. N.: Self-Confrontation in Psychotherapy Reviewed: Videotape Playback as a Clinical and Research Tool. *Amer. J. Psychother.*, 22:246-257, 1968.

DANET, B. N.: Impact of Audio-Visual Feedback on Group Psychotherapy. *J. Con. and Clin. Psychol.*, 33:632, 1969.

DANET, B. M.: Videotape Playback as a Therapeutic Device in Group Psychotherapy. *Intern. J. Group Psychother.*, 19:433-440, 1969.

DANIELS, R. S. and PROSEN, H.: The Contribution of Visual Observation to the Understanding of an Interview. *Int. J. Group Psychother.*, 12:230, 1962.

DAVIES, H.: Social Imitation: A Neglected Factor in Psychotherapy? *British J. Psychiat.*, 121:281-285, 1972.

DAVIES, T. S.: Closed-Circuit Television in a Mental Hospital. *Brit. Med. J.*, 5318: 1531-1532, 1962.

DEL REY, P.: The Effects of Video-Taped Feedback on Form, Accuracy, and Latency in an Open and Closed Environment. *J. Motor Behav.*, 3:281-287, 1971.

DINOFF, M. et al.: Reliability of Videotape Interviewing. *Psychol. Reports*, 27:275-278, 1970.

DINOFF, M., STENMARK, D. E., and SMITH, R. E.: Comparison of Videotape and Face-to-Face Interviewing. *Psychol. Reports*, 27:53-54, 1970.

DINOFF, M., FINCH, A. J., and SKELTON, H. M. A Circuit for Videotape Interviewing and its Recording Reliability. *J. Applied Behav. Analysis*, 5:203-207, 1972.

DOYLE, R. B., COLEMAN, R., and WILLIAMS, W. A Task Related Social Behavior Adjustment Program for Chronic Psychiatric Patients. *Newsl. for Research in Ment. Health and Behavioral Sci.*, 15:9-11, 1973.

DWYER, F. M.: The Effect of Image Size on Visual Learning. *J. Experim. Educat.*, 39: 36-41, 1970.

EDELSON, R. I. and SEIDMAN, E.: Use of Videotaped Feedback in Altering Interpersonal Perceptions of Married Couples: A Therapy Analogue. *J. Consul. Clin. Psychol.*, 43:244-250, 1975.

EISENBUD, J., et al.: Two Camera and Television Experiments with Ted Serios. *J. Amer. Soc. Psychical Research*, 64:261-276, 1970.

EISLER, R. M., HERSEN, M., and AGRAS, W. S.: Effects of Videotape and Instructional Feedback on Nonverbal Marital Interaction: An Analog Study. *Behav. Therapy*, 4:551-558, 1973.

EISLER, R. M., HERSEN, M., and AGRAS, W. S.: Videotape: A Method for the Controlled Observation of Nonverbal Interpersonal Behavior. *Behav. Therapy*, 4:420-25, 1973.

EISLER, R. M., HERSEN, M., and MILLER, P. M.: Shaping Components of Assertive Behavior with Instructions and Feedback. *Amer. J. Psychiat.*, 131:1344-7, 1974.

ESVELDT, K. C., DAWSON, P. C., and FORNESS, S. R.: Effect of Videotape Feedback on Children's Classroom Behavior. *J. Educ. Research*, 67:453-456, 1974.

EVANS, R. and CLIFFORD, A.: Captured for Consideration—Using Videotape as an

Aid to the Treatment of the Disturbed Child. *Child: Care, Health Dev.*, 2:129-137, 1976.

EVANS, L. A., SNIBBE, J. R., JOHNSON, C. W., and AMON, S.: Use of Videotaped Patient Interview Simulation in Psychiatric Medical Education. *J. of Biocommunicat.*, 4:3:5-8, 1977.

FECHTER, J. V., Jr.: Modeling and Environmental Generalization by Mentally Retarded Subjects of Televised Aggressive or Friendly Behavior. *Amer. J. Ment. Deficiency*, 76:266-267, 1971.

FEIGHNER, A. C. and FEIGHNER, J. P.: Multimodality Treatment of the Hyperkinetic Child. *Amer. J. Psychiat.*, 131:459-463, 1974.

FEINSTEIN, C., and TAMERIN, J. S.: Induced Intoxication and Videotape Feedback in Alcoholism Treatment. *Quart. J. Stud. Alcohol.*, 33:408-416, 1972.

FLINT, C.: Legal and Ethical Aspects of Proprietary Rights to Federally Funded Media Programs. *J. Biocommunicat.*, 4:3:9-17, 1977.

FORD, F. and HERRICK, J.: Family Rules: Family Life Styles. *Amer. J. Orthopsychiat.*, 44:61-69, 1974.

FORREST, D. V., RYAN, H., GLAVIN, R., and MERRITT, H. H.: Through the Viewing Tube: Videocassette Psychiatry. *Amer. J. Psychiat.*, 131:90-94, 1974.

FROELICH, R. E. and BISHOP, F. M.: One Plus One Equals Three. *Med. Biol. Illus.*, 19:15-18, 1969.

FULLER, F. and MANNING, B. A.: Self-Confrontation Reviewed: A Conceptualization for Video Playback in Teacher Education. *Review Educat. Research*, 43:469-528, 1973.

FURMAN, S., and FEIGHNER, A.: Video Feedback in Treating Hyperkinetic Children: A Preliminary Report. *Amer. J. Psychiat.*, 130:792-796, 1973.

GANT, H. M.: Studies of Closed-Circuit Television in Psychotherapy Yield Promising Results. *Psychiat. News*, 3:8-9, 1968.

GEERSTMA, R. H. and STOLLER, R. J.: The Objective Assessment of Clinical Judgment in Psychiatry. *Arch. Gen. Psychiat.*, 2:278-285, 1960.

GEERTSMA, R. H. and REIVICH, R. S.: Repetitive Self-Observation by Videotape Playback, *J. Nerv. Ment. Dis.*, 141:29-41, 1965.

GEERTSMA, R. H. et al.: Auditory and Visual Dimensions of Externally Medicated Self-Observation. *J. Nerv. Ment. Dis.*, 148:210-223, 1969.

GEERTSMA, R. H. et al.: Videotape Recording of Emergency Room Care. *Med. and Biolog. Illust.*, 20:13-17, 1970.

GELSO, C. J.: Effect of Audiorecording and Videorecording on Client Satisfaction and Self-Expression. *J. Consult. and Clin. Psychol.*, 3:455-461, 1973.

GERGEN, K. J.: Self Theory and the Process of Self-Observation. *J. Nerv. Ment. Dis.*, 148:437-448, 1969.

GERSZEWSKI, M. C.: The Effects of Focused Videotape Feedback Upon Group Expressions of Warmth, Hostility, and Flight. *Dissert. Abstracts Internat.*, 33:4832-4833, 1973.

GLADFELTER, J.: Videotape Supervision of Co-Therapists. In M. M. Berger (Ed.), *Videotape Techniques in Psychiatric Training and Treatment* (Chapter 7). New York: Brunner/Mazel, 1970.

GOIN, M. K., and KLINE, F. M.: Supervision Observed. *J. Nerv. Ment. Dis.*, 1958: 208-213, 1974.

GOIN, M. K. and KLINE, F. M.: Countertransference: A Neglected Subject in Clinical Supervision. *Amer. J. Psychiat.*, 133:41-44, 1976.

GOIN, M. K., KLINE, F. M. and ZIMMERMAN, W.: The Use of Videotape in Teaching Supervision. *J. Psychiat. Educat.*, 1977 (in press).

GOLDFIELD, M. D. and LEVY, R.: The Use of Television Videotape to Enhance the Therapeutic Value of Psychodrama. *Amer. J. Psychiat.*, 125:690-692, 1968.

GONEN, J. Y.: The Use of Psychodrama Combined with Videotape Playback on an Inpatient Floor. *Psychiatry,* 34:198-213, 1971.

GORDON, C.: Self-Conceptions Methodologies. *J. Nerv. Ment. Dis.,* 148:328-364, 1969.

GOULD, J. and SMITH, K. U.: Angular Displacement of Visual Feedback of Motion. *Percept. Motor Skills,* 17:699-710, 1963.

GOULD, J. and SMITH, K. U.: Sensory Feedback Analysis of Stereotelevision Pursuit Tracking. *J. Appl. Psychol.,* 48:152-160, 1964.

GREEN, J. H., et al.: Use of Videotape Recording and Live Closed-Circuit Television in Teaching Medical Students. *Brit. J. Med. Educ.,* 1:135-143, 1967.

GREER, M. and PRADO, W. M.: Stimulating Participation in an Alcohol Treatment Program Through Videotape Modeling. *Newsl. Research Ment. Health and Behav. Sci.,* 15:34-35, 1973.

GREER, R. M. and CALLIS, R.: The Use of Videotape Models in an Alcohol Rehabilitation Program. *Rehab. Couns. Bull.,* 18:154-159, 1975.

GRIFFITHS, R. D.: Videotape Feedback as a Therapeutic Technique: Retrospect and Prospect. *Behav. Res. Ther.,* 12:1-8, 1974.

GRIFFITHS, R. D. and HINKSON, J.: The Effect of Videotape Feedback on the Self-Assessments of Psychiatric Patients. *Brit. J. Psychiat.,* 123:223-224, 1973.

GRUENBERG, P. B., LISTON, E. H., and WAYNE, G. J.: Intensive Supervision of Psychotherapy with Videotape Recording. *Amer. J. Psychother.,* 23:98-105, 1969.

HAGGARD, E. A., HIKEN, J. R., and ISAACS, K. S.: Some Effects of Recording and Filming on the Psychotherapeutic Process. *Psychiatry,* 28:169-191, 1965.

HARRIS, J. J.: Television as an Educational Medium in Medicine: An Historical Purview. *J. Med. Ed.,* 41:1-19, 1966.

HARTSON, D. J. and KUNCE, J. T.: Videotape Replay and Recall in Group Work. *J. of Counsel. Psychol.,* 20:437-441, 1973.

HECKEL, R. V.: The Television Camera as Co-Therapist in Group Psychotherapy. *The Psychiat. Forum,* Winter, 1975.

HECTOR, W.: Closed-Circuit Television for Schools of Nursing. *Nurs. Times,* 66:136-138, 1970.

HEIDEL, S., DILLON, D., ENGSTROM, F., LEHMAN, A., and THARP, D. Medical Student Assessment of Videocassettes in Psychiatry. *J. Med. Educ.,* 50:908-910, 1975.

HELLER, S., and POLSKY, S.: Television Violence: Guidelines for Evaluation. *Arch. of Gen. Psychiat.,* 24:279-285, 1971.

HERZKA, H. S.: Self-Confrontation in the First Year of Life. A Contribution to the Anthropology of the Child. *Prax. Kinderpsychol.,* 16:15-18, 1967.

HILLIARD, J., et al.: New Approaches to Teaching Basic Interview Skills to Medical Students. *Am. J. Psychiat.,* 127:10, 1971.

HIRSH, H. and FREED, H.: Pattern Sensitization in Psychotherapy Supervision by Means of Videotape Recording. *Psychiat. Spect.,* 5:7-8, 1968.

HOGAN, P. and ALGER, I. Impact of Videotape Recording on Insight in Group Therapy. *Int. J. Group Psychother.,* 19:158-165, 1969.

HOGAN, P.: The Use of Videotape Playback as a Technique in Psychotherapy. In G. D. Goldman and D. S. Milman (Eds.), *Innovations in Psychotherapy.* Springfield, Ill.: Charles C Thomas, Chapt. XXII, p. 293, 1972.

HOLMES, D. J.: Closed Circuit Television in Teaching Psychiatry. *Univ. Mich. Med. Bull.,* 27:330-336, 1961.

HOLZMAN, P. S.: On Hearing and Seeing Oneself. *J. Nerv. Ment. Dis.,* 148:198-209, 1969.

HORAN, J. J., HERR, E. L., and WARNER, R. W.: Effects of Audio and Video Montoring on Interviewer Discomfort. *J. Employ. Counsel.,* 10:40-43, 1973.

HUNT, W., MACKINNON, R., and MICHELS, R.: A Clinical Clerkship in Psychiatry. *J. Med. Educ.,* 50:1113-1119, 1975.

HUTSON, T. and OSEN, D.: A Multi-Media Approach to Gifted Children in a High

380 Videotape in Psychiatric Training, Treatment

School Group Psychology-Counseling Seminar. *Gifted Child Quart.*, 14:186-190, 1970.

IVES, J. M.: A Strategy for Instructional Television Research. *Av. Communicat. Review*, 19:149-160, 1971.

IVEY, A. E.: Attending Behavior: The Basis of Counseling. *School Counsel.*, 18:117-120, 1970.

IVEY, A. E.: *Microcounseling: Innovations in Interviewing Training.* Springfield, Ill.: Charles C Thomas, 1971.

IVEY, A. E.: Media Therapy: Educational Change Planning for Psychiatric Patients. *J. Couns. Psychol.*, 20:338-343, 1973.

JONES, N. A., SWANSON, A., and JOHNSON, J.: Educational Materials Reviewed for AVLINE. *J. Med. Educ.*, 51:299-304, 1976.

KAGAN, N., KRATHWOHL, D. R., and MILLER, R.: Stimulated Recall in Therapy Using Videotapes: A Case Study. *J. Counsel. Psychol.*, 10:237-243, 1963.

KAGAN, N. and KRATHWOHL, D. R.: Studies in Human Interaction. (Final Report, Grant No. OE7-32-0410-270) Ed. Publ. Serv., Mich. St. Univ., East Lansing, 1967.

KAGAN, N., SCHAUBLE, P., RESNIKOFF, A., DANISH, S. J., and KRATHWOHL, D. R.: Interpersonal Process Recall. *J. Nerv. Ment. Dis.*, 148:365-374, 1969.

KANNER, J. H.: The Instructional Effectiveness of Color in Television: A Review of the Evidence. *Eric*, Stanford, Calif., Series 1, p. 9 (Jan.) 1968.

KASWAN, J. et al.: Confrontation as a Method of Psychological Intervention. *J. Nerv. Ment. Dis.*, 148:224-237, 1969.

KEATING, J. P. and LATANE, B.: Distorted Television Reception, Distraction and Attitude Change. *Proceedings of Annual Convention Amer. Psycholog. Assoc.*, 7: 141-142, 1972.

KENDELL, R. E.: Psychiatric Diagnosis in Britain and the United States. *Br. J. Psychiat.*, Spec. No. 9:453-461, 1975.

KNIGHT, J. A.: The Impact of Confrontation in Learning. *J. Med. Educ.*, 41:670-678, 1966.

KOGAN, K. L. and GORDON, B.: A Mother-Instruction Program: Documenting Change in Mother-Child Interactions. *Child Psychiat. Human Dev.*, 5:189-200, 1975.

KORNFELD, D. S. and KOLB, L. C.: The Use of Closed Circuit TV in the Teaching of Psychiatry. *J. Nerv. Ment. Dis.*, 138:452-459, 1964.

KRUGMAN, H. E.: Brain Wave Measures of Media Involvement. *J. Advertis. Research*, 11:3-9, 1971.

KRUMBOLTZ, J. D.: Evaluation of Programmed Instruction. In J. P. Lysaught (Ed.), *Programmed Instruction in Medical Education.* Rochester, N.Y.: The Rochester Clearing House, 139-149, 1965.

KRYSTAL, H.: Postgraduate Teaching in Psychiatry: Combining Television and FM-Radio with Seminars. *Psychosomatics*, 3:1-4, 1962.

KUBIE, L. S.: Some Aspects of the Significance to Psychoanalysis of the Exposure of a Patient to the Televised Audiovisual Reproduction of His Activities. *J. Nerv. Ment. Dis.*, 148:301-309, 1969.

LaBRUZZO, R.: The What and How of Video Hardware and Tape. In M. M. Berger (Ed.), *Videotape in Psychiatric Training and Treatment.* New York: Brunner/ Mazel, 1970.

LAMBERD, W. G., ADAMSON, J. D., and BURDICK, J. A.: A Study of Self-Image Experience in Student Psychotherapists. *J. Nerv. Ment. Dis.*, 155:184-191, 1972.

LAQUEUR, H. P.: Systems Therapy. *Curr. Psychiatr. Ther.*, 11:52-55, 1971.

LAQUEUR, H. P.: Multiple Family Therapy: Questions and Answers. *Semin. Psychiat.*, 5:195-205, 1973.

LAUTCH, H.: Videotape Recording as an Aid to Behaviour Therapy. *Brit. J. Psychiatr.*, 117:207-208, 1970.

LAZES, P. M. et al.: Community-Oriented Videotapes: A Low-Cost, Effective Teaching Tool. *Int. J. Health Educ.*, 20:68-70, 1977.

LAWRENCE, S. B.: Videotape and Other Therapeutic Procedures with Nude Marathon Groups. *Amer. Psychol.*, 24:476-479, 1969.

LAZARUZ, H. R. and BIENLEIN, D. K.: Soap Opera Therapy. *Int. J. Group Psychother.*, 17:2:252-256, 1967.

LIEBERT, R. M. and BARON, R. A.: Some Immediate Effects of Televised Violence on Children's Behavior. *Develop. Psychol.*, 6:469-475, 1972.

LOEB, F. F., Jr.: The Microscopic Film Analysis of the Function of a Recurrent Behavioural Pattern in a Psychotherapeutic Session. *J. Nerv. Ment. Dis.*, 147:605-618, 1968.

LOMBARDI, T. P. et al.: Utilization of Videosonic Equipment with Mentally Retarded. *Ment. Retard.*, 6:7-9, 1968.

LOVE, A. M. and RODERICK, J. A.: Teacher Nonverbal Communication: The Development and Field Testing of an Awareness Unit. *Theory Into Pract.*, 10:295-299, 1971.

LURIE, H. J.: The Actress as a Mental Health Teacher. *Psychat. in Med.*, 4:183-189, 1973.

LYSAUGHT, J. P. and WILLIAMS, C. M.: *A Guide to Programmed Instruction.* New York: John Wiley and Sons, Inc., 1963.

LYSAUGHT, J. P., SHERMAN, C. D., Jr., and WILLIAMS, C. M.: Utilization of Programmed Instruction in Medical Education. *J. Med. Ed.*, 39:769-779, 1964.

MACLAY, D. T.: Teaching Psychiatry by Closed-Circuit Television. *Brit. J. Psychiat.*, 114:918-919, 1968.

MACLEAN, U.: Edinburgh Experiments in the Use of Television in the Teaching of Social Medicine. *Brit. J. Prevent. and Social Med.*, 24:62, 1970.

McDERMOTT, J. F. and HARRISON, S. I.: Some Considerations in the Use of Television During the Clinical Years. *J. Med. Educ.*, 39:889, 1964.

McGILL, G. A. and THRASHER, J. W.: Videotapes: The Reel Thing of the Future. *Trial Mag.*, Sept.-Oct., 1975, pp. 43, 48, 49.

McGUIRE, F. L., MOORE, F. J., HARRISON, C. A. and RILEY, R. E.: The Efficiency of Television as Applied to the Use of Laboratory Demonstrations in Teaching. *J. Med. Educ.*, 36:715-716, 1961.

McGUIRE, F. L. and STIGALL, T. T. Psychotherapy by Television: A Research Paradigm. *Psychother.: Theory, Res., Pract.*, 3:159-162, 1966.

McKEACHIE, W. J.: Teaching Psychology on Television. *Amer. Psychol.*, VII:503-506, 1952.

McMILLAN, G. J.: Video-Stimulated Recall in Pastoral Psychotherapy Training. *J. of Pastoral Care*, 28:262-266, 1974.

MAGER, R. F.: *Preparing Objectives for Programmed Instruction.* San Francisco: Fearon Publishers, 1961.

MAGER, R. F.: Criteria for Evaluation. In J. P. Lysaught (Ed.), *Self-Instruction in Medical Education.* Rochester, N.Y.: Rochester Clearing House, 1967.

MARTIN, G. L. and OVER, H. R.: Therapy by Television. *Audiov. Commun. Review*, 4:119-130, 1956.

MARVIT, R. C., LIND, J. and McLAUGHLIN, D. G.: Use of Videotape to Induce Attitude Change in Delinquent Adolescents. *Amer. J. Psychiat.*, 131:996-999, 1974.

MASON, EDWARD A.: Filmed Case Material: Experience or Exposure? *Amer. J. Orthopsychiat.*, 39:99-105, 1969.

MARTIN, C. V. and BANKS, F. M.: Marathon Group Therapy. *Psychother. and Psychosomat.*, 20:191-199, 1972.

MARTIN, R. D. et al.: Videotape Equipment and Procedures in Group Settings. *Intern. J. Group Psychother.*, 20:230-234, 1970.

MELNICK, J. and TIMS, A. R., Jr.: Application of Videotape Equipment to Group Therapy. *Int. J. Group Psychother.*, 24:199-206, 1974.

MERRILL, I. R.: Closed-Circuit Television in Health Sciences Education. *J. of Med. Educ.*, 38:329-338, 1963.

MENOLASCINO, F. J. and OSBORNE, R. G.: Psychiatric Television Consultation for the Mentally Retarded. *Amer. J. Psychiat.*, 127:515-520, 1970.

MICHAUX, M. H., COHEN, M. J., and KURLAND, A. A.: Closed-Circuit Television in the Scientific Measurement of Psychopathology. *Med. Biol. Illus.*, 13:49-57, 1963.

MILLER, G. E., ALLENDER, J. S., and WOLF, A. V.: Differential Achievement with Programmed Text, Teaching Machine, and Conventional Instruction in Physiology. *J. Med. Educ.*, 40:817-831, 1965.

MILLER, M. F.: Responses of Psychiatric Patients to their Photographed Images. *Dis. Nerv. System*, 23:296-298, 1962.

MILLER, D.: The Effects of Immediate and Delayed Audio and Videotaped Feedback on Group Counseling. *Comparat. Group Studies*, 1:19-49, 1970.

MONOGHAN, R. R. and McCARTHY, K. E.: A Media-Directed Communication Learning Program. *Gr. Psychother. and Psychodrama*, 23:5-15, 1970.

MOORE, F. J., HANES, L. C., and HARRISON, C. A.: Improved Television, Stereo and the Two-Person Interview. *J. Med. Educ.*, 36:162-166, 1961.

MOORE, F. J., CHERNELL, E., and WEST, M. J.: Television as a Therapeutic Tool. *Arch. Gen. Psychiat.*, 12:217-222, 1965.

MOORE, F. J., RUSSELL, S. C., HUBBARD, O. E., DAVIS, C. G., STUART, B. R., and OVERALL, J. E.: Clinical Judgment: The Effectiveness of Television and Videotape for the Symptomatic Evaluation of Psychiatric Patients.

MORENO Z. T.: Psychodrama on Closed and Open Circuit Television. *Group Psychother.*, 21:106-109, 1968.

MORENO, J. L.: Television Videotape and Psychodrama. *Amer. J. Psychiat.*, 125:1453-1454, 1969.

MUSLIN, H. L.: Overview: The Use of Recordings as Evaluation Mechanisms in Psychiatry. In H. L. Muslin et al. (Eds.), *Evaluative Methods in Psychiatric Education*. Washington, D.C.: American Psychiatric Association, 1974.

MUSLIN, H. L. (Ed.): *Evaluative Methods in Psychiatric Education*. Washington, D.C.: American Psychiatric Association, 1974.

MUZEKARI, L. H. and KAMIS, E.: The Effects of Videotape Feedback and Modeling on the Behavior of Chronic Schizophrenics. *J. Clin. Psychol.*, 29:313-316, 1973.

MUZEKARI, L. H., WEINMAN, B., and KREIGER, P. A.: Self-Experiential Treatment in Chronic Schizophrenia. *J. Nerv. Ment. Dis.*, 157:420-427, 1973.

MUZEKARI, L. J.: The Effects of Videotape Models on the Behavior of Chronic Schizophrenics. *J. Clin. Psychol.*, 32:801-802, 1976.

NEILSON, F.: *Studies in Self-Confrontation: Viewing a Second Motion Picture of Self and Another Person in a Stressful Dyadic Interaction*. Copenhagen: Munskaard, 1962.

NICOLETTI, J. and FLATER, L.: A Community-Oriented Program for Training and Using Volunteers. *Comm. Ment. Health J.*, 11:58-63, 1975.

NEWMARK, C. S., DINOFF, M., and RAFT, D.: The Standardized Videotape Interview as an Objective Dependent Variable in Psychotropic Drug Research. *J. Nerv. Ment. Dis.*, 158:18-24, 1974.

ONDER, J. J.: The Use of Television in Psychiatric Treatment and Education. *J. Soc. Motion Pict. Telev. Engrs.*, 77:1034-1037, 1968.

ONDER, J. J.: A Review of Television Formats for Students of Psychiatry. *Health Sci. TV Bull.*, 6:1-6, 1969.

ONDER, J. J.: *Manual of Psychiatric Television*. Ann Arbor, Mich.: Maynard House, 1970.

OSBORN, D. K. and ENDSLEY, R. C.: Emotional Reactions of Young Children to TV Violence. *Child Dev.*, 42:321-331, 1971.

PADEN, R. C., et al.: Videotape Versus Verbal Feedback in the Modification of Meal Behavior of Chronic Mental Patients. *J. Consult. Clin. Psychol.*, 42:623, 1974.

PALMER, R. R., LUISADA, P. V., and PEELE, R.: Training Paraprofessionals: A Learning Experience for Psychiatric Residents. *Hosp. Community Psychiat.*, 26:286-288, 1975.

PAREDES, A. and CORNELISON, F. S.: Development of an Audiovisual Technique for the Rehabilitation of Alcoholics. *Quart. J. Stud. Alcohol.*, 29:84-92, 1968.

PAREDES, A., LUDWIG, K. D., HASSENFELD, I. N., and CORNELISON, F. S., Jr.: A Clinical Study of Alcoholics Using Audiovisual Self-Image Feedback. *J. Nerv. Ment. Dis.*, 148:449-456, 1969.

PAREDES, A., et al.: Behavioral Changes as a Function of Repeated Self-Observation. *J. Nerv. Ment. Dis.*, 148:287-299, 1969.

PASCAL, G. R., COTTRELL, T. B., and BAUGH, J. R.: A Methodological Note on the Use of Videotape in Group Psychotherapy with Juvenile Delinquents. *Int. J. Group Psychother.*, 17:248-251, 1967.

PAULSON, F.: Live Versus Televised Observations of Social Behavior. *Proc. of Annual Conv. of Amer. Psychol. Assoc.*, 7 (Pt. 1):135-136, 1972.

PETERSON, M. H., EATON, M. T., Jr., and STRIDER, F. D.: Use of Programmed Instruction in Teaching the Defense Mechanisms. (Abstract) *J. Med. Ed.*, 42:874-875, 1967.

PETERSON, M. H. and STRIDER, F. D.: Confrontation Anxiety in Medical Students During Mirror-Room and Videotaped Interviews. In H. J. Conrad (Ed.), *Health Sciences TV Source Book.* Durham, N.C.: Duke University Medical Center, 1968.

PETERSON, M. H. and STRIDER, F. D.: Institutional Differences in Students Using a Programmed Text. In J. P. Lysaught (Ed.), *Individualized Instruction in Medical Education.* Rochester, N.Y.: The Rochester Clearing House, 1968.

RAMEY, J. W.: Teaching Medical Students by Videotape Simulation. *J. Med. Educ.*, 43:55-59, 1968.

RAWLS, J. R. et al.: Evaluation of Closed Circuit Television in Teaching Educational Psychology. *Psychol. Rep.*, 22:1041-1044, 1968.

REIVICH, R. S. and GEERTSMA, R. H.: Observational Media and Psychotherapy Training. *J. Nerv. Ment. Dis.*, 148:310-327, 1969.

REIVICH, R. S. et al.: Television and Psychiatry. Observation Media in Psychiatry: The Concept of a Learning Laboratory. *J. Kansas Med. Soc.*, 70:101-104, 1969.

RESNIKOFF, A., et al.: Acceleration of Psychotherapy Through Stimulated Videotape Recall. *Amer. J. Psychotherap.*, 24:102-111, 1970.

RESNIK, H. L., DAVISON, W. T., SCHUYLER, D., and CHRISTOPHER, P.: Videotape Confrontation After Attempted Suicide. *Amer. J. Psychiat.*, 130:460-463, 1973.

RICHTER, H. E.: Television Transmission of Psychoanalytic Interviews. 1-19, 1969.

ROGERS, A. H.: Videotape Feedback in Group Psychotherapy. *Psychother. Theory, Res., Pract.*, 5:1:37-40, 1968.

ROME, H. P.: Therapeutic Films and Group Psychotherapy. *Group Psychotherapy, A Symposium.* New York: Beacon House, 1945, pp. 247-254.

ROME, H. P.: Motion Pictures as a Medium of Education. *Ment. Hyg.*, 30:9-20, 1946.

RUHE, D. S., GUNDEL, S., LAYBOURNE, P. D., FORMAN, L. D., JACOBS, M., and EATON, M. T.: Television in Teaching Psychiatry. *J. Med. Educ.*, 35:916-927, 1960.

RUHE, D. S. and GENTRY, K. C.: Ten Years of Television at the University of Kansas Medical Center. *J. Kansas Med. Soc.*, 62:94-99, 1961.

RYAN, J.: Teaching and Consultation by Television: II. Teaching by Videotape. *Ment. Hosp.*, 16:101-104, 1965.

SCHEFLEN, A., KENDON, A., and SCHAEFFER, J.: On the Choices of Audiovisual

Media. In M. M. Berger (Ed.), Videotape Techniques in Psychiatric Training and Treatment. New York: Brunner/Mazel, 1970.

SCHERER, S. E. and FREEDBERG, E. J.: Effects of Group Videotape Feedback on Development of Assertiveness Skills in Alcoholics: A Follow-up Study. Psychol. Rep. 39:983-992, 1976.

SCHIFF, S. B. and REIVICH, R. S.: Use of Television as an Aid to Psychotherapy Supervision. Arch. Gen. Psychiatr., 10:84-88, 1964.

SCHNEIDER, J. M., ADDIS, B. M., and ADDIS, M.: Films in the Behavioral Science: An Annotated Catalog. Behav. Sci. Media Lab., Univ. of Oklahoma Med. School, 1970.

SCHNEIDER, J. M. and ENELOW, A. J.: Assessment of Medical Students in Psychiatry: Applications of Film and Videotape. In H. L. Muslin et al. (Eds.), Evaluative Methods in Psychiatric Education. Washington, D.C.: American Psychiatric Association, 1974.

SCHWARTZ, M. S. and SCHWARTZ, C. G.: Problems in Participant Observation. Amer. J. Soc., 60:343-353, 1955.

SCLARE, A. B. et al.: The Use of Closed Circuit Television in Teaching Psychiatry to Medical Students. Brit. J. Med. Educ., 2:226-228, 1968.

SCOTT, M.: Television Hypnosis. JAMA, 193:4:854-855, 1965.

SERBER, M.: Videotape Feedback in the Treatment of Couples with Sexual Dysfunction. Arch. Sex. Behav., 3:377-380, 1974.

SERBER, M.: Shame Aversion Therapy. J. of Behav. Ther. and Exper Psychiat., 1: 213-215, 1970.

SETHNA, E. R. and NEAL, C. D.: Television in Psychotherapy. Brit. Med. J. 5457364, 1965.

SHAFFER, M. K. and PFEIFFER, D. Television Can Improve Instruction. J. Nurs. Educ., 15:3-8, 1976.

SHOSTROM, E. L.: Witnessed Group Therapy on Commercial Television. Amer. Psychol., 23:207-209, 1968.

SIGAL, J. J., GUTTMAN, H. A., CHAGOYA, L., and LASRY, J. C.: Predictability of Family Therapists' Behavior. Can. Psychiat. Assoc. J., 18:199-202, 1973.

SILK, S.: The Use of Videotape in Brief Joint Marital Therapy. Amer. J. Psychother., 26:417-424, 1972.

SMITH, K. U., GOULD, J., and WARGO, L.: Sensory Feedback Analyses of Visual Behavior. A New Theoretical-Experimental Foundation of Physiological Optics. Amer. J. Optom. Arch. Amer. Acad. Opt., 40:365-417, 1963.

SMITH, K. U. and GOULD, J.: Sensory-Feedback Analysis of Behavior in Stereo-Televised Visual Fields. J. Appl. Psychol., 48:361-368, 1964.

SMITH, K. U. and SMITH, T. J.: Systems Theory of Therapeutic and Rehabilitative Learning with Television. J. Nerv. Ment. Dis., 148:386-429, 1969.

SPENCER, D. A. and SCHIFFER, P. L.: List of Descriptive Cataloging Elements for Use in Bibliographic Control of Nonprint Materials. J. Biocommunic., 4:3:18-23, 1977.

SPIVACK, J. D.: Interpersonal Process Recall: Implications for Psychotherapy. Psychotherapy: Theory, Research and Practice, 11:235-238, 1974.

STOLLER, F. H.: Therapeutic Concepts Reconsidered in Light of Videotape Experience. Comp. Group Stud., 1:5-17, 1970.

STOLLER, F. H. and LAPOLLA, H.: TV and the Patient's Self-Image. Roche Report: Frontiers of Hosp. Psychiat., 2:7, 1965.

STOLLER, F. H.: Group Psychotherapy on Television. An Innovation with Hospitalized Patients. Amer. Psychol., 22:158-162, 1967.

STOLLER, F. H.: The Long Weekend. Psychol. Today, 1:28-33, 1967.

STOLLER, F. H.: Accelerated Interaction: A Time-Limited Approach Based on the Brief Intensive Group. Int. J. Group Psychother., 18:220-258, 1968.

STOLLER, F. H.: Focused Feedback with Videotape: Extending the Groups Functions. In G. M. Gazda (Ed.), *Basic Innovations in Group Psychotherapy and Counseling.* Springfield, Ill.: Charles C Thomas, 1968.

STOLLER, F. H.: Use of Videotape (Focused Feedback) in Group Counseling and Group Therapy. *J. Res., Develop. Educ.,* 1:30-44, 1968.

STOLLER, F. H.: Videotape Feedback in the Group Setting. *J. Nerv. Ment. Dis.,* 148:457-466, 1969.

SUESS, J. F.: Teaching Clinical Psychiatry with Closed Circuit Television and Videotape. *J. Med. Educ.,* 41:483-488, 1966.

SUESS, J. F.: Teaching Psychodiagnosis and Observation by Self-Instructional Programmed Videotapes. *J. Med. Educat.,* 48:676-683, 1973.

TALBERT, E. E., WILDEMANN, D. G., and ERICKSON, M. T.: Teaching Non-Professionals Three Techniques to Modify Children's Behavior. *Psychol. Reports,* 37s 1243-1252, 1975.

Television in the New Charcot Amphitheatre of the Salpêtrière in Paris. *Presse Méd.,* 76:350, 10 Feb. 1968 (Fr.).

THELEN, M. H., FRY, E. A., DOLLINGER, S. J., and PAUL, S. J.: Use of Videotaped Models to Improve the Interpersonal Adjustment to Delinquents. *J. Consult. Clin. Psychol.,* 44:492, 1976.

THE MEDIA CENTER. Preparing a Teleclass: A Case Study. *Nurs. Outlook,* 23:681, 1975.

The Sound Camera: Breakthrough in Research, Training, Therapy. *Front. Clin. Psychiat.,* Vol. 6 (No. 14): pp. 1, 2, 5, 6, 8, 11, Sept. 1, 1969.

THOMPSON, J. W., NASH, L. R., and EMMITT, T.: Closed-Circuit TV Used for Psychotherapy. *Mod. Hosp.,* 105:60-61, 1965.

TOEMAN, Z.: Audience Reactions to Therapeutic Films. Group Psychotherapy: A Symposium. New York: Brown House, 255-259, 1945.

TARKELSON, L. O. and ROMANO, M. T.: Self-Confrontation by Videotape: A Remedial Measure in Teaching Diagnostic Evaluation. *JAMA,* 201:773-775, 1967.

TRETHOWAN, W. H.: Teaching Psychiatry by Closed Circuit Television. *Brit. J. Psychiat.,* 114:517-522, 1968.

TRULL, S. G.: California Medical Team Videotapes Sessions. *Med. Tribune,* 10, 1966.

ULETT, F. A., AKPINAR, S. and ITIL, T. M.: Hypnosis By Video Tape. *Intern. J. Clin. and Expert. Hypnosis.,* 20:46-51, 1972.

VAN ZOOST, B.: Premarital Communication Skills Education With University Students. *Family Coordinator,* 22:187-191, 1973.

VERWOERDT, A., NOWLIN, J. B. and AGNELLO, S. A.: A Technique for Studying Effects of Self-Confrontation in Cardiac Patients. *Health Sci. TV Bull.,* 2:1-6, 1965.

Video Gives Patients Clearer View of Themselves. *J. Rehab.,* 33:24-25, 1967.

Videotape Aids Psychiatric Therapy. *Med. Hosp.* 110:172, 1968.

VTR Plays a Key Role in Rehabilitating Addicts. *Canad. Hosp.,* 46:36-37, 1969.

WALDRON, J.: Teaching Communication Skills In Medical School. *Amer. J. Psychiat.,* 130:579-581, 1973.

WALKENSHAW, M. R.: An Investigation Into The Possible Therapeutic Usefulness of Videotape Self-Confrontation. *Dissertation Abstracts Intern.,* 33: (12-A), 6759, 1973.

WALTER, G. A. and MILES, R. E.: Changing Self-Acceptance: Task Groups and Videotape Feedback or Sensitivity Training? *Small Group Behav.,* 5:356-364, 1974.

WARD, W. D. and BENDAK, S.: The Response of Psychiatric Patients to Photographic Self-Image Experience. *Newsl. for Res. in Psychol., Vet. Admin.* 6:29-30, 1964.

WARREN, F. Z.: Medical Television: An Evaluation. *J. Med. Educ.,* 31:418, 1956.

WATTERS, W. W., ELDER, P., SMITH, S. L. and CLEGHORN, J.: Psychotherapy Supervision-A Videotape Technique. *Canad. Psychiat. Assoc. J.,* 16:367-368, 1971.

WATTS, J. C.: Closed-Circuit TV in Psychiatric Hospitals: An Aid to Nursing. *Nurs. Times*, 60:15-17, 1964.

WAXER, P. H.: Therapist Training in Nonverbal Communication. II. Nonverbal Cues for Depression. *J. Clin. Psychol.* 30:215-218, 1974.

WEIR, W. D.: Clinical Psychiatry Videotest. *Biomed. Communicat.* 3:5, 1975.

WILMER, H. A.: Role of Psychiatrist in Consultation and Some Observations on Videotape Learning. *Psychosomatics,* 8:193-195, 1967.

WILMER, H. A.: Practical and Theoretical Aspects of Videotape Supervision in Psychiatry. *J. Nerv. Ment. Dist.,* 145:123-130, 1967.

WILMER, H. A.: Technical and Artistic Aspects of Videotape in Psychiatric Teaching. *J. Nerv. Ment. Dis.,* 144-207-223, 1967.

WILMER, H. A.: You Know. Observations on Interjectory, Seemingly Meaningless Phrases in Group Psychotherapy. *Psychiat. Quart.,* 41:296-323, 1967.

WILMER, H. A.: Innovative Usess of Videotape on a Psychiatric Ward. *Hosp. Comm. Psychiat.,* 19:129-133, 1968.

WILMER, H. A.: The Undisguised Camera in Videotape Teaching of Psychiatry. *Visual/Sonic Med.,* 3:5-11, 1968.

WILMER, H. A.: Television as Participant Recorder. *Amer. J. Psychiat.,* 124:1157-1163, 1968.

WILMER, H. A.: Use of the Television Monologue With Adolescent Psychiatric Patients. *Amer. J. Psychiat.* 126:1760-1766, 1970.

Witnessed Group Therapy on Television: Therapeutic or Not? *Amer. Psychol.,* 23:759-761, 1968.

WILMER, H. A.: Murder, You Know. *Psychiat. Quart.,* 43:414-447, 1969.

WITTSON, C. and DUTTON, R. A.: New Tool in Psychiatric Education. *Ment. Hosp.,* 7:11-14, 1956.

WOODY, R. H., et al.: Stimulated Recall in Psychotherapy Using Television and Videotape. *Amer. J. Clin. Hypn.,* 7:234-241, 1965.

WOODY, R. H.: Teaching Hypnosis with Videotapes. *Amer. J. Clin. Hypnosis,* 8:111-113, 1965.

WOODY, R. H.: Clinical Suggestion and the Videotaped Vicarious Desensitization Method. *Amer. J. Clin. Hypn.,* 11:239-244, 1969.

WOODY, R. H. and SCHAUBLE, P. G.: Videotaped Vicarious Desensitization Methodology and Research. *J. Nerv. Ment. Dis.,* 148:281-286, 1969.

WOODY, R. H. and SCHAUBLE, P. G.: Desensitization of Fear by Videotapes. *J. Clin. Psychol.,* 25:102-103, 1969.

WOODY, R. H.: Clinical Suggestion in Videotaped Psychotherapy: A Research Progress Report. *Amer. J. Clin. Hypn.,* 14:32-37, 1971.

YOUNGE, K. A.: The Use of Closed Circuit Television for the Teaching of Psychotherapeutic Interviewing to Medical Students. *Can. Med. Assoc. J.,* 92:747-751, 1965.

ADDITIONAL SIGNIFICANT REFERENCES FOR THE USERS OF VIDEOTAPE

TOWARD IMPROVED LEARNING. Library of Congress Catalog Card No. 67-60029. Vol. I. (April 1967). Volume II is currently in press and both volumes will soon be on sale from the U.S. Government Printing Office. Inquiries and orders can be addressed to: Miss Katherine Skogstad, Information and Publications Officer, National Medical Audiovisual Center, Atlanta, Georgia 30333.

TV IN PSYCHIATRY NEWSLETTER. Send $10.00 to L. Tyhurst, M.D., Ed., Dept. of Psychiatry, Univ. British Columbia, Vancouver, B.C., Canada V6T 1W5.

JOURNAL OF NERVOUS AND MENTAL DISEASES. Volume 148, Nos. 3 and 4, March-April, 1969. Two complete issues devoted to Videotape.

AMERICAN PSYCHOLOGIST, Vol. 10:10, 1955. Entire issue devoted to psychological implications of television.

ANNOTATED BIBLIOGRAPHY ON TELEVISION AND VIDEOTAPE IN PSYCHIATRY. Brigitte L. Kenney, Research Associate, TV Project Staff, University of Mississippi Medical Center, Department of Psychiatry, Jackson, Mississippi. April, 1969.

SOUTH BEACH PSYCHIATRIC CENTER. Media Catalogue of fifty-five videotapes. Write to Media Coordinator, South Beach Psychiatric Center, 777 Seaview Avenue, Staten Island, New York 10305.

BOGEN, B. Guidelines for Producers and Distributors of Media for the Health Sciences. *J. Biocommunic.*, 4:3:24-29, 1977.

CATALOGING NON-PRINT AT NMAC: A Guide for the Medical Librarian. National Medical Audiovisual Center, Atlanta, 1974.

EDUCATIONAL TECHNOLOGY: Definition and Glossary of Terms, Vol. I, Assoc. Educ'al Communications and Technology Task Force on Definition and Terminology, Washington, D.C. AECT, 1977.

SELECTED TECHNICAL REFERENCES ON VIDEO

BENSINGER, CHARLES and the Editors of *Photographic Magazine: Petersen's Guide to Videotape Recording.* Los Angeles, Calif.: Petersen Publishing Co., 1973.

DIAMANT, LINCOLN, (Ed.): *The Broadcast Communications Dictionary.* New York: Hastings House, Publishers, 1974.

GTE SYLVANIA: *Lighting Handbook 6th Edition for Television, Theatre, Professional Photography.* Danvers, Mass.: GTE Sylvania Inc., 1977.

JONES, PETER: *The Technique of the Television Cameraman.* New York: Hastings House Publishers, Inc., 1971.

KYBETT, HARRY: *How to Use Video Tape Recorders.* Indianapolis: Howard W. Sams & Co., Inc. and The Bobbs-Merrill Co., Inc., 1974.

KYBETT, HARRY: *Videotape Recorders.* Indianapolis: Howard W. Sams & Co., Inc., and The Bobbs-Merrill Co., Inc., 1974.

MATTINGLY, GRAYSON and SMITH, WELBY: *Introducing the Single Camera System.* Washington, D.C.: S & M Productions, Ltd., 1971.

MILLERSON, GERALD: *The Technique of Lighting for Television and Motion Pictures.* London and New York: Focal Press, 1972.

MILLERSON, GERALD: *The Technique of Television Production.* New York: Hastings House Publishers, Inc., 1972.

NISBETT, ALEC: *The Technique of the Sound Studio.* New York: Hastings House Publishers, Inc., 1974.

NISBETT, ALEC: *The Use of Microphones.* New York: Hastings House Publishers, Inc., 1974.

PFANNKUCH, ROBERT: *The Television Signal.* Norwalk, Conn.: Audio Video Industries, Inc., 1968.

RAY, SIDNEY: *The Lens in Action.* New York: Hastings House Publishers, Inc., 1976.

ROBINSON, JOSEPH F.: *Videotape Recording.* New York: Hastings House Publishers, Inc., 1975.
The Focal Encyclopedia of Film and Television. New York: Hastings House Publishers, Inc., 1969.
TREMAINE, HOWARD M.: *Audio Cyclopedia.* Indianapolis: Howard W. Sams & Co., Inc., and The Bobbs-Merrill Co., Inc., 1973.
WEINER, PETER: *Making the Media Revolution.* New York: Macmillan Publishing Co., Inc., 1973.
ZETTL, HERBERT: *Television Production Handbook.* Belmont, Calif.: Wadsworth Publishing Company, Inc., 1968.

Periodicals:

Educational and Industrial Television. Ridgefield, Conn.: C. S. Tepfer Publishing Co., Inc.
Videography. New York: United Business Publications, Inc.

TECHNICAL AND PRODUCTION GLOSSARY

ADAPTORS-AUDIO—Compact metal and or plastic assemblies for interconnecting 2 audio cables or a single cable to a reocrding machine or panel with differing connectors to form a complete circuit or line. Common types of audio adaptors are:
¼" phone (female) to mini (male);
mini (female) to ¼' phone (male);
¼" phone (female) to RCA phono (male);
RCA phono (female) to ¼" phone (male);
mini (female) to sub-mini (male);
mini (female) to RCA phono (male);
RCA phono (female) to mini (male);
XLR (female) to ¼" phone (male);
¼" (female) to XLR (male).

ADAPTORS-VIDEO—Compact metal assemblies for interconnecting 2 video cables or a single cable to a recording machine or panel with differing connectors to form a complete circuit or line. Common types of video adaptors are:
UHF (female) to BNC (male);
BNC (female) to UNF (male);
F (female to BNC (male);

AFTRA—Acronym for the American Federation of Television and Radio Artists, the union for artists in live and taped TV and radio.

AMBIENT LIGHT—The natural existing illumination in a given space. The inexperienced cameraman will not notice it, but the camera will arrange to carry it onto the tape (unfortunately).

AMBIENT SOUND—The complete indirect and natural aural effect of a given space, including decay time, frequency emphasis, feeling of "presence," etc. . . *not* including any direct sound from any source (musicians, speakers, electronic devices, etc.). This is the most common cause for poor sound in non-commercial, psychiatric video productions (doors slamming, telephone rings, radiators hissing, people talking or laughing in the background, sirens going by).

ANGLE-SHOT—A camera shot from other than the "straight on" to the subject position (e.g., a 45 degree angle from perpendicular to the subject's face). It is of value in offering the subject and the viewer another "view-point" and in creation of a split-screen dialogue-interaction shot.

APERTURE—The lens opening—a determining factor in how much light will strike the video, movie or still camera's light sensitive material. The aperture's size is described in "f-stops"; the lower the number (e.g., f 1.4, 1.8, 2.0), the wider the aperture. Conversely, the higher the number (e.g., f 8.0, 11, 16, etc.), the narrower the aperture will be. Accordingly, wider apertures allow *more* and narrower apertures allow *less* of the existing, reflected light to pass through the lens optics.

ASPECT RATIO—The height-to-width ratio of a television picture, e.g. 3 units high x 4 units wide. An important factor in visualizing scripts, framing shots and preparing graphics.

AUDIO—Synonym for sound. The audio portion of a video program contains the music, speech, sound effects of that program and also the usually disturbing, discordant and unwanted ambient sounds previously noted.

AUDIO LEVEL—The volume of the sound portion of a program (also see "line level"). In preparing a program made up of segments recorded at different times, it is important to pay major attention to the sound levels of the segments so that the edited production will come through on a more equal sound level.

AUDIO MIXER (S)—An electronic device designed to allow for the combination and independent control of separate sound sources. The mixer ideally allows the operator to control the sound or audio levels of microphones, tape recorders, 16mm film projectors, etc. Less expensive mixers often mix only two, three or four microphones and perhaps a line level input. Mixers can piggyback on each other. The optimal inexpensive mixer has switch-selectable inputs for mixing either line or mike level inputs (see chapter 28, section on sound).

AUDIO TRACKS (S)—That portion of the videotape on which the sound information is recorded. Videotape recorders may have several audio tracks to permit stereo and the recording of multilingual productions with English on one track and Spanish, for example, on the other, with the recorder being able to select either track for playback.

BLOOMING—In certain types of low light level cameras, when an extremely bright (by contrast to the rest of the scene) object appears in the field of view, blooming is the visual effect at the point of the spectacular highlight. The phenomenon, although visually irritating, causes no damage to the pick-up tubes under normal conditions and appears like a gaseous explosion.

BRIDGES—Aural and or visual continuity elements that are intended to provide a connection between or a transition from preceding and upcoming program, segments or clips. In actual practice, a voiceover can bridge from one segment to another in a very smooth fashion with the assistance of a graphic as the video picture component or an audience shot in the background can allow for voice content continuity.

BURN (VIDICON TUBE)—The temporary or permanent image retention by the vidicon pick-up tube caused by excessively bright (often by contrast with the rest of the scene) object in the camera's field of view. Burn appears as a darkened image of the bright object in the video rasteran image that remains fixed even if the camera is moved, irised down or capped. Severe burn can be permanent; lesser burns can often be flushed out by pointing the defocused camera at a white card (the card covers the entire field of view of the camera) for an appropriate length of time. To avoid vidicon tube burns, remember to keep the camera from facing a bright light for any extended length of time.

BUSY (PICTURE)—An image in which there is an excess of competing details which create visual distraction from the intended source of interest. E.g. a set in which the background props, through placement and/or quantity, vie with the talent for the viewer's attention; or a jacket or coat of design sufficient to cause moiré, crawl, or apparent oscillation in the picture. Solid color clothing and background of sets help to avoid a too busy picture and allow the viewer to concentrate on the activity of the interpersonal interaction.

CAMERA (VIDEO)—An electronic device that produces either a black and white or color representation of a given subject. This electronic portrait is customarily displayed on a television set. The camera is a conduit to bring a picture from a reality situation to a recording videotape or closed circuit system so it can be viewed elsewhere simultaneously and/or at a later time.

CANDELA—Replace ancient term "candle" as basic unit of measurement of light. (Also see "lumen".) (1.02 candela = 1.0 candle).

CARTRIDGE—In video, generally a shell in which one supply reel of tape is housed. Tape is usually threaded automatically by the videotape recorder from the cartridge and onto a permanent takeup reel in the machine. It is common to interchange—incorrectly—the names cartridge and cassette, although one cannot be physically compatible with the other (a ½" cartridge cannot fit into or be played by a ½" cassette video recorder-reproducer).

CASSETTE-AUDIO—A module in which both the supply and take-up reel of ⅛" wide audio tape are housed.

CASSETTE-MINI VIDEO—The ¾" U-matic format video cassette developed for mobile field production and news gathering portable U-matic video cassette recorders. This cassette, physically smaller than the full size video cassette, is usually supplied in 15- to 20-minute tape lengths. Although not immediately apparent, this smaller video cassette can be used with confidence in full-size video cassette recorder-players.

CASSETTE-VIDEO—A shell in which is housed a supply and a take-up reel of video tape (commonly either ½" or ¾" in width). The video tape recorder utilizing the cassette format is equipped with automatic threading.

CATV—The acronym for Community Antenna Television or "Cable" TV, a process in which subscribers receive, through a special direct cable hook-up, any number of national, regional and local telecasts, usually 3 or 4 times the number of such telecast channels normally available to non-cable, open circuit ("roof antenna" types) TV receivers.

CCTV—The acronym for Closed Circuit Television, often used interchangeably with CATV although CCTV systems are generally local to one or several buildings or locations: hospitals, college campus, businesses, hotels and the like. CCTV systems are often "specialty" systems dedicated to limited programming—from the "instant replay" of a race at the track to the live telecast of surgery to a conference of physicians.

CHROMA—The technical, general name for "color."

CINCHING—Buckled—or worse—loops of tape folded over one another on a take-up or supply reel. This destructive phenomenon usually occurs when the videotape recorder stops abruptly or when one reel is momentarily caught while the other continues to spool tape onto it. It is more likely to occur with reel-to-reel equipment than with cassette machines. It can happen when the control buttons are too rapidly moved from forward to stop to rewind to forward or fast forward.

CLEANING—The essential process of removing dust, oil, oxide, etc. from vital tape contacts and other electronic and mechanical parts in any electronic device (specifically: video, audio tape recorders, switchers, mixers and the like). To assure proper operation, a regular cleaning and preventive maintenance program for equipment must be set up and executed. The signs of oxide particle build-up should be learned so the situation can be dealt with before a major equipment breakdown occurs. Head cleaner should always be kept available.

CLOSED CIRCUIT—See CCTV

CO-AXIAL CABLE—Typically, the type of internal conductor/insulator configuration commonly found in video cable. The wire strands and mesh-shields share the same axis as do the insulators giving a cross section of the cable the appearance of concentric circles with the center conductor on the common axis. The most common type of coaxial video cable is the RG-59U.

CONNECTORS-AUDIO—Small metal and/or plastic assemblies of specific shape affixed by crimping (pressure) or soldering to audio cable for the purpose of mating with complementary fixtures, thus completing a circuit or line. Common types of audio connectors are: (available in either male or female)
  ¼" phone;
  mini phone;
  sub mini phone;
  RCA phone;
  XLR (often called ITT or Cannon).

CONNECTORS-VIDEO—Mental and/or plastic assemblies of specific shape affixed by crimping (pressure) or soldering to video cable for the purpose of mating with complementary fixtures, thus completing a circuit or line. Common types of video connectors are (available in either male or female form):
  UHF (sometimes called PL-259);
  BNC;
  "F."

CONTROL TRACK—That band on a videotape on which is recorded the timing or sync information necessary to the production or reproduction of a stable black and white or color video picture.

CONVERSION—The process of transferring a television program from one format to another format. Conversion can simply mean, for example, dubbing to ½" open reel from a ¾" master, or, in a far more sophisticated sense, the transfer from NTSC standard to PAL or SECAM standard for international exchange of programs.

CUE—The electronic and/or mechanical signal prompting a performer and/or a device that an action is to be performed. Hand cues, for example, keep the performer on time, on the action. Electronic editing systems utilize pulses and other operator-initiated cues to execute program assembly.

CUT—The signal to stop or the operation which stops an action. Also, the process of abruptly changing video (as opposed to the gradual changes in dissolves or fades). In editing, this process is called cutting; the same technique—when performed *live* at the time of the original recording—is called "taking."

DECIBEL (dB)—An arbitrary unit of measurement of signal intensity or strength.

DEFINITION (VIDEO CAMERAS)—The ability to reproduce fine detail in a picture as measured in T.V. lines.

DEPTH OF FIELD—At any given aperture and point of focus (e.g., an F 5.6 at 8 ft.), that "zone" in which objects will be perceived as "in focus"; objects closer to or farther away than the near/far parameters of the zone will be out of focus, appearing blurred.

DISC: VIDEO—The video playback device using laser or electron beam and advanced platter technology to record and reproduce television picture and sound images on discs (limilar to LP albums) rather than magnetic tape.

DISSOLVE—The process of fading out one picture as a second picture is faded in, causing an "overlapping" of the two images as one picture "becomes" another. Holding the overlapping images or slowing the dissolve are significant techniques in psychiatric videotaping as they convey the interactional process.

DISTRACTIONS: VISUAL—Elements, usually in the background, that create competing centers of interest for a viewer. (Also see "Busy.") Previewing the set on taped replay may help you in spotting and eliminating these distractions.

DROPOUT—A streak or dash visible in the reproduced picture from a videotape; dropout of the signal at these points and sections of the image may be caused by imperfections on the magnetic tape record/playback surface. Sources of dropout are: improper handling of tape (dust, dirt, oil from hands, etc.) and manufacturer error (defective tape or tape oxide coating). Dropout is measured in number per minute—the fewer, the better. Many new videotape recorders have automatic dropout compensators in their playback circuitry. These compensators—by sensing a dropout and re-inserting a line of the previous video—all but eliminate the visual disturbance caused by dropout.

DUB— (see DUBBING)

DUBBING—The common name for the transfer of a program from one tape or disc to another. The copy resulting is called a "dub." The dubs closest to the original or edited master are better in quality than dubs from dubs from dubs from dubs on into infinity.

ECU—The acronym for "extreme close-up"— a "tight view" of one element in a scene. A director may say to a cameraman, "I want an ECU of the patient" or "ECU her hands."

EDITING: VERTICAL INTERVAL—That method of glitch-free editing that produces cuts or edits free from vertical or horizontal disturbance. All editing should be of the vertical-interval type.

EFP—Acronym for "electronic field production," the method of taping on location with the lower cost ENG-type video equipment.

EIA—Acronym for Electronics Industry Association, the American standard-setting body for U.S. made electronic instruments.

EIAJ—Acronym for Electronics Industry Association of Japan, the Japanese standard-setting group for electronic instruments made in Japan.

ELECTRONIC EDITING—The process of assembling or reordering audio and/or video information by electronic rather than physical techniques. Older forms of editing required that tape be cut if different, out-of-sequence events were to be joined; with contemporary technology, physical cutting of the tape is rarely, if ever, done.

ENG—Acronym for "electronic news gathering," a system developed by CBS and Ikegami to use portable video (and not film) cameras for location news coverage.

ERASE—To "wipe" or degauss a tape, thus rendering it free of any previously recorded material.

ESSENTIAL AREA (IN A VIDEO PICTURE)—That portion of the picture which is always seen by all television sets in normal working condition. It is the portion in which all graphic material may be placed and all essential visual information can be located without fear that on some TV sets a head may but cut off or a graphic may appear too long.

ESTABLISHING SHOT—That view which sets the context for the program. This is often a wide angle shot of the entire "scene" and it is often selected for the "head" of the tape (sometimes carrying titles over it) and/or for the end.

FADE IN—To come in slowly to an audio or video source. (Fade ins come from silence in audio and from "black" in video.)

FADE OUT—To go out slowly from an audio or video source. (Fade out goes to silence in audio and to "black" in video.)

FADER—A volume or intensity control for the regulation of a signal.

FIELD—One half of a frame; an image appearing for about 17 milliseconds on alternate scan lines (262.5 odd number and 262.5 even number) which is interlaced with its complement to produce one full 525-line video frame every 1/30th of a second.

FILM TRANSFER—The 16mm film copy of a videotaped program. Commonly called kinescopes, the film transfer traditionally was of poor-to-fair quality. The process of reconstituting the video image created by Image Transform has given the film transfer computer-assisted precision and striking quality; this process of film transfer is called "image transform" after the company which developed the excellent system.

FRAME—One full (two-field) 525-line video picture. In the United States and Japan, there are 30 frames per second.

FREEZE FRAME— (See SLO-MO)

F-STOP—Common name for the aperture of the lens iris. "F" is the accepted symbol for the mathematical relationship between aperture and the lens focal length. The lower the F-stop number (e.g., F 1.4, F 2.8), the wider the aperture; the higher the F-stop number (e.g., F 16, F 22), the narrower the aperture.

GAFFER TAPE—A gray pressure-sensitive tape of high durability commonly used in television and theater production to fasten all manner of objects, or to wipe out the shine of metal surfaces.

GAIN—Generally, audio signal level or volume. Sometimes used to refer to any level (video, lighting, etc.).

GENERATION—The stage of a recording: the first recording is the first generation; a copy of that original recording is the second generation; a dub of that copy is the third generation, etc. Every generation represents some deterioration in audio/video quality as compared with the previous generation; the degree of deterioration (usually expressed in dB of signal-to-noise loss) varies with the quality and condition of the dubbing machines.

HEAD—The beginning of a program. Also tape recorder component for video or audio "writing" of electronic picture or sound information. It is vital for you to know where the head on your recorder is located and how to clean it. A "dirty head" can ruin an elegantly planned program.

HEADROOM—The distance between the top of a subject and the top edge of the picture monitor. Always leave enough headroom when "shooting" until you get familiar with the spatial requirements of the camera you are using.

HEAD SHOT—A view of the performer in which only the head and sometimes the shoulders are shown. It is advisable to vary your shots from time to time to maintain interest and context so you don't produce a "head show."

HELICAL SCAN— (Slant Track) Method of "writing" the video information (in long diagonal lines on the tape), common in most popularly available portable 1", ¾" and ½" videotape. At first a "stepchild" to studio quadruplex videotape equipment, the helical scan video tape recorders have achieved impressive image quality and transport stability making them the excellent studio and field production instruments they are today.

HERTZ (Hz)—A unit of measurement of the frequency of a waveform; 1 Hz equals one cycle per second.

IMAGE RETENTION—An undesirable characteristic of certain types of television pick-up tubes where an after image remains as the subject and/or camera head is moved. The retention of the image in a ghost-like effect is often called lag.

IMAGE TRANSFORM—(See FILM TRANSFER)

INTERCOM—The private line for communication between members of a production crew (camera operators, director, producer, etc.).

IRIS—An assembly of overlapping leaves that effectively controls the aperture of a lens.

JACK—The common name for the receptacle among audio and video connectors. Also known (oddly, yet quite popularly) as the "female" contact or connector. Jacks are usually found mounted in panels behind electronic devices, although in-line jacks for mating with other in-line plugs are also frequently used.

JUMP CUT—The clumsy error of assemble editing two clips of the same subject in nearly the same position so that the tape, when reviewed, shows a snapping or jerking of the subject at the point of the edit.

LAG—(See IMAGE RETENTION)

LENS—A barrel-like housing in which various glass or acrylic elements are set to gather light reflected from an object and to focus that light onto a target (in the video camera, a photoconductive plate.)

LENS EXTENDER—An adaptor barrel that, although it reduces the speed of the lens, effectively increases its focal length or telephoto capability. A 2x telextender (lens extender), for example, converts a standard 12.5mm to 75mm zoom lens to a 25mm to 150mm zoom lens.

LIMBO—A lighting technique in which the space surrounding the subject(s) is allowed to seem endless, giving the viewer no frame of reference.

LINE LEVEL—An input/output to an audio device where the input/output impedance is 600 ohms. Sometimes called "audio in" or "audio out."

LINE MONITOR—That video monitor displaying the program picture (often a composite of a number of pictures seen on small monitors from a number of cameras) to be aired, viewed, or recorded on tape.

LOG—The process of noting in and out cues as well as the content of a given tape, usually for the purpose of editing.

LUMEN—Equals one candela (cd) of light over one square foot. (See LUX)

LUX—The metric measurement equal to one lumen per square meter of area.

MCU—Acronym for "medium close-up," a framed shot showing the performer from top of head to waist.

MIXER—The audio or video device which is capable of combining a number of sources to produce—often with enhancement or special effects—a single, composite whole. Also, the individual operating the device.

MOS—Colloquially, "mit-out sound," a film term originally. Now taken also in video to mean a program element in which there is picture *without* sound. (Silent.)

NAB—National Association of Broadcasters (broadcast radio and television station standards-setting group.)

NABET—National Association of Broadcast Employees and Technicians (union for broadcast technicians).

NOISE—Unwanted interference in sound or picture. Often referred to as "snow" in video because it appears as grains, or white specs throughout the screen.

NTSC—National Television Standards Committee, the establishing body and name of the system for black and white and color television image specifications in the United States. The systems, devised in the 1940s and 50s, of 525-line scanning is inferior in resolution and color phase error to the newer PAL and SECAM systems in use throughout most of the world.

ORIGINAL—The first recording of a program, the "raw" footage or original production material. The higher the quality of machine on which you tape-record your original (e.g. 1" is higher than ½"), the better quality your edited master tape will be.

PAL—Phase alternate line system of creating the television image. Although demanding greater technical accuracy, this 625-line system is less subject to color shifting than the American NTSC system. The PAL system is used widely in Western Europe (except France which uses SECAM), England, South Africa, Mid-East, Australia ,and Scandinavia.

PATCH BAY—A rack devoted to panels in which are mounted audio, video or AC/DC jacks to enable relatively easy interconnection of a number of electronic or electrical components. Many audio and video patch bays are replaced today by the pushbutton activated switch matrix.

PLUG—The popular name for the "male" connector used on uadio and video cables. This connector will properly mate with the appropriately configured jack to form a complete circuit.

POT—Abbreviated version of potentiometer or variable resistor (rheostat) for the control of signal levels (e.g., a volume control on an audio mixer.)

QUADRUPLEX VTR—A transverse scan videotape recorder utilizing 2" wide videotape to produce high quality video programs. The 2" Quad has been the standard for broadcast, but new 1" helical scan decks, a tightening economy, and the need for system versatility have initiated an erosion of the Quad's dominance.

RESOLUTION— (See DEFINITION)

SECAM—Séquential couleur à mémoire, the French, Eastern European and Russian 625-line color television system, is a far simpler system than PAL and most resistant of all three systems (PAL, SECAM, NTSC) to color distortion.

SEGUÉ—The smooth transition from one point to another.

SIGNAL—Generally, the name given to the electronic pulses representative of the physical images and sounds telecast or taped by video equipment.

SIGNAL-TO-NOISE RATIO—That proportion between the amplitude of the desired signal and the undesired noise in a television or sound reproduction.

SLANT TRACK— (See HELICAL SCAN)

SLO-MO—Abbreviation for slow-motion, usually achieved by a video disc (although successfully done with the Ampex V 1″ helical scan videotape recorder) and often used in conjunction with freeze frame and reverse actions effects. In freeze frame, the disc or deck is parked and reading one full frame of video information.

SPLICE—The physical joining of new segments or the rejoining of the damaged pieces of a segment of tape or film. Splicing of videotape is not an accepted practice since there is a high probability of visual disturbance at and after the splice.

SPLIT SCREEN—An electronic effect in which, through the use of a video special effects generator, the inputs of two carefully positioned cameras are combined to achieve a divided frame with a specific section of each camera's full shot isolated and juxtaposed for clinical and/or artistic purposes, to bring together in an enlarged picture the faces of two people who are geographically distant or to convey interpersonal interaction.

SMPTE—Society of Motion Picture and Television Engineers, a group of professional Engineers who set technical parameters for the AV professions. The SMPTE time code is popular at this time.

SYNC—The regulated (in broadcast by EIA-RS-170 spec) electronic control of the television picture. Replay Synchronization is accomplished by accurately timed pulses which are recorded on the "sync track" of the videotape deck being played back to the reproducing system.

TAKE—In live production, the abrupt transition from one camera shot to another.

TRACKING—The process of adjusting (in many cases automatic) the playback videotape recorder to "read" the sync pulses encoded with the picture and sound information on the prerecorded tape.

TRIPOD—A camera mounting device characterized by three adjustable legs. The tripod often includes wheels for moving the camera easily on floors.

VIDEO TAPE—A mylar or polyester based tape in various widths which is impregnated with oxide particles on which are stored magnetically the picture, sound and synchronizing information necessary for the replay of a television image.

ZOOM LENS—A variable focal length lens in which the continuous adjustment of effective lens length realizes, theoretically, an infinite number of focal lengths (from wide angle to telephoto) without the need to change lenses. A 1:10 zoom lens offers many options for the cameraman.

SUBJECT INDEX

NAME INDEX

404